Accession no.
3623 5668

D1394091

Clinical Dilemmas in

Inflammatory
Bowel Disease

JET LIBRARY

Clinical Dilemmas in

Inflammatory Bowel Disease

New Challenges

Second Edition

EDITED BY

Peter M. Irving MD, MRCP

Consultant Gastroenterologist
Department of Gastroenterology
Guy's and St Thomas' Hospitals
London, UK

Corey A. Siegel MD, MS

Assistant Professor of Medicine and The Dartmouth Institute for Health Policy and Clinical Practice;
Dartmouth Medical School
Director, Inflammatory Bowel Disease Center
Dartmouth–Hitchcock Medical Center
Section of Gastroenterology and Hepatology
Lebanon, NH, USA

David S. Rampton DPhil, FRCP

Professor of Clinical Gastroenterology
Centre for Digestive Diseases
Barts and The London School of Medicine and Dentistry
London, UK

Fergus Shanahan MD

Professor and Chair
Department of Medicine
Director, Alimentary Pharmabiotic Centre
University College Cork
National University of Ireland
Cork, Ireland

LIS - LIBRARY

Date	Fund
5/3/18	rep – LEI

Order No.

285188x

University of Chester

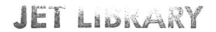

WILEY-BLACKWELL

A John Wiley & Sons, Ltd., Publication

JET LIBRARY

This edition first published 2011 © 2006, 2011 Blackwell Publishing Ltd.

Blackwell Publishing was acquired by John Wiley & Sons in February 2007. Blackwell's publishing program has been merged with Wiley's global Scientific, Technical and Medical business to form Wiley-Blackwell.

Registered office: John Wiley & Sons, Ltd, The Atrium, Southern Gate, Chichester, West Sussex, PO19 8SQ, UK

Editorial offices: 9600 Garsington Road, Oxford, OX4 2DQ, UK
The Atrium, Southern Gate, Chichester, West Sussex, PO19 8SQ, UK
111 River Street, Hoboken, NJ 07030-5774, USA

For details of our global editorial offices, for customer services and for information about how to apply for permission to reuse the copyright material in this book please see our website at www.wiley.com/wiley-blackwell

The right of the author to be identified as the author of this work has been asserted in accordance with the UK Copyright, Designs and Patents Act 1988.

All rights reserved. No part of this publication may be reproduced, stored in a retrieval system, or transmitted, in any form or by any means, electronic, mechanical, photocopying, recording or otherwise, except as permitted by the UK Copyright, Designs and Patents Act 1988, without the prior permission of the publisher.

Designations used by companies to distinguish their products are often claimed as trademarks. All brand names and product names used in this book are trade names, service marks, trademarks or registered trademarks of their respective owners. The publisher is not associated with any product or vendor mentioned in this book. This publication is designed to provide accurate and authoritative information in regard to the subject matter covered. It is sold on the understanding that the publisher is not engaged in rendering professional services. If professional advice or other expert assistance is required, the services of a competent professional should be sought.

The contents of this work are intended to further general scientific research, understanding, and discussion only and are not intended and should not be relied upon as recommending or promoting a specific method, diagnosis, or treatment by physicians for any particular patient. The publisher and the author make no representations or warranties with respect to the accuracy or completeness of the contents of this work and specifically disclaim all warranties, including without limitation any implied warranties of fitness for a particular purpose. In view of ongoing research, equipment modifications, changes in governmental regulations, and the constant flow of information relating to the use of medicines, equipment, and devices, the reader is urged to review and evaluate the information provided in the package insert or instructions for each medicine, equipment, or device for, among other things, any changes in the instructions or indication of usage and for added warnings and precautions. Readers should consult with a specialist where appropriate. The fact that an organization or Website is referred to in this work as a citation and/or a potential source of further information does not mean that the author or the publisher endorses the information the organization or Website may provide or recommendations it may make. Further, readers should be aware that Internet Websites listed in this work may have changed or disappeared between when this work was written and when it is read. No warranty may be created or extended by any promotional statements for this work. Neither the publisher nor the author shall be liable for any damages arising herefrom.

Library of Congress Cataloging-in-Publication Data

Clinical dilemmas in inflammatory bowel disease : new challenges / edited by Peter Irving ... [et al.]. – 2nd ed.
    p. ; cm.
  Includes bibliographical references and index.
  ISBN-13: 978-1-4443-3454-8 (pbk. : alk. paper)
  ISBN-10: 1-4443-3454-9 (pbk. : alk. paper)
  ISBN-13: 978-1-4443-4254-3 (ePDF)
  ISBN-13: 978-1-4443-4257-4 (e-ISBN-10: : Wiley Online Library) [etc.]
 1. Inflammatory bowel diseases.   2. Inflammatory bowel diseases–Decision making.
 I. Irving, Peter, 1970-
  [DNLM: 1. Inflammatory Bowel Diseases. WI 420]
  RC862.I53C553 2011
  616.3′44–dc22

                                                           2011007515

A catalogue record for this book is available from the British Library.

This book is published in the following electronic formats: ePDF 9781444342543; Wiley Online Library 9781444342574; ePub 9781444342550; Mobi 9781444342567
Set in 8.75 /12pt Minion by Aptara® Inc., New Delhi, India
Printed and bound in Singapore by Fabulous Printers Pte Ltd

01   2011

Contents

Contributors

Ashwin N. Ananthakrishnan
MD, MPH
Instructor in Medicine
Harvard Medical School
Gastrointestinal Unit
Massachusetts General Hospital
Boston, MA, USA

Donna Appleton MD, MRCS
Specialist Registrar
Department of General and Colorectal
    Surgery
Stafford General Hospital
Stafford, UK

Judith E. Baars MSc, PhD
Medical Student
Erasmus University
Rotterdam, The Netherlands
Department of Gastroenterology and
    Hepatology
Erasmus MC Hospital
Rotterdam, The Netherlands

Jacques Belaiche PhD
Professor of Gastroenterology
Department of gastroenterology
CHU Liège and GIGA Research University
    of Liège
Liège, Belgium

David G. Binion MD
Visiting Professor of Medicine
Division of Gastroenterology, Hepatology,
    and Nutrition
University of Pittsburgh School of Medicine
Pittsburgh, PA, USA

Wojciech Blonski MD, PhD
Research Scholar
Division of Gastroenterology
University of Pennsylvania
Philadelphia, PA, USA;
Department of Gastroenterology
Medical University
Wroclaw, Poland

Brian Bressler MD, MS, FRCPC
Clinical Assistant Professor of Medicine
Division of Gastroenterology
University of British Columbia
Vancouver, BC, Canada

Emma Calabrese MD, PhD
University of Rome "Tor Vergata"
Rome, Italy

Adam S. Cheifetz MD
Assistant Professor of Medicine;
Clinical Director, Center for Inflammatory
    Bowel Disease
Division of Gastroenterology
Beth Israel Deaconess Medical Center and
    Harvard Medical School
Boston, MA, USA

Dorothy K.L. Chow MBChB,
MD, MRCP
Clinical Assistant Professor (Honorary)
Department of Medicine and Therapeutics
Prince of Wales Hospital
The Chinese University of Hong Kong
Hong Kong SAR, China

Miranda Clark BSc(Hons)
Clinical Trials Coordinator
University Hospital
Queen's Medical Centre
Nottingham, UK

Norman R. Clark III MD
Division of Gastroenterology
Vanderbilt University Medical Center
Nashville, TN, USA

Morven Cunningham
MA(Hons), MBBS, MRCP
Clinical Research Fellow
Blizard Institute of Cell and Molecular
    Science
Barts and The London School of Medicine
    and Dentistry
Queen Mary, University of London
UK

Andrew S. Day MB,ChB, MD,
FRACP, AGAF
Associate Professor
Department of Paediatrics
University of Otago
Dunedin, Otago, New Zealand;
Pediatric Gastroenterology
Christchurch Hospital
Christchurch, New Zealand

Alan N. Desmond MB, BCh,
BAO, BMedSc, MRCPI
Specialist Registrar
Department of Gastroenterology and
    General Internal Medicine
Cork University Hospital
Wilton, Cork, Ireland

Shane M. Devlin MD, FRCPC
Clinical Assistant Professor
Division of Gastroenterology
Inflammatory Bowel Disease Clinic
The University of Calgary
Calgary, AB, Canada

Geert D'Haens MD, PhD
Professor of Medicine
Academic Medical Centre
Amsterdam, The Netherlands

Axel Dignass MD, PhD, FEBG, AGAF
Professor of Medicine
Head, Department of Medicine I
Markus Hospital
Frankfurt/Main, Germany

Glen A. Doherty MB, PhD, MRCPI
Consultant Gastroenterologist
Centre for Colorectal Disease
St Vincent's University Hospital/University College Dublin
Dublin, Ireland

Marla C. Dubinsky MD
Associate Professor of Pediatrics
Director, Pediatric IBD Center
Cedars Sinai Medical Center
Los Angeles, CA, USA

Tim Elliott MBBS, FRACP
Specialist Registrar
Department of Gastroenterology
Guys and St Thomas' Hospitals
London, UK

Marc Ferrante MD, PhD
Consultant Gastroenterologist
Department of Gastroenterology
University Hospital Gasthuisberg
Leuven, Belgium

Laurie N. Fishman MD
Assistant Professor of Pediatrics
Center for Inflammatory Bowel Disease
Division of Gastroenterology and Nutrition
Children's Hospital Boston
Harvard Medical School
Boston, MA, USA

Phillip Fleshner MD, FACS, FASCRS
Program Director, Colorectal Surgery Residency
Los Angeles, CA, USA;
Clinical Professor of Surgery
UCLA School of Medicine
Los Angeles, CA, USA

Anna Foley MBBS(Hons), FRACP
Consultant Gastroenterologist
Department of Gastroenterology and Hepatology
Box Hill Hospital
Melbourne, VIC, Australia

Graham R. Foster FRCP, PhD
Professor of Hepatology
Blizard Institute of Cell and Molecular Science
Barts and The London School of Medicine and Dentistry
Queen Mary, University of London
London, UK

Richard B. Gearry MB, ChB, PhD, FRACP
Associate Professor of Medicine
Consultant Gastroenterologist
Department of Medicine
University of Otago
Dunedin, Otago, New Zealand;
Department of Gastroenterology
Christchurch Hospital
Christchurch, New Zealand

Peter Gibson MD, FRACP
Professor of Medicine and Consultant Gastroenterologist
Department of Gastroenterology and Hepatology
Eastern Health Clinical School
Monash University, Melbourne
VIC, Australia

James Goodhand BSc(Hons), MBBS, MRCP
Clinical Research Fellow
Barts and the London School of Medicine and Dentistry
Queen Mary's University of London
London, UK

Richard J. Grand MD
Professor of Pediatrics
Harvard Medical School
Director Emeritus, Center for Inflammatory Bowel Diseases
Division of Gastroenterology and Nutrition
Children's Hospital Boston
Boston, MA, USA

Gauree Gupta MD
Staff Physician
Department of Medicine
Cedars Sinai Medical Center and David Geffen School of Medicine at UCLA
Los Angeles, CA, USA

Elizabeth J. Hait MD, MPH
Center for Inflammatory Bowel Disease
Division of Gastroenterology and Nutrition
Children's Hospital Boston
Harvard Medical School
Boston, MA, USA

Stephen B. Hanauer MD
Professor of Medicine and Clinical Pharmacology
Section of Gastroenterology, Hepatology, and Nutrition
University of Chicago Medical Center
Chicago, IL, USA;
Chief, Section of Gastroenterology, Hepatology, and Nutrition
University of Chicago Medical Center
Chicago, IL, USA

Catherine A. Harwood
Centre for Cutaneous Research
Blizard Institute of Cell and Molecular Science
Barts and The London School of Medicine and Dentistry
Queen Mary University of London
London, UK

Christopher J. Hawkey DM, FRCP
Professor of Gastroenterology
University Hospital
Queen's Medical Centre
Nottingham University Hospitals NHS Trust
Nottingham, UK

A. Barney Hawthorne DM, FRCP
Consultant Gastroenterologist
Department of Medicine
University Hospital of Wales
Cardiff, UK

Michael Hershman DHMSA, MSc(Hons), MS(Hons), FRCS (Eng, Ed, Glas & Irel), FICS
Consultant Surgeon
Department of General Surgery
Stafford Hospital
Stafford, UK

Rob Horne
Professor of Behavioural Medicine
Director, Centre for Behavioural Medicine
The School of Pharmacy
University of London
London, UK

Peter M. Irving MD, MRCP
Consultant Gastroenterologist
Department of Gastroenterology
Guy's and St Thomas' Hospitals
London, UK

Jennifer L. Jones MD, MSc, FRCPC
Director, MDIBD Clinic and IBD Clinical Trials
Assistant Professor
Departments of Medicine and Community Health Sciences and Epidemiology
University of Saskatchewan
Royal University Hospital
Saskatoon, SK, Canada

Ahmed Kandiel MD, MPH
Staff Gastroenterologist
Department of Gastroenterology and Hepatology
Digestive Disease Institute
Cleveland Clinic
Cleveland, OH, USA

Sunanda Kane MD, MSPH
Professor of Medicine
Mayo Clinic College of Medicine
Rochester, MN, USA

Gilaad Kaplan MD, MPH, FRCPC
Assistant Professor
Departments of Medicine and Community Health Sciences
Teaching Research and Wellness Center
University of Calgary
Calgary, AB, Canada

Michael D. Kappelman MD, MPH
Assistant Professor
Division of Pediatric Gastroenterology
Department of Pediatrics
University of North Carolina Chapel Hill
Chapel Hill, NC, USA

Louise Langmead BSc(Hons), MD
Consultant Gastroenterologist
Endoscopy Unit
Barts and the London NHS Trust
The Royal London Hospital
London, UK

Bret Lashner MD, MPH
Professor of Medicine
Department of Gastroenterology and Hepatology
Digestive Disease Institute
Cleveland Clinic
Cleveland, OH, USA

Joanna K. Law MD, MA [Ed], FRCP(C)
Clinical Instructor, Division of Gastroenterology
University of British Columbia
Vancouver, BC, Canada

Ian Craig Lawrance MBBS(Hons), PhD, FRACP
Professor, School of Medicine and Pharmacology
University of Western Australia
Perth, WA, Australia;
Director, Centre for Inflammatory Bowel Diseases
Fremantle Hospital
Fremantle, WA, Australia

Keith Leiper MD, FRCP
Consultant Gastroenterologist
Royal Liverpool University Hospital
Liverpool, UK

Rupert W.L. Leong MBBS, MD, FRACP
Associate Professor of Medicine (Conjoint)
The University of New South Wales
Sydney, NSW, Australia;
Director of Endoscopy
Department of Gastroenterology and Liver Services
Sydney South West Area Health Service
Concord and Bankstown Hospitals
Sydney, NSW, Australia

John Leung MD
Instructor
Division of Gastroenterology
Tufts Medical Center
Boston, MA, USA

L. Campbell Levy MD
Assistant Professor of Medicine
Dartmouth Medical School
Section of Gastroenterology and Hepatology
Dartmouth–Hitchcock Medical Center
Lebanon, NH, USA

Gary R. Lichtenstein MD
Professor of Medicine
Division of Gastroenterology
University of Pennsylvania
Philadelphia, PA, USA

Ming Valerie Lin MD
Department of Internal Medicine
Pennsylvania Hospital
University of Pennsylvania Health System
Philadelphia, PA, USA

Keith D. Lindor MD
Professor of Medicine
Division of Gastroenterology and Hepatology
Mayo Clinic
Rochester, MN, USA;
Dean, Mayo Medical School
Mayo Clinic
Rochester, MN, USA

James O. Lindsay PhD, FRCP
Consultant and Senior Lecturer in Gastroenterology,
Digestive Diseases Clinical Academic Unit
Barts and the London NHS Trust
The Royal London Hospital
Whitechapel, London, UK

Richard Logan MB, ChB, MSc, FFPH, FRCP
Professor of Clinical Epidemiology/Consultant Gastroenterologist
Division of Epidemiology and Public Health
Queens Medical Centre
Nottingham University Hospitals
Nottingham, UK

Edouard Louis MD, PhD
Professor of Gastroenterology
Department of Gastroenterology
CHU Liège and GIGA Research University of Liège
Liège, Belgium

Mark Lust MBBS, FRACP, PhD
Senior Clinical Fellow in Gastroenterology
Translational Gastroenterology Unit
John Radcliffe Hospital
Oxford, UK

Michael M. Maher MD
Professor
Department of Radiology
Alimentary Pharmabiotic Centre
University College Cork
National University of Ireland
Cork, Ireland

Robert G. Maunder MD
Associate Professor and Staff Psychiatrist
Mount Sinai Hospital and University of
    Toronto
Toronto, ON, Canada

Jane M. McGregor MA, MB
BChir, FRCP, MD
Senior Lecturer and Honorary Consultant
    Dermatologist
Barts and the London NHS Trust
London, UK;
Centre for Cutaneous Research
Blizard Institute of Cell and Molecular
    Science
Barts and The London School of Medicine
    and Dentistry
Queen Mary University of London,
    London, UK

Simon D. McLaughlin MD,
MRCP
Consultant Gastroenterologist
Department of Gastroenterology
Royal Bournemouth Hospital
Bournemouth, UK

Tina A. Mehta
Department of Gastroenterology
Bristol Royal Infirmary
Bristol, Avon, UK

Gil Y. Melmed MD, MS
Assistant Clinical Professor of Medicine
Cedars Sinai Medical Center and David
    Geffen School of Medicine at UCLA
Los Angeles, CA, USA

Owen J. O'Connor MD,
FFR(RCSI), MRCSI
Radiology Lecturer
Department of Radiology
University College Cork
National University of Ireland
Cork, Ireland

Tom Øresland MD, PhD
Professor
Department of GI Surgery
Akershus University Hospital
University of Oslo
Lørenskog, Norway

Helen M. Pappa MD, MPH
Instructor in Pediatrics
Harvard Medical School
Staff, Center for Inflammatory Bowel
    Diseases
Division of Gastroenterology and Nutrition
Children's Hospital Boston
Boston, MA, USA

Miles Parkes MA, DM, FRCP
Consultant Gastroenterologist
Addenbrooke's Hospital and University of
    Cambridge
Cambridge, UK

Kiran K. Peddi MBBS, MRCP (UK)
Department of Gastroenterology
Specialist Registrar and Fellow in
    Gastroenterology
Fremantle Hospital
Fremantle, WA, Australia

Conal M. Perrett MB, ChB,
MRCP(UK), PhD
Consultant Dermatologist and Honorary
    Senior Lecturer
University College London Hospitals
London, UK

Chris S.J. Probert MD, FRCP,
FHEA
Professor of Gastroenterology
Bristol Royal Infirmary
Bristol, UK

David S. Rampton DPhil, FRCP
Professor of Clinical Gastroenterology
Centre for Digestive Diseases
Barts and The London School of Medicine
    and Dentistry
London, UK

Catherine Reenaers MD, PhD
Department of Gastroenterology
CHU Liège and GIGA Research University
    of Liège
Liège, Belgium

Jonathan M. Rhodes MD, FRCP,
FMedSci
Division of Gastroenterology
School of Clinical Sciences
University of Liverpool and Royal Liverpool
    University Hospital
Liverpool, UK

Emile Richman BSc(Hons), MSc,
PGCE
Specialist Gastroenterology Dietitian
Department of Nutrition and Dietetics
Royal Liverpool University Hospital
Liverpool, UK

David T. Rubin MD
Associate Professor of Medicine
Codirector, Inflammatory Bowel Disease
    Center
Program Director, Fellowship in
    Gastroenterology, Hepatology, and
    Nutrition
University of Chicago Medical Center
Chicago, IL, USA

Matthew D. Rutter MBBS, MD,
FRCP
Consultant Gastroenterologist and Trust
    Endoscopy Lead
University Hospital of North Tees
Stockton-on-Tees, Cleveland, UK;
Clinical Director, Tees Bowel Cancer
    Screening Centre
University Hospital of North Tees
Stockton-on-Tees, Cleveland, UK

Jeremy D. Sanderson MBBS,
MD, FRCP
Consultant Gastroenterologist
Department of Gastroenterology
St Thomas' Hospital
London, UK;
Senior Clinical Research Fellow
Nutritional Sciences Research
Kings College London
London, UK

Hermann Schulze Dr.med.
Frankfurter Diakonie-Kliniken
Markus-Krankenhaus
Frankfurt, Germany

David A. Schwartz MD
Associate Professor of Medicine
Director, IBD Center
Division of Gastroenterology
Vanderbilt University Medical Center
Nashville, TN, USA

Ernest G. Seidman MDCM, FRCPC, FACG
Professor of Medicine and Pediatrics
Division of Gastroenterology
McGill University Health Center
Faculty of Medicine
McGill University
Montreal, QC, Canada

Christian P. Selinger MRCP
Salford Royal Hospital
Department of Gastroenterology
Salford, UK

Raanan Shamir MD
Chairman, Institute of Gastroenterology, Nutrition, and Liver Diseases
Schneider Children's Medical Center
Petach-Tikva, Israel;
Professor of Pediatrics
Sackler Faculty of Medicine
Tel-Aviv University
Tel-Aviv, Israel

Fergus Shanahan MD
Professor and Chair
Department of Medicine
Director, Alimentary Pharmabiotic Centre
University College Cork
National University of Ireland
Cork, Ireland

Bo Shen MD
Professor of Medicine
Department of Gastroenterology
Cleveland Clinic Lerner College of Medicine
Case Western Reserve University
Cleveland, OH, USA;
Staff Gastroenterologist
Department of Gastroenterology
Cleveland ClinicCleveland, OH, USA

Corey A. Siegel MD, MS
Assistant Professor of Medicine and The Dartmouth Institute for Health Policy and Clinical Practice;
Dartmouth Medical School
Director, Inflammatory Bowel Disease Center
Dartmouth–Hitchcock Medical Center
Section of Gastroenterology and Hepatology
Lebanon, NH, USA

Emmanouil Sinakos MD
Research Fellow
Division of Gastroenterology and Hepatology
Mayo Clinic
Rochester, MN, USA

Melissa A. Smith
BSc(Hons), MB, ChB, MA, MRCP
Specialist Registrar
Department of Gastroenterology
St Thomas' Hospital
Guy's and St Thomas' NHS Foundation Trust
London, UK

Ing Shian Soon MD
Resident
Division of Gastroenterology
Department of Pediatrics and Community Health Sciences
University of Calgary
Calgary, AB, Canada

Miles Sparrow MBBS, FRACP
Consultant Gastroenterologist
Department of Gastroenterology
The Alfred Hospital
Melbourne, VIC, Australia

A. Hillary Steinhart MD, FRCP(C)
Inflammatory Bowel Disease Centre
Mount Sinai Hospital
Toronto, ON, Canada;
Associate Professor of Medicine
University of Toronto
Toronto, ON, Canada

Venkataraman Subramanian MD, DM, MRCP (UK)
Academic Clinical Lecturer (Gastroenterology)
Nottingham Digestive Diseases Centre
Queens Medical Centre
Nottingham University Hospitals NHS Trust
Nottingham, UK

Simon Travis DPhil, FRCP
Consultant Gastroenterologist
Translational Gastroenterology Unit
John Radcliffe hospital
Oxford, UK

William J. Tremaine MD
Maxine and Jack Zarrow Professor
Division of Gastroenterology and Hepatology
Mayo Clinic
Rochester, MN, USA

C. Janneke van der Woude MD, PhD
Gastroenterologist Department of Gastroenterology and Hepatology
Erasmus MC Hospital
Rotterdam, The Netherlands

Séverine Vermeire MD, PhD
Assistant Professor
Department of Gastroenterology
University Hospital Gasthuisberg
Leuven, Belgium

Joel V. Weinstock MD
Professor in Gastroenterology
Division of Gastroenterology
Tufts Medical Center
Boston, MA, USA

Jonathan M. Wilson MBCh B, FRCS(Edin), PhD
Specialist Registrar in Colorectal Surgery
Department of Colorectal Surgery
University College London Hospitals
London, UK

Alastair Windsor MD, FRCS, FRCS (Ed), FRCS (Glas)
Consultant SurgeonUniversity College London Hospitals
London, UK

Henit Yanai MD
University of Chicago Medical Center
Chicago, IL, USA

Preface

In 2006, three of us published a short book containing about 60 pithy and sometimes provocative chapters on controversial topics in IBD. These were selected with the aim of covering areas that commonly cause clinicians difficulties in decision-making. The book was well received but because of its subject matter has inevitably, at least in some chapters, become a bit out of date. Therefore, we have now produced a new book guided by the same principles as the first. A few of the chapters in this book are updates of their predecessors, but most are entirely new, reflecting the changing challenges faced by gastroenterologists at the beginning of the millennium's second decade. Our authors are almost all acknowledged experts in their fields and work wherever IBD is common in the world. To help widen the appeal of the book, for this edition we have engaged both a US coeditor (CS) and more US-based contributors than previously.

As before, we have deliberately chosen some tricky topics, and should point out that as editors we do not necessarily agree with all that is written here; if we did the book might be dull. Again, we hope the book will appeal both to senior and trainee gastroenterologists, as well as other members of the IBD team, and that readers will find that it provides a useful distillation and analysis of a wide range of current management dilemmas.

We are very grateful to all our coauthors, almost all of whom delivered their chapters on time and with minimal hassling. We are particularly grateful too to the team at Blackwell's, especially Oliver Walter for his support for the project and Jennifer Seward for her editorial work.

PMI, CS, DSR, FS July 2011

PART I:
Genes and Phenotype in IBD

Which will take us further in IBD—study of coding variation or epigenetics?

Miles Parkes

Department of Gastroenterology, Addenbrooke's Hospital and University of Cambridge, Cambridge, UK

LEARNING POINTS

- Genome-wide association scans have revealed many genetic risk factors for Crohn's disease and ulcerative colitis.

- As with environmental risk factors, some of the genetic risk is shared and some is specific to either Crohn's disease or ulcerative colitis.

- Only about 20% of the variance in heritability has been accounted for by known genetic loci.

- The study of genetic variants is valuable because it reveals insights into disease pathogenesis.

- Increasing evidence suggests that much of the host susceptibility to IBD may be epigenetic, lying at the level of the regulation of gene expression.

- Epigenetic risk is heritable through mitosis and possibly meiosis, and many of the known environmental or lifestyle risk factors may operate at an epigenetic level by influencing gene transcription.

Genetic susceptibility to inflammatory bowel disease (IBD) is complex. While genome-wide association scans (GWAS) have pushed Crohn's disease (CD) to the front of the field of complex disease genetics, the recognition that only 20% of the variance in heritability has so far been accounted for provides a salutary reminder of the challenges ahead [1]. The main achievement of GWAS has been to highlight a number of previously unsuspected pathogenic pathways for IBD and to provide a stable base-camp from which to explore the genetic higher ground—defining causal variants at each of the loci identified, accounting for the remaining 80% of heritability and exploring functional implications.

This chapter discusses what is understood regarding causal mechanisms in IBD genetics, particularly the relative contributions of simple variation in DNA coding sequence and epigenetic regulation of gene transcription. For some readers, epigenetic regulation of gene transcription may be an unfamiliar concept: it involves changes in gene expression resulting from mechanisms such as chromatin packaging, histone acetylation (affecting electrostatic charge and hence DNA binding), and DNA methylation.

Gene expression: sequence variation versus epigenetic factors

The human genome is thought to encode some 23,000 protein-coding genes, comprising just 1.5% of the total of 3 billion base pairs. Sequence variation can take many forms from single nucleotide polymorphisms (SNPs) to indels (insertion–deletion polymorphisms) to copy number variants, where segments up to thousands of base pairs long can be deleted or duplicated. SNPs are the commonest variant. They occur approximately every 200 base pairs, but less frequently in coding sequence because of potential for adversely affecting protein function and hence incurring negative selection pressure.

Genes comprise exons (the coding sequence) and introns, which are removed prior to mRNA being translated to protein. Gene density varies considerably, with lengthy tracts of noncoding sequence, formerly and erroneously

Clinical Dilemmas in Inflammatory Bowel Disease: New Challenges, Second Edition. Edited by P. Irving, C. Siegel, D. Rampton and F. Shanahan.
© 2011 Blackwell Publishing Ltd. Published 2011 by Blackwell Publishing Ltd.

referred to as "junk DNA," being interposed. Increasingly, it is recognized that much of the complexity of human biology derives not from the coding sequence, but from the complex, networked regulation of gene transcription by a host of epigenetic mechanisms. These include alternative exon splicing and control of mRNA stability by microRNAs, as well as DNA methylation and histone binding. These mechanisms (reviewed in [2]) allow dynamic activation or silencing of genes, and are heritable in being transmissible at mitosis, for example, to maintain tissue-specificity of gene expression, but they are not related to changes in DNA sequence.

Genetic variation in IBD

What forms of genetic variation contribute to IBD? The answer is likely to be "all of them," to a greater or lesser extent, perhaps including mechanisms yet to be characterized. Extrapolation from monogenic disease initially suggested that coding variation was likely to be most relevant, and its obvious impact on protein structure and function supported this intuition. Further, the three relatively common causal variants in NOD2, the first IBD gene to be identified, were all coding variants [3]. Thus, early genome-wide genotyping arrays, which could accommodate relatively few SNPs, focussed only on "nonsynonymous" SNPs. Although some interesting results were obtained, particularly in identifying the importance of ATG16L1 and autophagy in CD, the yield was unimpressive [4].

Truly hypothesis-free GWAS studies have followed, interrogating most if not all common variations (allele frequency >5%) genome-wide. Interestingly, the yield from these "proper" GWAS studies has been much greater than from nonsynonymous SNP scans and many lessons have been learned.

One remarkably consistent feature of GWAS studies has been the number of "gene deserts" showing association across a range of complex diseases. The supposition is that these loci contain elements that regulate transcription, and there is now evidence that sequence variation influences transcription for many genes. Thus, epigenetic regulation is itself a heritable trait and may be the key factor contributing to phenotypic variation in humans [5].

Several "gene desert" associations have been seen in IBD: indeed in the first meta-analysis plus replication of CD GWAS studies from the international IBD genetics con-

sortium, 6 out of the 32 confirmed loci mapped to gene deserts. More than this, our now detailed knowledge of all common sequence variations genome-wide allowed us to identify how many of the CD susceptibility loci correlated with *any* known coding variation. The answer, rather startlingly, was just 9 [1]. To emphasize this point, coding variation has to date been confirmed as causal for just two loci—NOD2 and ATG16L1, with one other at IL23R strongly implicated.

Regulation of gene expression in IBD

Accepting the indirect evidence that regulatory effects are important, is there any direct evidence? The answer is emphatically yes. In the Belgian CD GWAS, the strongest association was seen with a 1.25-Mb gene desert on chromosome 5. Using publicly available expression quantitative trait loci (eQTL) data, Libioulle et al. showed that these same SNPs that showed association with CD also correlated strongly with expression of the prostaglandin receptor gene EP4 270 Kb away [6]. The international CD meta-analysis study identified a number of other such correlations [1], and in its most recent analysis identified association at a DNA methyltransferase gene, emphasizing the importance of epigenetic regulation and its interrelationship with sequence variation in CD susceptibility.

Evidence from basic research corroborates the importance and potential complexity of epigenetic effects. Thus, the toll-like receptor-induced inflammatory response in mouse macrophages is regulated at a gene-specific level by transient chromatin modification, with Th2 "bias" being conferred by a transcriptional regulator of IL-4 called Mina. Highlighting the interplay of sequence variation with epigenetics, production of Mina is itself strongly correlated with SNP haplotypes in its promoter [7].

Identifying correlation between IBD association signals and gene expression hints at functional regulatory elements, but usually does not explain the mechanism. The expectation is that genome-wide assays for DNA methylation, ChIP seq, histone binding, and DNA tertiary structure (e.g., chromatin conformation capture or 3C), will provide some answers over the next few years [8]. They should allow both a better understanding of the mechanisms underlying current GWAS signals and also permit de novo genome-wide studies.

Limitations of current studies of epigenetic mechanisms in IBD

At present, difficulties in defining which cell type to target for expression analyses are limiting. The relevance of this comes from the recognition that many gene regulatory effects are cell-type specific—as seen for the CD-associated allele of IRGM which affects expression in opposite directions in different cell types [9]. Further concerns relate to the confounding effects of inflammation and drug therapy. Nonetheless, the evidence that epigenetic mechanisms are crucial in regulating gene transcription and thereby affecting susceptibility to disease will drive development of the appropriate resources to tackle these questions.

Epigenetic regulation is also significantly influenced by environmental factors, including diet, smoking, and infection—all of which are implicated in IBD pathogenesis. For example, aryl hydrocarbon receptor (AhR) agonists, which are present in substances as varied as cigarette smoke and *Brassica* vegetables, can strongly influence COX-2 expression. The effect may be related to AhR acting directly as a transcriptional regulator and also by regulating histone acetylation and hence chromatin structure [10]. The AhR also plays a key role in modulating Th17 lymphocyte development through epigenetic mechanisms [11]. The suggestion that some epigenetic regulatory influences may be transmissible through meiosis to the next generation adds particular interest to this story [12].

Conclusions

At present, GWAS studies are being widely deployed not because they provide all the answers, but rather because they are technologically tractable and provide robust and reproducible data. More technologically challenging and complex studies will follow to advance our knowledge of the epigenetic regulation of gene transcription and its contribution to inflammatory disease [13].

The suspicion is that many of the pathways highlighted by GWAS studies will also be flagged as important for IBD pathogenesis by other techniques. A case in point might come from the confirmed association of noncoding SNPs adjacent to IL-10 with IBD [14], plus the recent observation that IL-10 gene expression in antigen-presenting cells is strongly regulated by the histone deacetylase HDAC11 [15]. Perhaps these findings are directly correlated, or maybe the GWAS signal is flagging a pathway influenced by many epigenetic and other mechanisms that themselves regulate IL-10 transcription and thereby influence IBD susceptibility.

All of these studies represent work in progress, and despite recent exciting developments this remains a field in its infancy. Nonetheless, current evidence suggests that for most individuals with IBD, coding variation is likely to have made only a modest contribution to their disease risk, while epigenetic regulation of gene transcription, perhaps influenced by environmental factors such as smoking, bacteria, and diet, play a much more important role.

References

1. Barrett JC, Hansoul S, Nicolae DL, Cho JH, Duerr RH, Rioux JD, et al. Genome-wide association defines more than 30 distinct susceptibility loci for Crohn's disease. *Nat Genet* 2008; **40**(8): 955–962.

2. Bernstein BE, Meissner A, Lander ES. The mammalian epigenome. *Cell* 2007; **128**(4): 669–681.

3. Hugot JP, Chamaillard M, Zouali H, Lesage S, Cezard JP, Belaiche J, et al. Association of NOD2 leucine-rich repeat variants with susceptibility to Crohn's disease. *Nature* 2001; **411**(6837): 599–603.

4. Hampe J, Franke A, Rosenstiel P, Till A, Teuber M, Huse K, et al. A genome-wide association scan of nonsynonymous SNPs identifies a susceptibility variant for Crohn disease in ATG16L1. *Nat Genet* 2007; **39**(2): 207–211.

5. Dixon AL, Liang L, Moffatt MF, Chen W, Heath S, Wong KC, et al. A genome-wide association study of global gene expression. *Nat Genet* 2007; **39**(10): 1202–1207.

6. Libioulle C, Louis E, Hansoul S, Sandor C, Farnir F, Franchimont D, et al. Novel Crohn disease locus identified by genome-wide association maps to a gene desert on 5p13.1 and modulates expression of PTGER4. *PLoS Genet* 2007; **3**(4): e58.

7. Okamoto M, Van Stry M, Chung L, Koyanagi M, Sun X, Suzuki Y, et al. Mina, an Il4 repressor, controls T helper type 2 bias. *Nat Immunol* 2009; **10**(8): 872–879.

8. Parker SC, Hansen L, Abaan HO, Tullius TD, Margulies EH. Local DNA topography correlates with functional noncoding regions of the human genome. *Science* 2009; **324**(5925): 389–392.

9. McCarroll SA, Huett A, Kuballa P, Chilewski SD, Landry A, Goyette P, et al. Deletion polymorphism upstream of IRGM associated with altered IRGM expression and Crohn's disease. *Nat Genet* 2008; **40**(9): 1107–1112.

10. Degner SC, Papoutsis AJ, Selmin O, Romagnolo DF. Targeting of aryl hydrocarbon receptor-mediated activation of cyclooxygenase-2 expression by the indole-3-carbinol metabolite 3,3′-diindolylmethane in breast cancer cells. *J Nutr* 2009; **139**(1): 26–32.

11. Veldhoen M, Hirota K, Westendorf AM, Buer J, Dumoutier L, Renauld JC, et al. The aryl hydrocarbon receptor links TH17-cell-mediated autoimmunity to environmental toxins. *Nature* 2008; **453**(7191): 106–109.

12. Jirtle RL, Skinner MK. Environmental epigenomics and disease susceptibility. *Nat Rev Genet* 2007; **8**(4): 253–262.

13. Wilson AG. Epigenetic regulation of gene expression in the inflammatory response and relevance to common diseases. *J Periodontol* 2008; **79**(Suppl. 8): 1514–1519.

14. Franke A, Balschun T, Karlsen TH, Sventoraityte J, Nikolaus S, Mayr G, et al. Sequence variants in IL10, ARPC2 and multiple other loci contribute to ulcerative colitis susceptibility. *Nat Genet* 2008; **40**(11): 1319–1323.

15. Villagra A, Cheng F, Wang HW, Suarez I, Glozak M, Maurin M, et al. The histone deacetylase HDAC11 regulates the expression of interleukin 10 and immune tolerance. *Nat Immunol* 2009; **10**(1): 92–100.

IBD in different ethnic groups: same or different?

Rupert W.L. Leong[1], Dorothy K.L. Chow[2], and Christian P. Selinger[3]

[1] Department of Gastroenterology and Liver Services, Sydney South West Area Health Service, Concord and Bankstown Hospitals, Sydney, NSW, Australia
[2] Department of Medicine and Therapeutics, Prince of Wales Hospital, The Chinese University of Hong Kong, Hong Kong SAR, China
[3] Department of Gastroenterology, Salford Royal Hospital, The University of Salford, Manchester, UK

LEARNING POINTS

- There are many genotypic but few phenotypic differences in IBD in different ethnic groups.

- In relation to genotypic differences:

  - the NOD2 and IL23R gene polymorphisms highly linked to Crohn's disease (CD) in Caucasians appear to be absent in Asians;

  - few genes show homologous risk susceptibility in Asians and Caucasians: these include the tumor necrosis factor superfamily 15 (TNFSF15) gene for CD and the HLA region for ulcerative colitis;

  - among genes known to confer risk of IBD, there may be unidentified polymorphisms in Asians.

- The few phenotypic differences in different ethnic groups include a male preponderance of IBD in Asians and primary sclerosing cholangitis being rare in Asians.

Introduction

Inflammatory bowel disease (IBD) occurs worldwide but predominates in Western countries. However, in recent years there has been a marked rise in the incidence of IBD in developing countries, especially in Asia from where most non-Western IBD data are derived. Whether IBD in different ethnicities is the same disease is not certain. Disease similarities may be studied according to a compari-

son of their genotypes and phenotypes and help confirm analogous pathogeneses, natural histories, and responses to treatment. Comparing diseases may validate the generalization of IBD research and clinical practice across different populations.

Genotype

IBDs are polygenic diseases of variable penetrance that require a complex interaction with the environment and the intestinal microflora for phenotypic manifestation. Familial clustering of IBD differs in the West (up to 40% [1]) and Asia (0–7% [2]), but there are few data on twins, IBD concordance, and phenotypic concordance in low-prevalence ethnicities.

While there has been a vast increase in research in IBD genetics, especially using genome-wide association scans in Western populations, similar large-scale studies need to be replicated in non-Western populations. Data from Asian populations have been derived mainly from tertiary institutions as case-control samples, often through single nucleotide polymorphism (SNP) testing. What research has been done has highlighted differences in the genetic makeup of IBD in different ethnic populations, and while an extensive review of this area is beyond the scope of this chapter, NOD2 and IL-23R are used as examples.

Clinical Dilemmas in Inflammatory Bowel Disease: New Challenges, Second Edition. Edited by P. Irving, C. Siegel, D. Rampton and F. Shanahan.
© 2011 Blackwell Publishing Ltd. Published 2011 by Blackwell Publishing Ltd.

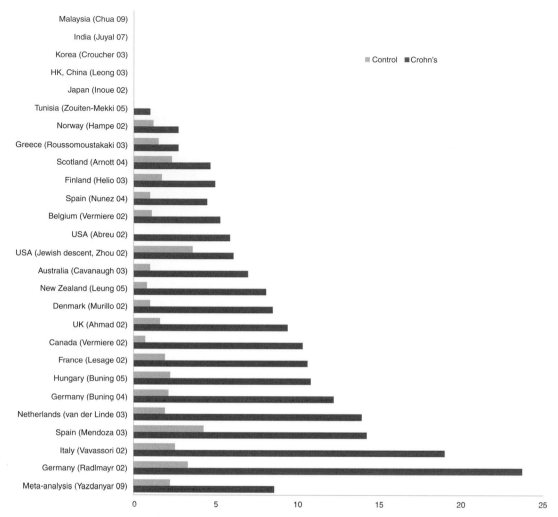

FIGURE 2.1 The percentage allelic frequencies of the 1007fs frameshift (SNP13) polymorphism of the NOD2 gene in Crohn's disease (CD) and controls from different countries, with author and year of publication.

The NOD2 Gene

Approximately 30% of patients of European ancestry have at least one of three SNPs linked to the development of CD. In contrast, the prevalence of NOD2 mutations in Asian IBD and non-IBD conditions is negligible at around 0% in the Chinese, Japanese, and Korean populations [4], although gene-sequencing studies have occasionally revealed rare novel NOD2 mutations of uncertain significance in Asians. While SNP8, SNP12, and SNP13 have been most closely linked to CD in Caucasians, SNP5 has been linked to the development of both UC (odd ratio (OR) 1.72, 95% con-

fidence interval (CI) 1.17–2.52) and CD in India [5]. Figure 2.1 demonstrates the heterogeneity of the allelic frequencies of the 1007fs frameshift gene (SNP13) polymorphism in CD and controls from different countries.

The Interleukin 23 Receptor

The interleukin 23 receptor (IL-23R) and Th17 pathway mediates microbial defense and intestinal inflammation [6]. Multiple genes along the IL-23 signaling pathway are associated with both CD and UC. The Arg381Gln SNP of the IL-23R on chromosome 1p31 was found to protect against the development of CD in Caucasians

[7]. However, in the Japanese population there was no association with CD in a study of ten IL-23R SNPs in 484 CD patients and 439 controls [8]. The same study also found that some SNPs that are found in Caucasians are entirely absent in the Japanese population, further demonstrating the genetic divergence between different ethnicities. Using DNA direct sequencing on a Chinese cohort, T allele carriers at the rs11465788 marker of the nontranscribed intron were significantly lower in 134 CD patients (75%) compared with 131 controls (91%, $P < 0.0005$) [9]. As the DNA intron region does not code amino acids, epigenetic factors may influence IBD pathogenesis (see Chapter 1). The CD phenotype of this polymorphism (nonstricturing, nonpenetrating) did not match that of CD Caucasian patients (ileal, stricturing), and a larger replication study needs to be performed. However, the study suggests that different gene polymorphisms affecting similar pathogenic pathways may occur in different racial populations.

Phenotype

IBD phenotypes differ between and within populations, and there are no distinguishing phenotypes that separate Western from Asian IBD. Male predominance of CD is a common feature of IBD in developing countries, but smoking may be a confounding factor [10]. CD and UC behavior and extent appear similar in Asian and Western IBD. Despite the genotypic differences between Western and Asian IBD, the lack of phenotypic differences supports the concept that IBD is a heterogenous collection of diseases that are not race-specific. These findings, plus the rapid increase in disease incidence, suggest that environmental factors also play a crucial role in the development of IBD.

Age

The age of diagnosis of CD in Asia is similar to, or older than that of Western countries. A younger age of diagnosis

of CD in Asia is associated with a worse prognosis, with greater number of flares and requirement for azathioprine. In Caucasians, a younger age of diagnosis of CD is also associated with a worse outcome with earlier stricturing and penetrating complications and requirement for surgery.

In a cohort of Chinese UC patients from Hong Kong, the median age at diagnosis was 37 years (range 12–85) with an equal distribution of men (52%) and women [11]. In comparison a review of studies of North American populations found a slight predominance of females (48–65%) and that age of diagnosis ranged from 33 to 39 years [12].

Behavior

The behavior of CD in Asia resembles that in Western countries. Despite the negligible contribution of the NOD2 SNPs in Asian CD, terminal ileal stricturing disease is still apparent but in lower proportions than Western CD, suggesting that these gene polymorphisms are not necessary for the development of tCD features.

The evolution of CD behavior with time leads to a progressive increase in patients developing stricturing or penetrating phenotypes in both Western and Chinese populations [13].

Location

The location of CD remains relatively stable over time in both Asians and Caucasians. In one cohort of Chinese CD patients, 19% of patients had gastrointestinal involvement proximal to the terminal ileum . However, isolated small bowel disease is uncommon in Chinese patients (4%) in comparison with Western patients (24–45%); Table 2.1 compares the location of CD in the Hong Kong Chinese with Western series. For UC, the extent of inflammation in Asia is similar to Western studies when similar patient recruitment methodologies are employed [18,19].

TABLE 2.1 A comparison of the locations of Crohn's disease (CD) in percent in different countries based on the Vienna classification

Crohn's disease (CD) location	Hong Kong [4]	Stockholm Sweden [14]	Perth Australia [15]	Vancouver Canada	Liege Belgium [16]	New York USA [17]
Terminal ileum	4	28	24	25	45	26
Colon	30	52	42	27	27	39
Ileocolon	44	14	34	35	24	22
Upper gastrointestinal tract	19	6	0	13	4	12

Dysplasia in UC

A recent multicenter study from Korea revealed a high cumulative rate of colorectal cancer (CRC) in UC patients over time [20]. The cumulative risk of UC-associated CRC was 0.7%, 7.9%, and 33.2% after 10, 20, and 30 years of disease, respectively. Whether the particularly high rate of CRC with long disease duration relates to differences in disease behavior or is a result of other factors, such as knowledge about and use of screening and chemoprevention or perhaps methodological issues with the study, is unclear.

Extraintestinal Manifestations

In general, the proportion of patients having extraintestinal manifestations (EIM) in Asia is similar to Western series with 6–35% of IBD patients having at least one EIM [16,21]. However, the incidence of primary sclerosing cholangitis is much lower in Asian IBD patients [22,23].

Conclusions

Geographic variance in IBD prevalence is related both to genotypic variations and environmental risk factors suppressing or promoting phenotypic expression. Recently, there has been an increase in the incidence of IBD in many parts of the world, the phenotype occurring being remarkably similar to that of Western IBD populations in terms of disease location, severity, behavior, and complications. EIM and mucosal dysplasia in chronic colitis also occur. Overall, there are more differences in IBD phenotype within a race than between races. Therefore, similar IBD pathogenic pathways and responses to treatment could be expected in different ethnicities.

However, the genotype of Asian IBD differs markedly to that of Western IBD. The near absence of NOD2 and IL-23R gene polymorphisms in Asians may indicate alternative polymorphism locations that are currently not tested for on SNP studies. There is a need to perform high-quality genome-wide association (GWA) studies in non-Caucasian populations to confirm this. On the other hand, it is possible that a complex interaction between genes, cytokines, signaling molecules, and the gene epistasis means that mechanisms of intestinal inflammation that differ between ethnicities may result in common clinical manifestations.

References

1. Lashner BA, Evans AA, Kirsner JB, et al. Prevalence and incidence of inflammatory bowel disease in family members. *Gastroenterology* 1986; **91**: 1395–1400.
2. Yang SK, Loftus EV, Jr, Sandborn WJ. Epidemiology of inflammatory bowel disease in Asia. *Inflamm Bowel Dis* 2001; **7**: 260–270.
3. Leong RW, Lau JY, Sung JJ. The epidemiology and phenotype of Crohn's disease in the Chinese population. *Inflamm Bowel Dis* 2004; **10**: 646–651.
4. Cho JH, Weaver CT. The genetics of inflammatory bowel disease. *Gastroenterology* 2007; **133**: 1327–1339.
5. Juyal G, Amre D, Midha V, Sood A, Seidman E, Thelma BK. Evidence of allelic heterogeneity for associations between the NOD2/CARD15 gene and ulcerative colitis among North Indians. *Aliment Pharmacol Ther* 2007; **26**(10): 1325–1332.
6. McGeachy MJ, Cua DJ. The link between IL-23 and Th17 cell-mediated immune pathologies. *Semin Immunol* 2007; **19**: 372–376.
7. Duerr RH, Taylor KD, Brant SR, et al. A genome-wide association study identifies IL23R as an inflammatory bowel disease gene. *Science* 2006; **314**(5804): 1461–1463. Epub Oct 26, 2006.
8. Yamazaki K, Onouchi Y, Takazoe M, Kubo M, Nakamura Y, Hata A. Association analysis of genetic variants in IL23R, ATG16L1 and 5p13.1 loci with Crohn's disease in Japanese patients. *J Hum Genet* 2007; **52**(7): 575–583.
9. Bin C, Zhirong Z, Xiaoqin W, et al. Contribution of rs11465788 in IL23R gene to Crohn's disease susceptibility and phenotype in Chinese population. *J Genet* 2009; **88**(2): 191–196.
10. APDW2004 Chinese IBD Working Group. Retrospective analysis of 515 cases of Crohn's disease hospitalization in China: nationwide study from 1990 to 2003. *J Gastroenterol Hepatol* 2006; **21**: 1009–1015.
11. Chow DK, Leong RW, Tsoi KK, et al. Long-term follow-up of ulcerative colitis in the Chinese population. *Am J Gastroenterology* 2009; **104**(3): 647–654.
12. Loftus EV, Jr, Schoenfeld P, Sandborn WJ. The epidemiology and natural history of Crohn's disease in population based patient cohorts from North America: a systematic review. *Aliment Pharmacol Ther* 2002; **16**: 51–60.
13. Chow DK, Leong RW, Lai LH, Wong GL, Leung WK, Chan FK, Sung JJ. Changes in Crohn's disease phenotype over time in the Chinese population: validation of the Montreal classification system. *Inflamm Bowel Dis* 2008; **14**(4): 536–541.
14. Lapidus A. Crohn's disease in Stockholm County during 1990-2001: an epidemiological update. *World J Gastroenterol* 2006; **12**: 75–81.

15. Lawrance IC, Murray K, Hall A, Sung JJ, Leong R. A prospective comparative study of ASCA and pANCA in Chinese and Caucasian IBD patients. *Am J Gastroenterol* 2004; **99**(11): 2186–2194.

16. Louis E, Collard A, Oger AF, Degroote E, Aboul Nasr El Yafi FA, Belaiche J. Behaviour of Crohn's disease according to the Vienna classification: changing pattern over the course of the disease. *Gut* 2001; **49**: 777–782.

17. Dorn SD, Abad JF, Panagopoulos G, Korelitz BI. Clinical characteristics of familial versus sporadic Crohn's disease using the Vienna Classification. *Inflamm Bowel Dis* 2004; **10**: 201–206.

18. Sood A, Midha V, Sood N, Bhatia AS, Avasthi G. Incidence and prevalence of ulcerative colitis in Punjab, North India. *Gut* 2003; **52**: 1587–90.

19. Jiang Li, Xia Bing, Li Jin, et al. Retrospective survey of 452 patients with inflammatory bowel disease in Wuhan city, central China. *Inflamm Bowel Dis* 2006; **12**: 212–217.

20. Kim BJ, Yang SK, Kim JS, et al. Trends of ulcerative colitis-associated colorectal cancer in Korea: A KASID study. *J Gastroenterol Hepatol* 2009; **24**(4): 667–671.

21. Kochhar R, Mehta SK, Nagi B, et al. Extraintestinal manifestations of idiopathic ulcerative colitis. *Indian J Gastroenterol* 1991; **10**: 88–89.

22. Park SM, Han DS, Yang SK, et al. Clinical features of ulcerative colitis in Korea. *Korean J Intern Med* 1996; **11**: 9–17.

23. Thia KT, Loftus EV, Jr, Sandborn WJ, Yang SK. An update on the epidemiology of inflammatory bowel disease in Asia. *Am j Gastroenterol* 2008; **103**: 3167–3182.

PART II:
Bugs and IBD—Good, Bad, or Indifferent?

3 How does the risk of infection influence management of IBD around the world?

Kiran K. Peddi[1] and Ian Craig Lawrance[2,3]

[1] Department of Gastroenterology, Fremantle Hospital, Alma Street, Fremantle, WA, Australia
[2] The Centre for Inflammatory Bowel Diseases, Fremantle Hospital, Fremantle, WA, Australia
[3] School of Medicine and Pharmacology, University of Western Australia, WA, Australia

LEARNING POINTS

- Infections endemic to a given geographic location should be taken into consideration when managing patients with IBD.

- An infective cause must be excluded at initial presentation and with each flare of IBD.

- Immunomodulators used in the treatment of IBD, especially when used in combination with corticosteroids, increase the risk of opportunistic infections.

- In parts of the world where TB is common, particular care should be taken when using immunomodulators, steroids, or anti-TNF (antitumor necrosis factor) therapy.

- The possibility of reactivation of hepatitis B and varicella zoster should be considered when starting immunomodulator and/or anti-TNF agents and treatment or vaccination offered to appropriate patients.

Introduction

Crohn's disease (CD) was considered to occur primarily in countries of the developed western world, but over the last decade evidence has emerged that the number of cases in the developing world is also increasing. Data from China, Hong Kong, and the Asian subcontinent all suggest that as the standard of living rises and the population becomes more urbanized, the risk of developing CD increases. It would also appear that as the CD risk increases, the rate of ulcerative colitis (UC) decreases.

Current practice promotes the use of early and aggressive therapy, and evidence suggests that the use of biological agents early in CD may improve the long-term outcomes of the disease. However, this must be tempered with the risk of adverse events. As steroids, immunomodulators and biological therapy can result in the development of serious infections, the endemic nature of various infections in each country may require modification of the medical management of the inflammatory bowel diseases (IBDs).

Acute bacterial and parasitic infections mimicking IBD flare

Infection must be considered at the initial presentation, and at each flare, of IBD. In the United Kingdom, acute gastroenteritis was associated with a 2.5-fold increased risk of developing IBD [1] suggesting that an acute infective gastroenteritis might provoke the chronic intestinal inflammatory changes in genetically susceptible individuals [2]. Many bacterial infections can also result in the relapse of IBD. Clostridium difficile infection has particularly been implicated with disease flares in developed countries [3], and may be difficult to diagnose. Thus, multiple stool specimens are recommended in patients having a disease flare.

Parasite infections also require exclusion. *Strongyloides stercoralis* is endemic in the tropics and subtropics with sporadic localization in temperate regions. Hyperinfection leading to alveolar hemorrhage and disseminated disease can occur in immunosuppressed patients [4] and should be excluded in endemic regions before such therapy is started.

Clinical Dilemmas in Inflammatory Bowel Disease: New Challenges, Second Edition. Edited by P. Irving, C. Siegel, D. Rampton and F. Shanahan.
© 2011 Blackwell Publishing Ltd. Published 2011 by Blackwell Publishing Ltd.

Toxoplasma gondii can also present with focal encephalitis in the immunocompromised, while amoebic dysentery, best identified by sending a hot fresh stool for prompt microscopy, requires differentiation from the new diagnosis of IBD in tropical countries and in returning travelers. This is particularly important as the use of corticosteroids can be dangerous in these patients [5].

Influence of IBD therapies on the risk of infection

Corticosteroids, azathioprine (AZA), 6-mercaptopurine (6-MP), and the anti-TNF (antitumor necrosis factor) medications all increase the risk of infection, which itself varies with the geographic region. One case-control study undertaken in the developed world demonstrated that the use of two or more immunosuppressive medications in combination increased the risk of opportunistic infections by 14.5-fold [6]. In this study, the majority of the risk occurred with the addition of corticosteroids to thiopurines and anti-TNF agents. The TREAT registry collected almost 24,600 CD patient years of follow-up, again in the developed world, and identified that infliximab-treated patients had an increased risk of serious infections. However, this was also noted to be independently associated with the use of prednisone and not infliximab [7]. Thus, although the independent risk of infection with thiopurines and anti-TNF agents has been variable, the risk of serious infections in association with corticosteroid therapy has been consistently demonstrated.

TNF is involved in the regulation of cellular immunity with a particular role in eradication of intracellular pathogens like *Mycobacterium tuberculosis* (TB). TNF also plays a key role in clearance of the hepatitis B virus (HBV). Therefore, reactivation of TB and increased HBV replication can be associated with anti-TNF medications [8]. Thus, the use of immunosuppressive medications must be tempered by the potential risks in the various regions of the world.

Tuberculosis

The use of anti-TNF agents increases the risk of TB infection. However, even before the anti-TNF era TB in the United Kingdom was more common in IBD patients taking immunomodulators, particularly with corticosteroid use [9]. Unfortunately, a primary infection that develops during anti-TNF therapy is usually extrapulmonary, or disseminated, making diagnosis difficult. Reactivation of latent

TB frequently occurs in the first few weeks after initiating anti-TNF therapy and requires clinical surveillance.

The risk for primary TB is dependent on its prevalence in the community (Figure 3.1). In Spain, TB prevalence was 21/100,000, while patients receiving anti-TNF therapy demonstrated a 90-fold increased risk [10]. In the United States, where the prevalence was lower at 6.8/100,000, the risk with anti-TNF therapy increased 8-fold. In Australia, the prevalence of TB is 0.9/100,000 in the nonindigenous Australian-born population and the risk with anti-TNF therapy is lower still [11]. However, screening is required for all patients prior to anti-TNF therapy, particularly in high-risk regions. Screening includes a detailed medical history, physical examination, chest X-ray, Mantoux test, and/or interferon gamma release assay (Quantiferon gold) [7]. Following the introduction in Spain of routine screening prior to starting anti-TNF therapy, a 74% reduction in the rate of TB cases was observed [12]. Patients identified with latent or active TB can then be treated according to the local guidelines in consultation with an expert in pulmonary or infectious diseases. Screening could also be considered prior to the use of corticosteroids and other immunomodulators in regions of high endemicity, although efficacy of this has not been demonstrated.

Hepatitis B (see also Chapter 5)

HBV is a ubiquitous virus with a global distribution. It is highly endemic in all of Africa, parts of South America, Eastern Europe, Eastern Mediterranean, Southeast Asia, China, and the Pacific Islands where 5–15% of the population are chronically infected carriers (Figure 3.1). HBV can persist after serological recovery from acute infection, and TNF plays a key role in HBV clearance from infected hepatocytes. Treatment with anti-TNF agents can promote HBV replication and lead to life-threatening flares because of rebound of the body's immune response on ceasing anti-TNF therapy [13]. Recommendations in Australia, and the European Crohn's and Colitis Organization (ECCO), suggest that HBV serology should be performed on all IBD patients prior to starting anti-TNF therapy. Individuals with negative serology could then be considered for vaccination.

This is of even greater importance in regions of high HBV endemicity. Those patients who require immunosuppression or anti-TNF therapy, and have chronic active HBV, should receive treatment with nucleotide/nucleoside analogs such as lamivudine. Unfortunately, this requires

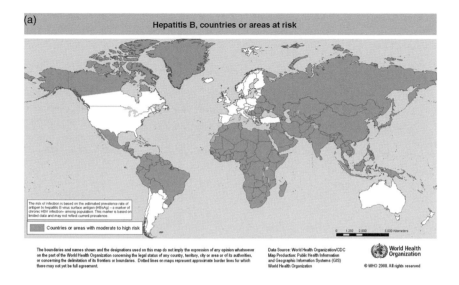

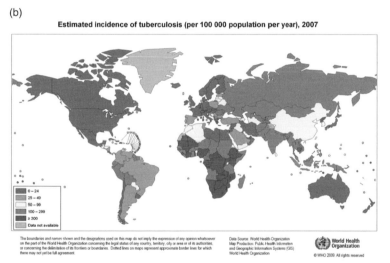

FIGURE 3.1 World distribution of TB and hepatitis B. (Modified from the WHO websites: http://gamapserver.who.int/mapLibrary/ Files/Maps/Global_MDG6_TBincidence_2007.png; http://gamapserver.who.int/mapLibrary/Files/Maps/Global_HepB_ITHRiskMap.png.)

medical resources that may not be readily available in some countries. For those patients who are HBSAg –ve and anti-HBc +ve, monitoring by regular liver function tests and HBV serology while on immunosuppression is also recommended [4]. Unfortunately, the interferon medications can cause CD to flare and should be avoided when treating coexisting HBV infections [14].

In contrast to HBV, hepatitis C Virus (HCV) has a broadly similar prevalence throughout the world. Treatment with immunomodulators is considered to be safe

in patients with HCV, but many authorities still advocate monitoring the disease activity while on these therapies.

Herpes zoster virus

Infection with herpes viruses is common and not localized to a single region. Following initial infection, the viruses can be latent in neural tissue. Varicella zoster virus (VZV) has been identified as a common anti-TNF-associated opportunistic infection [4,6,11], and both primary infection with and subsequent reactivation of VZV can be avoided in

VZV-naïve patients by vaccination. However, the VZV vaccine is a live virus and is not recommended for people on immunomodulators [4]. Thus, consideration should be given to assessment of a patient's VZV status prior to commencement of any immunosuppressive therapy with a view to the immunization of naïve patients. Typically, a delay in initiating immunosuppressive therapy of at least 1 month is required after live vaccination with VZV (see Chapter 10).

Conclusion

Corticosteroids, immunomodulators, and anti-TNF agents play a major role in the current management of IBD. However, the potential benefits should be weighed against the infection risk, which varies in different parts of the world. Acute enteric infections, the incidence of which again varies geographically, are common triggering factors for disease flares and must be excluded. Screening for TB, hepatitis, and herpes zoster is important prior to immunosuppressive therapy, and appropriate preventive measures should be undertaken.

References

1. Alberto L, Rodriguez G, Ruigomez A, Panes J. Acute gastroenteritis is followed by an increased risk of inflammatory bowel disease. *Gastroenterol* 2006; **130**(6): 1588–1594.
2. Irving PM, Gibson PR. Infections and IBD. *Nat Clin Pract Gastr* 2008; **5**(1): 18–27.
3. Rodemann JF, Dubberke ER, Reske KA, Seo DH, Stone CD. Incidence of clostridium difficile infection in inflammatory bowel disease. *Clin Gastroenterol Hepatol* 2007; **5**(3): 339–344.
4. Rahier JF, Ben-Horin S, Chowers Y, et al. European evidence-based consensus on the prevention, diagnosis and management of opportunistic infections in inflammatory bowel disease. *J Crohns Colitis* 2009; **3**(2): 47–91.
5. Abbas MA, Mulligan DC, Ramzan NN, et al. Colonic perforation in unsuspected amebic colitis. *Digest Dis Sci* 2000; **45**(9): 1836–1841.
6. Toruner M, Loftus EV, Harmsen WS, et al. Risk factors for opportunistic infections in patients with inflammatory bowel disease. *Gastroenterology* 2008; **134**(4): 929–936.
7. Lichtenstein GR, Cohen R, Feagan B, et al. Safety of infliximab and other Crohn's disease therapies-TREAT registry data with nearly 24,575 patient years of follow-up. *Am J Gastroenterology* 2008; **104**(S1): 5436.
8. Keane J, Gershon S, Wise RP, et al. Tuberculosis associated with infliximab, a tumor necrosis factor (alpha)-neutralizing agent. *N Engl J Med* 2001; **345**(15): 1098–1104.
9. Aberra FN, Stettler N, Brensinger C, Lichtenstein GR, Lewis JD. Risk for active tuberculosis in inflammatory bowel disease patients. *Clin Gastroenterol Hepatol* 2007; **5**(9): 1070–1075.
10. Gomez-Reino JJ, Carmona L, Valverde VR, Mola EM, Montero MD. Treatment of rheumatoid arthritis with tumor necrosis factor inhibitors may predispose to significant increase in tuberculosis risk—a multicenter active-surveillance report. *Arthritis Rheum* 2003; **48**(8): 2122–2127.
11. Lawrance IC, Bampton PA, Sparrow M, et al. Serious infective complications associated with anti-TNF alpha therapy in inflammatory bowel disease. *J Gastroenterol Hepatol* 2008; **23**(Suppl. 4): A195.
12. Carmona L, Gomez-Reino JJ, Rodriguez-Valverde V, et al. Effectiveness of recommendations to prevent reactivation of latent tuberculosis infection in patients treated with tumor necrosis factor antagonists. *Arthritis Rheum* 2005; **52**(6): 1766–1772.
13. Nathan DM, Angus PW, Gibson PR. Hepatitis B and C virus infections and anti-tumor necrosis factor-alpha therapy: guidelines for clinical approach. *J Gastroenterol Hepatol* 2006; **21**(9): 1366–1371.
14. Scherzer TM, Staufer K, Novacek G, et al. Efficacy and safety of antiviral therapy in patients with Crohn's disease and chronic hepatitis C. *Aliment Pharmcol Ther* 2008; **28**(6): 742–748.

Traveling with IBD

Ing Shian Soon[1] and Gilaad Kaplan[2]

[1]Division of Gastroenterology, Departments of Pediatrics and Community Health Sciences, University of Calgary, Calgary, AB, Canada
[2]Departments of Medicine and Community Health Sciences, Teaching Research and Wellness Center, University of Calgary, Calgary, AB, Canada

LEARNING POINTS

- Advanced planning is important for traveling with IBD.

- Routine immunizations should be up to date and additional vaccines considered depending on travel destinations, type of activities, and duration of travel.

- Live vaccines are contraindicated in patients on immunosuppressive therapies.

- Differentiating traveler's diarrhea from an acute flare of IBD can be difficult. Thus, IBD patients should seek medical attention if symptoms develop.

- IBD patients should be educated about food safety and self-treatment of traveler's diarrhea.

- Standard prophylactic measures against venous thromboembolism should be used on long flights.

- Several Web sites (e.g., Centers of Disease Control) can assist the traveling IBD patient.

Introduction

Traveling can be challenging for people with inflammatory bowel disease (IBD) because of concerns about disease recurrence and the complexity of using immune-suppressing medications: this is especially true for travel to countries where the risk of infection is high. However, with advanced planning and appropriate precautions, travel for IBD patients can be routine. In this chapter, we outline the measures that patients with IBD should take to make their traveling as rewarding, trouble-free, and enjoyable as possible.

IBD, infections, and vaccination

IBD patients are often prescribed immunosuppressive therapies and consequently are at increased risk of infection. Hence, protection against vaccine-preventable diseases is important. Prior to traveling abroad, healthcare providers should ensure that IBD patients are up to date with their routine immunization, and that they comply with country-specific immunization requirements [1].

Endemic infections

Traveling requires the consideration of additional vaccines depending on the destination, type of activities, and duration of travel. For example, hepatitis A virus immunization is recommended for travel to countries with highly endemic rates of hepatitis A infection. Typhoid fever, caused by *Salmonella typhi*, is usually spread through contaminated food and water, and typhoid vaccine is recommended for people traveling to countries where there is a risk of typhoid fever (e.g., the Indian subcontinent, Latin America, the Middle East, and Africa) [2]. Preexposure rabies immunization should be considered for those who will be traveling to areas where they may encounter wild or domestic animals, or where they may engage in activities involving increased risk of rabies transmission [3]. Japanese encephalitis virus, spread by *Culex* species mosquitoes, is a risk in Southeast Asia, China, eastern Russia, and the Indian subcontinent. Vaccination is recommended for travelers with prolonged residence in areas where Japanese encephalitis is endemic during the transmission season and for travelers who will engage in high-risk activities with extensive outdoor exposure [4]. Meningococcal disease, caused by

Clinical Dilemmas in Inflammatory Bowel Disease: New Challenges, Second Edition. Edited by P. Irving, C. Siegel, D. Rampton and F. Shanahan.
© 2011 Blackwell Publishing Ltd. Published 2011 by Blackwell Publishing Ltd.

Neisseria meningitidis, is transmitted via close contact with respiratory secretions or saliva. The incidence of meningococcal disease is highest in sub-Saharan Africa with periodic epidemics during the dry season (December through June). Travelers to the meningitis belt with prolonged contact with local populations are at highest risk and should be vaccinated [5].

Vaccination in patients on immunosuppressive therapy

Live bacteria and virus vaccines are contraindicated in IBD patients on immunosuppressive agents: these include prednisone at a dose > 20 mg/day; immunomodulators such as 6-mercaptopurine (6-MP), azathioprine, and methotrexate; and biologics such as infliximab, adalimumab, certolizumab pegol, and natalizumab [6]. For example, yellow fever vaccine is a live-attenuated virus vaccine that is recommended for persons aged 9 months and older, who are traveling to or living in areas where yellow fever infection is officially reported (i.e., Africa and South America). Yellow fever is transmitted by *Aedes aegypti* mosquitoes and the clinical spectrum ranges from subclinical infection to overwhelming pansystemic disease. Some countries require documentation of yellow fever vaccine as a condition of entry, including travelers arriving from regions with endemic infection. If IBD patients must travel to a yellow fever endemic zone, then patients should be advised of the risks posed by such travel, instructed in methods for avoiding vector mosquitoes, and supplied with vaccination waiver letters by their physicians. Other live vaccines that should be avoided include intranasal influenza vaccine, mumps, measles, and rubella (MMR), varicella, oral rotavirus, and Bacillus Calmette-Guérin (BCG). Persons with anaphylactic allergy to eggs or egg products should also avoid yellow fever and influenza vaccines.

For destination specific immunization requirements and health considerations, please visit the Centers of Disease Control Web site: http://wwwnc.cdc.gov/travel/destinations/list.aspx.

Malaria

Travelers to the tropics may be exposed to other diseases, such as malaria, which can be life-threatening. Malaria can be avoided by using antimalarial chemoprophylaxis and prevention of mosquito bites. The appropriate chemoprophylactic regimen depends on the areas to be visited and the risk of exposure to chloroquine-resistant *Plasmodium*

falciparum. Antimalarial agents should begin 1 week before arrival in the area with endemic infection and be taken weekly for the duration of exposure and for 4 weeks after departure from the areas. IBD patients traveling to areas where malaria is endemic should be advised to use personal protective measures similar to all other travelers [7].

Travelers' diarrhea

Travelers' diarrhea is a particularly significant potential problem in patients with IBD. It may be mitigated by paying attention to foods and beverages ingested and by drinking bottled water. Chemoprophylaxis generally is not recommended. Educating families about self-treatment is critical, this includes oral rehydration salts and antimicrobial agents for treatment of severe diarrheal symptoms. As bacterial causes of travelers' diarrhea are more common than other microbial etiologies, empiric treatment with an antibiotic directed at enteric bacterial pathogens is the best therapy for travelers' diarrhea. Single-dose or one-day therapy of ciprofloxacin can be used for travelers' diarrhea, while azithromycin is an alternative for children [8]. Patients should pack oral rehydration salts and antibiotics for travelers' diarrhea.

Differentiating travelers' diarrhea from an acute flare of underlying IBD can be difficult; furthermore, enteric infections can potentially exacerbate IBD [9]. Acute onset of diarrhea and high fever are more suggestive of travelers' diarrhea than IBD flare [10]. In travelers with an apparent exacerbation of their IBD, infections should be ruled out by organizing stool microscopy and cultures prior to the administration of corticosteroids or other immunosuppressive therapy. Patients should seek medical attention if they have bloody diarrhea or fluid depletion.

Tuberculosis

Reactivation of tuberculosis has been associated with the use of antitumor necrosis factor (anti-TNF) agents in IBD. Hence, patients on these drugs should take special precautions when traveling to endemic countries. Patients traveling for a prolonged period to a moderately or highly endemic area, and those who anticipate prolonged exposure to tuberculosis (e.g., close contact with hospital, prison, or homeless shelter populations) should be advised to have a two-step tuberculin skin test or interferon-gamma release assay before departure. If negative, it should be repeated approximately 8–10 weeks after returning [11]. Patients with IBD on immunomodulators and anti-TNF agents should avoid contact with tuberculosis patients.

Consultation with the travel medicine clinic is strongly recommended as the need for immunizations and preventative medications differ between destinations, duration, and purpose of the travel. Ideally, this should be done at least 6 months prior to travel. Furthermore, it is important to obtain a travel history of previous visits to a region where tuberculosis is endemic to risk stratify patients prior to initiation of anti-TNF agents.

Pretravel preparation

A checklist for IBD patients prior to traveling is outlined in Table 4.1.

Travel letter

Prior to travel, patients with IBD should consult their family physician or gastroenterologist to assess whether they are fit for travel and to obtain information on pretravel preparation, as well as their risk of disease flare. A travel letter outlining the patient's diagnosis, current medications, and dosage, known allergies as well as plans for an acute

TABLE 4.1 Checklist prior to travel

Family physician or gastroenterologist visit for assessment of fit to travel
Travel letter including the following items:

- Summary of IBD care: diagnosis, current medications and dosages, allergy
- Fit to travel
- Syringe, needles, and medication if on injection medications

Refill of current medications and medical supplies to ensure adequate supply of medications for the length of travel.
Emergency contacts for local gastroenterology clinic and travel destinations
Research on destination and route of travel, including bathroom accessibility
Immunizations:

- Ensure routine immunizations are up to date
- Special immunization depends on travel destination, type of activities, and duration of travel

Consultation with travel medicine clinic
Oral rehydration packs and antibiotics for traveler's diarrhea
Travel insurance

flare would be helpful to healthcare providers in case of emergency and may be needed by some airlines.

Medication supply

Patients should have an adequate supply of all current medications for the length of travel plus an extra week in case of unpredictable circumstances. For patients who are on injection medications, a medical letter outlining the purposes of the syringe, needles, and liquid medication may be needed for airport security. All medications and medical supplies should be packed in the hand carry bag, and extra clothing, toilet paper, and wipes may be useful. Patients prescribed medications that require refrigeration, including infliximab, adalimumab, and certolizumab pegol, should bring a cooler or ensure that they have access to a refrigerator on the airplane.

Journey planning

IBD patients are recommended to research their travel destinations and plan their itineraries prior to travel. Patients on infliximab should try to plan their trip around infusions. However, if this is not possible, identification of an infusion clinic at the destination should be done in advance. For travel by road, the availability of toilet facilities on public transport, on the route, and at the destination should be assessed. An aisle seat on the plane may allow easier access to the toilet. In view of the increased risk of venous thromboembolism in patients with IBD, prophylactic measures should be taken on long flights. Patients on methotrexate should pay attention to sunscreen, as photosensitivity is a potential side effect.

Travel insurance

Individuals should be covered for medical expenses, in the case of emergency during travel, either through their current medical insurance or travel insurance. IBD patients should be aware of any restrictions associated with their travel insurance.

Alert bracelets and contact details

Patients who are on corticosteroids should wear a medical alert bracelet to ensure prompt treatments such as stress-dose steroids in emergencies. Details of contacts for local clinic resources at travel destinations including IBD foundations, gastroenterologists, and hospitals should be taken by traveling IBD patients. IBD patients are recommended to review the Crohn's and Colitis Foundation of America's

Web site for additional information on travel specific needs: http://www.ccfa.org/info/links under International organizations. Additionally, the International Association for Medical Assistance to Travelers (www.iamat.org) coordinates a network of doctors and clinics around the world that will help IBD patients identify qualified English-speaking doctors, hospitals, and healthcare centers.

References

1. Melmed GY, Ippoliti AF, Papadakis KA, Tran TT, Birt JL, Lee SK, *et al.* Patients with inflammatory bowel disease are at risk for vaccine-preventable illnesses. *Am J Gastroenterol* 2006; **101**(8): 1834–1840.

2. Brunette GW, Kozarsky PE, Magill AJ, Shlim DR. Centers for Disease Control and Prevention. CDC Health Information for International Travel 2010. Atlanta: U.S. Department of Health and Human Services, Public Health Service, 2009.

3. Manning SE, Rupprecht CE, Fishbein D, Hanlon CA, Lumlertdacha B, Guerra M, *et al.* Human rabies prevention–United States, 2008: recommendations of the advisory committee on immunization practices. *MMWR Recomm Rep* 2008; **57**(RR-3): 1–28.

4. Inactivated Japanese encephalitis virus vaccine. Recommendations of the Advisory Committee on Immunization Practices (ACIP). *MMWR Recomm Rep* 1993; **42**(RR-1): 1–15.

5. Bilukha OO, Rosenstein N, National Center for Infectious Diseases CfDC, Prevention. Prevention and control of meningococcal disease. Recommendations of the Advisory Committee on Immunization Practices (ACIP). *MMWR Recomm Rep* 2005; **54**(RR-7): 1–21.

6. Sands BE, Cuffari C, Katz J, Kugathasan S, Onken J, Vitek C, *et al.* Guidelines for immunizations in patients with inflammatory bowel disease. *Inflammatory Bowel Diseases* 2004; **10**(5): 677–692.

7. Centers of Disease Control and Prevention. Measures to prevent bites from mosquitoes, ticks, fleas and other insects and arthropods. [Online]; 2007. Available from: http://wwwnc.cdc.gov/travel/content/mosquito-tick.aspx (accessed Jan 10, 2010).

8. Diemert DJ. Prevention and self-treatment of traveler's diarrhea. *Clinical Microbiology Reviews* 2006; **19**(3): 583–594.

9. Weber P, Koch M, Heizmann WR, Scheurlen M, Jenss H, Hartmann F. Microbic superinfection in relapse of inflammatory bowel disease. *J Clin Gastroenterol* 1992; **14**(4): 302–308.

10. Schumacher G, Kollberg B, Ljungh A. Inflammatory bowel disease presenting as travellers' diarrhoea. *Lancet* 1993; **341**(8839): 241–242.

11. Centers for Disease Control and Prevention, ed. *CDC Health Information for International Travel 2010*. Atlanta: US Department of Health and Human Services, Public Health Service, 2009; 2010.

5 What to do about hepatitis B and hepatitis C in patients with IBD

Morven Cunningham and Graham R. Foster

Blizard Institute of Cell and Molecular Science, Barts and The London School of Medicine and Dentistry, Queen Mary, University of London, London, UK

LEARNING POINTS

- All patients with IBD should be screened for hepatitis B infection (HBV), and there is a strong argument for screening for hepatitis C infection (HCV).

- In patients with chronic viral hepatitis and IBD requiring immunosuppressive therapy:

  o Those with HBV infection and HBsAg positivity should receive carefully supervised prophylactic therapy with a nucleoside analogue.

  o Those with previous or occult HBV infection do not require antiviral prophylaxis, but should be monitored closely for recurrent viremia.

  o As no effective prophylaxis currently exists for patients with chronic HCV who are immunosuppressed, such patients should be monitored by 3-yearly liver biopsies.

- Data on the safety of interferon-alpha in patients with IBD are limited:

  o It can be avoided in HBV by use of other agents.

  o In HCV, it appears safe in well-controlled ulcerative colitis, but should be used with caution in Crohn's disease.

Introduction

Chronic infection with hepatotropic viruses—either hepatitis B (HBV) or hepatitis C (HCV)—is common and many patients with inflammatory bowel disease (IBD) will have past or ongoing infection. Here we discuss the relationship between viral hepatitis and IBD before reviewing the complex interactions between the different treatments for these disorders.

IBD and chronic viral hepatitis

Patients with IBD have an increased risk of acquiring HBV or HCV infection, with a prevalence of up to 25% in one series [1]. The excess risk has been attributed to greater exposure to surgery and blood transfusion, and may now be reducing as effective screening of blood products is introduced [2]. Cell-mediated immunity driven by Th-1 cytokines is a feature of Crohn's disease (CD), while ulcerative colitis (UC) may be more Th-2 cytokine driven. Th-2 responses may contribute to the development of chronic HCV infection; however, no studies to date have examined the natural history of chronic viral hepatitis in conjunction with IBD.

Effect of treatment for IBD on viral hepatitis

Treatment of malignancy with immunosuppressive chemotherapy is a recognized cause of potentially fatal HBV reactivation [3]. Thus, the treatment of IBD with immunomodulatory drugs raises concerns regarding their effect on coexistent viral hepatitis.

Several case reports have described HBV reactivation following anti-TNF therapy for IBD, including one consequent fatality [4]. By contrast, short courses of anti-TNF agents do not seem to lead to an increase in HCV RNA or

Clinical Dilemmas in Inflammatory Bowel Disease: New Challenges, Second Edition. Edited by P. Irving, C. Siegel, D. Rampton and F. Shanahan.
© 2011 Blackwell Publishing Ltd. Published 2011 by Blackwell Publishing Ltd.

transaminase activity in patients with chronic HCV [5], but safety over the longer term is not established.

HBV contains a glucocorticoid responsive element that stimulates viral replication, and long-term corticosteroid treatment results in increased expression of viral antigens [6]. Increases in liver inflammation due to HBV (disease "flare") have been observed following corticosteroid treatment for IBD, in one instance leading to hepatic failure [7]. In chronic HCV infection, corticosteroids may increase viremia with a concomitant decrease in transaminases, presumably reflecting a reduction in immune-mediated liver inflammation. In renal transplant patients, this is associated with an increased rate of fibrosis progression [8].

There are few reports of the effect of other immunosuppressants such as thiopurines, methotrexate, and cyclosporin on viral hepatitis. Thiopurines may induce disease recurrence and reactivation in patients with past or chronic HBV infection. When used with infliximab in rheumatoid arthritis, methotrexate reactivates HBV [9], and the same effect is likely in IBD. In relation to chronic HCV, immunosuppression with low dose corticosteroids and azathioprine in renal transplant patients increased both viremia and the rate of fibrosis progression. It is probable that thiopurine monotherapy will have similar effects.

The effect of cyclosporin on HCV replication is controversial. Cyclophilins (intracellular cyclosporin targets) are necessary for HCV replication, and drug inhibitors of the HCV-cyclophilin interaction are under evaluation as therapeutic agents [10]. However, the effects of cyclosporin A on HCV replication appear modest, although there is some evidence of clinical benefit in the liver transplant setting [11].

Finally, while 5-aminosalicylate drugs have little effect on hepatotropic viruses, they can induce chronic hepatitis. Thiopurines and methotrexate are also hepatotoxic. Therefore, changes in liver inflammation in patients with chronic viral hepatitis receiving these medications should be investigated by liver biopsy.

Treatment of IBD in patients with HBV

Given the likelihood that individuals with IBD will require immunosuppressive therapy, universal screening for HBV is recommended, with vaccination for those who are seronegative. Response should be ensured as booster doses may be required.

Immunosuppressive medications are associated with increased viral replication in those with previous or chronic HBV infection. Disease flares are often seen on reduction or withdrawal of therapy, coincident with immune reconstitution and destruction of infected hepatocytes. Prophylaxis with the nucleoside analogue (NA) lamivudine prior to cancer chemotherapy results in a reduction in HBV reactivation and HBV-related mortality [12]. Case reports in patients with IBD and chronic HBV support the notion that lamivudine prophylaxis prior to immunosuppressive therapy is superior to a "watch and wait" policy in control of viral reactivation. The European Crohn's and Colitis Organization (ECCO) recommend that HBV surface antigen (HBsAg) positive patients should receive a prophylactic NA 2 weeks prior to commencing immunosuppressive therapy for IBD [13], and current recommendations from the European Association for the Study of the Liver (EASL) are to continue prophylactic NA therapy for 12 months following cessation of immunosuppressants [14].

Although the evidence for efficacy is limited, NA prophylaxis should be given to IBD patients with chronic HBV receiving any immunosuppressive agent. Considering the relatively high rate of resistance associated with prolonged use of lamivudine, agents such as entecavir or tenofovir should be considered. Most authorities now agree that lamivudine should not be used as a first-line therapy in patients with significant amounts of detectable HBV DNA [13].

Reactivation of HBV in patients with occult infection (HBsAg negative, but HBV core antibody and/or HBV surface antibody positive) occurs infrequently following immunosuppressive therapy. Routine prophylaxis is not currently recommended; however close monitoring for viremia is advised so that NA therapy can be instigated promptly if indicated, prior to a detectable rise in transaminases [13,14].

Treatment of IBD in patients with HCV

While flares of HCV have not been documented following immunosuppression with anti-TNF agents, their safety profile in longer term use remains to be established. The observation of increased viremia and worsening liver fibrosis with corticosteroid and azathioprine use in renal transplant recipients with chronic HCV tells a cautionary tale. No direct inhibitors of HCV replication currently exist for use as prophylaxis, although developments in this area are moving rapidly and new, direct-acting antivirals are anticipated within the next 2 years [15]. While present guidelines do not advocate against the use of immunosuppressants in patients with IBD and coexistent HCV [13], the doses should be minimized and the drug discontinued as soon as possible. Regular liver biopsies (e.g., every 3 years) should be considered for these patients, with biopsy-proven fibrosis progression prompting a review of the therapeutic options.

Treatment of viral hepatitis—effect of interferon on IBD

Interferon-alpha (IFN-α) is widely used to treat viral hepatitis. Pegylated IFN-α combined with ribavirin is the current standard treatment of chronic HCV. The immunomodulatory effects of IFN are complex, with both immunostimulatory and immunoinhibitory functions. It is believed that the context and dose have a major effect on the outcome of IFN-α therapy, but its contradictory effects make it impossible to predict its impact in patients with IBD. In the few studies that have examined IFN-α treatment for HCV in patients with IBD, IFN-α appears as efficacious in IBD patients as controls [16]. The risk of a flare of bowel disease while receiving IFN-α may be greater in CD than in well-controlled UC [16,17]. IFN-α should not be used in HBV, as safer drugs with greater potency are available.

Conclusions

We recommend that all patients with IBD should have viral hepatitis screening. Patients with chronic HBV infection requiring immunosuppression should receive carefully supervised NA therapy. Those with high-level viremia or likely to require prolonged therapy should receive a third-generation agent (entecavir or tenofovir), while patients with undetectable or barely detectable viremia may be successfully managed with lamivudine. Those with inactive or previous HBV infection should be monitored closely for viral reactivation. In the absence of effective therapeutic options, patients with chronic HCV infection who require immunosuppression for IBD should be monitored with liver biopsies every 3 years.

IFN-α appears safe in patients with well-controlled UC, although safety in CD is less established. IFN-α can be avoided in HBV by use of other agents, and, when necessary in HCV, should be used with caution.

References

1. Biancone L, Pavia M, Del Vecchio Blanco G, et al. Hepatitis B and C virus infection in Crohn's disease. *Inflamm Bowel Dis* 2001; **7**(4): 287–294.
2. Loras C, Saro C, Gonzalez-Huix F, Minguez M, et al. Prevalence and factors related to hepatitis B and C in inflammatory bowel disease patients in Spain: a nationwide, multicenter study. *Am J Gastroenterol* 2009; **104**(1): 57–63.
3. Dillon R, Hirschfield GM, Allison ME, Rege KP. Fatal reactivation of hepatitis B after chemotherapy for lymphoma. *BMJ* 2008; **337**: a423.
4. Esteve M, Saro C, Gonzalez-Huix F, Suarez F, Forne M, Viver JM. Chronic hepatitis B reactivation following infliximab therapy in Crohn's disease patients: need for primary prophylaxis. *Gut* 2004; **53**(9): 1363–1365.
5. Zein NN. Etanercept as an adjuvant to interferon and ribavirin in treatment-naive patients with chronic hepatitis C virus infection: a phase 2 randomized, double-blind, placebo-controlled study. *J Hepatol* 2005; **42**(3): 315–322.
6. Perrillo RP. Acute flares in chronic hepatitis B: the natural and unnatural history of an immunologically mediated liver disease. *Gastroenterology* 2001; **120**(4): 1009–1022.
7. Zeitz J, Mullhaupt B, Fruehauf H, Rogler G, Vavricka SR. Hepatic failure due to hepatitis B reactivation in a patient with ulcerative colitis treated with prednisone. *Hepatology* 2009; **50**(2): 653–654.
8. Zylberberg H, Nalpas B, Carnot F, et al. Severe evolution of chronic hepatitis C in renal transplantation: a case control study. *Nephrol Dial Transplant* 2002; **17**(1): 129–133.
9. Ostuni P, Botsios C, Punzi L, Sfriso P, Todesco S. Hepatitis B reactivation in a chronic hepatitis B surface antigen carrier with rheumatoid arthritis treated with infliximab and low dose methotrexate. *Ann Rheum Dis* 2003; **62**(7): 686–687.
10. Flisiak R, Feinman SV, Jablkowski M, et al. The cyclophilin inhibitor Debio 025 combined with PEG IFNalpha2a significantly reduces viral load in treatment-naive hepatitis C patients. *Hepatology* 2009; **49**(5): 1460–1468.
11. Rayhill SC, Barbeito R, Katz D, et al. A cyclosporine-based immunosuppressive regimen may be better than tacrolimus for long-term liver allograft survival in recipients transplanted for hepatitis C. *Transplant Proc* 2006; **38**(10): 3625–3628.
12. Katz LH, Fraser A, Gafter-Gvili A, Leibovici L, Tur-Kaspa R. Lamivudine prevents reactivation of hepatitis B and reduces mortality in immunosuppressed patients: systematic review and meta-analysis. *J Viral Hepat* 2008; **15**(2): 89–102.
13. Rahier J, Ben-Horin S, Chowers Y, et al. (2009) European evidence-based Consensus on the prevention, diagnosis and management of opportunistic infections in inflammatory bowel disease. *J Crohn's and Colitis* 2009; **3**(2): 47–91.

14. European Association for the Study of the Liver. EASL clinical practice guidelines: management of chronic hepatitis B. *J Hepatol* 2009; **50**(2): 227–242.

15. McHutchison JG, Everson GT, Gordon SC, et al. (2009) Telaprevir with peginterferon and ribavirin for chronic HCV genotype 1 infection. *N Engl J Med* 2009; **360**(18): 1827–1838.

16. Bargiggia S, Thorburn D, Anderloni A, et al. Is interferon-alpha therapy safe and effective for patients with chronic hepatitis C and inflammatory bowel disease? A case-control study. *Aliment Pharmacol Ther* 2005; **22**(3): 209–215.

17. Scherzer TM, Staufer K, Novacek G, et al. Efficacy and safety of antiviral therapy in patients with Crohn's disease and chronic hepatitis C. *Aliment Pharmacol Ther* 2008; **28**(6): 742–748.

6 CMV in IBD—passenger or pathogen?

Ahmed Kandiel and Bret Lashner

Department of Gastroenterology and Hepatology, Digestive Disease Institute, Cleveland Clinic, Cleveland, OH, USA

LEARNING POINTS

- Cytomegalovirus (CMV) infection can worsen IBD flares, but the presence of CMV replication does not necessarily imply a causative role in patients with steroid refractory disease.

- CMV infection is best diagnosed with flexible sigmoidoscopy with biopsies and immunohistochemical staining of tissue, and CMV blood DNA levels

- In steroid-refractory cases with evidence of active CMV infection, antiviral treatment with IV ganciclovir should be initiated; immunosuppression can be cautiously continued.

- Future research is needed to help differentiate pathogenic from nonpathogenic strains of CMV.

Introduction

Cytomegalovirus (CMV) is a member of the herpes-virus family and is a common viral infection in humans, occurring in 40–100% of adults [1]. The principal reservoirs of CMV are fibroblasts, myeloid cells, and endothelial cells [2], and the virus is excreted in body fluids and transmitted via close personal contact [3]. A primary infection of CMV is most often followed by a period of viral latency from which the virus may be reactivated. CMV reactivation can be triggered by tumor necrosis factor (TNF), interferon-γ (IFN-γ), catecholamines, proinflammatory prostaglandins, and medications such as steroids, cyclosporine, tacrolimus, and sirolimus [4]. When a patient is admitted with a flare of inflammatory bowel disease (IBD), a superimposed active CMV infection needs to be considered, especially if the patient has been on recent immunosuppressive medications.

Diagnosis of CMV infection

There are several available tests for diagnosis of CMV infection (Table 6.1). However, it is important to distinguish between a latent CMV infection, which is simply presence of the virus without active replication, and active infection leading to CMV disease.

Active disease is defined as detectable viral replication in peripheral blood or end organs in the presence of clinical signs and symptoms such as fever, leukopenia, or organ inflammation [2]. CMV infection can be diagnosed with endoscopy accompanied by histologic examination, serologic testing, viral culture, antigen testing, or DNA testing. The most commonly used tests are endoscopy accompanied by histologic examination, and blood CMV DNA testing.

Endoscopy with biopsy and immunohistochemical staining (more sensitive than hematoxylin and eosin (H&E) staining) is considered the gold standard for diagnosis of active CMV infection. However, immunohistochemical staining takes additional time to perform, and is not available in all centers. Since up to 30% of cases of CMV colitis exclusively involve the right colon [5], a flexible sigmoidoscopy will miss some cases, but a complete colonoscopy is often too risky to perform in the setting of severe colitis. The endoscopic appearance of CMV colitis is difficult to distinguish from a noninfectious flare of IBD colitis since both show colonic ulceration, erythema, loss of vascular pattern, and friability of the mucosa. Biopsies of ulcer beds will maximize the chance of detecting CMV disease, if present.

Clinical Dilemmas in Inflammatory Bowel Disease: New Challenges, Second Edition. Edited by P. Irving, C. Siegel, D. Rampton and F. Shanahan.
© 2011 Blackwell Publishing Ltd. Published 2011 by Blackwell Publishing Ltd.

Test	Sensitivity (%)	Specificity (%)
Histology (H&E)	10–87	92–100
Histology (Immunohistochemistry)	78–93	92–100
CMV culture	45–78	89–100
CMV antigen test	60-100	83–100
CMV DNA test	65–100	40–92

TABLE 6.1 Diagnostic tests for detecting CMV infection

H&E, hematoxylin and eosin.

CMV DNA testing is limited by two main factors. First, different assays are used in different centers. Second, standardized CMV DNA cut-off values for determining clinically significant CMV infection have not been determined. In this context, an analysis of cut-off values used in studies in the transplant literature seems to indicate that >5000 copies/mL for plasma assays or >25,000 copies/mL for whole blood assays is likely to be associated with clinically significant CMV infection and should be treated [6].

Passenger or pathogen?

When significant CMV viral replication is detected in the setting of an IBD flare, the challenge is determining whether the virus is just a passenger or so called "innocent bystander," or is actually playing an active role in the patient's symptomatic colitis. This distinction is not always easy to make. Some experimental studies have shown that rapidly proliferating cells in granulation tissue are susceptible to CMV infection. Perhaps, the virus is simply attracted to areas of IBD colitis, and does not in and of itself cause worsening inflammation [7]. This theory is supported by the observation that histologic evidence of CMV infection and CMV antigenemia in the setting of an IBD flare are not always associated with steroid resistance, and some of these patients improve with standard IBD care without the need for antiviral therapy [8].

However, many patients with steroid-refractory IBD flares and superimposed CMV have poor outcomes, with rates of up to 15% for toxic dilation, 62% for colectomy, and 44% for mortality [9]. In these cases, antiviral therapy, with or without modification of immunosuppression, appears to improve outcomes [1]. Currently, the most widely held theory is that CMV infects areas of active IBD and causes further colonic injury in these cases. It is thought that increased TNF-α and IFN-γ production in IBD patients with a flare causes reactivation of latent CMV infection. This subsequently causes more tissue injury and necrosis, and

liberation of proinflammatory cytokines, such as IL-6, that further exacerbate the IBD colitis [10,11]. Prospective studies have shown that the detected incidence of active CMV infection in acute severe ulcerative colitis (UC) is 21–34%, and in steroid-refractory colitis is 33–36% [8,12–15].

CMV treatment

Active CMV infection is treated with ganciclovir 5 mg/kg IV every 12 hours for 2–3 weeks. If there is improvement in symptoms after 3–5 days of IV treatment, then switching to oral treatment with valganciclovir 900 mg by mouth twice daily to complete a 2–3 week course can be considered. Bone marrow suppression is the most limiting side effect of ganciclovir and occurs in up to 40% of patients [16]. Foscarnet 90 mg/kg IV every 12 hours or 60 mg/kg IV every 8 hours for 2–3 weeks can be used in patients with ganciclovir resistance or intolerance. Up to a third of patients given foscarnet develop side effects such as nephrotoxicity, electrolyte abnormalities (such as hypocalcemia, hypophosphatemia, hyperphosphatemia, hypokalemia, or hypomagnesemia), or neurological problems [16]. Specific treatment of active CMV infection in patients with IBD leads to remission rates of 67–100% [1,8,12,13,17].

Conclusions and recommendations

Superimposed CMV infection should always be considered when IBD patients are admitted with severe colitis flares. Prospective studies have reported a significant incidence of CMV infection in the setting of severe flares, and antiviral treatment can lead to improved outcomes and decrease morbidity and mortality. A subset of patients with severe colitis and evidence of active CMV infection may do well with standard IBD care without the need for antiviral treatment, these patients may be infected with a less virulent CMV strain, a possibility warranting further research.

For IBD patients admitted to the hospital with severe colitis who do not respond to IV steroids after 48 hours, we recommend an unprepared flexible sigmoidoscopy with random biopsies to evaluate for CMV with H&E and immunohistochemistry, as well as checking blood CMV DNA levels. Evidence of CMV infection seen on blood CMV DNA testing or colon biopsies in patients whose symptoms are not improving warrants antiviral treatment. Data from previous reports suggest that immunosupprssion can be cautiously continued in these situations [1,8,12,13,17].

References

1. Papadakis KA, Tung JK, Binder SW, et al. Outcome of cytomegalovirus infections in patients with inflammatory bowel disease. *Am J Gastroenterol* 2001; **96**(7): 2137–2142.
2. Rowshani AT, Bemelman FJ, van Leeuwen EM, et al. Clinical and immunologic aspects of cytomegalovirus infection in solid organ transplant recipients. *Transplantation* 2005; **79**(4): 381–386.
3. Galiatsatos P, Shrier I, Lamoureux E, et al. Meta-analysis of outcome of cytomegalovirus colitis in immunocompetent hosts. *Dig Dis Sci* 2005; **50**(4): 609–616.
4. Pereyra F, Rubin RH. Prevention and treatment of cytomegalovirus infection in solid organ transplant recipients. *Curr Opin Infect Dis* 2004; **17**(4): 357–361.
5. Streetz KL, Buhr T, Wedemeyer H, et al. Acute CMV-colitis in a patient with a history of ulcerative colitis. *Scand J Gastroenterol* 2003; **38**(1): 119–122.
6. Kandiel A, Lashner B. Cytomegalovirus colitis complicating inflammatory bowel disease. *Am J Gastroenterol* 2006; **101**(12): 2857–2865.
7. Pfau P, Kochman ML, Furth EE, et al. Cytomegalovirus colitis complicating ulcerative colitis in the steroid-naive patient. *Am J Gastroenterol* 2001; **96**(3): 895–899.
8. Criscuoli V, Casa A, Orlando A, et al. Severe acute colitis associated with CMV: A prevalence study. *Dig Liver Dis* 2004; **36**(12): 818–820.
9. Hommes DW, Sterringa G, van Deventer SJ, et al. The pathogenicity of cytomegalovirus in inflammatory bowel disease: a systematic review and evidence-based recommendations for future research. *Inflamm Bowel Dis* 2004; **10**(3): 245–250.
10. Rahbar A, Bostrom L, Lagerstedt U, et al. Evidence of active cytomegalovirus infection and increased production of IL-6 in tissue specimens obtained from patients with inflammatory bowel diseases. *Inflamm Bowel Dis* 2003; **9**(3): 154–161.
11. Soderberg-Naucler C, Fish KN, Nelson JA. Interferon-gamma and tumor necrosis factor-alpha specifically induce formation of cytomegalovirus-permissive monocyte-derived macrophages that are refractory to the antiviral activity of these cytokines. *J Clin Invest* 1997; **100**(12): 3154–3163.
12. Cottone M, Pietrosi G, Martorana G, et al. Prevalence of cytomegalovirus infection in severe refractory ulcerative and crohn's colitis. *Am J Gastroenterol* 2001; **96**(3): 773–775.
13. Wada Y, Matsui T, Matake H, et al. Intractable ulcerative colitis caused by cytomegalovirus infection: A prospective study on prevalence, diagnosis, and treatment. *Dis Colon Rectum* 2003; **46**(Suppl. 10): S59–S65.
14. Kishore J, Ghoshal U, Ghoshal UC, et al. Infection with cytomegalovirus in patients with inflammatory bowel disease: prevalence, clinical significance and outcome. *J Med Microbiol* 2004; **53**(Pt. 11): 1155–1160.
15. Domenech E, Vega R, Ojanguren I, et al. Cytomegalovirus infection in ulcerative colitis: A prospective, comparative study on prevalence and diagnostic strategy. *Inflamm Bowel Dis* 2008; **14**(10): 1373–1379.
16. de la Hoz RE, Stephens G, Sherlock C. Diagnosis and treatment approaches of CMV infections in adult patients. *J Clin Virol* 2002; **25**(Suppl. 2): S1–12.
17. Vega R, Bertran X, Menacho M, et al. Cytomegalovirus infection in patients with inflammatory bowel disease. *Am J Gastroenterol* 1999; **94**(4): 1053–1056.

Clostridium difficile in IBD: impact, prevention, and treatment

Ashwin N. Ananthakrishnan[1] and David G. Binion[2]

[1]Gastrointestinal Unit, Harvard Medical School, Massachusetts General Hospital, Boston, MA, USA
[2]Division of Gastroenterology, Hepatology, and Nutrition, University of Pittsburgh School of Medicine, Pittsburgh, PA, USA

LEARNING POINTS

- *Clostridium difficile* infection (CDI) is increasingly common in patients with IBD and is associated with significant morbidity and mortality.

- Antibiotic exposure and prior healthcare contact are no longer considered essential risk factors for the acquisition of CDI.

- The range of presentation can vary from asymptomatic carriage to fulminant colitis.

- As symptoms of CDI frequently mimic an IBD flare, a high index of suspicion is essential to institute appropriate testing through stool toxin assays.

- Oral vancomycin and metronidazole are the two drugs of choice in the treatment of CDI, with oral vancomycin being preferred in those with severe disease.

- Attention should be paid to hand-washing and environmental decontamination to prevent person-to-person transfer and recurrent infection.

Introduction

Clostridium difficile (*C. difficile*) is a gram-positive anaerobe first described in antibiotic-associated pseudomembranous colitis [1]. Recent reports have highlighted its emergence as an important cause of nosocomial diarrhea with an estimated doubling of incidence over the last decade in short-stay hospitals in North America and accounting for up to $3 billion dollars in healthcare costs in the United States annually. There has also been a change in the epidemiology of *C. difficile* infection (CDI) from a predominantly antibiotic or healthcare-associated infection to one which is often community-acquired in patients without recent such exposure.

Several studies have also documented an increasing frequency of CDI in patients with inflammatory bowel disease (IBD)—Crohn's disease (CD), ulcerative colitis (UC)[2–4]. In addition to increasing rates of infection, there also seems to be significant morbidity, and even mortality, associated with CDI in patients with IBD. The relatively similar clinical presentation of an IBD flare and superimposed CDI, but markedly divergent treatment algorithms for these two scenarios, makes it essential for the treating physicians to have a high index of suspicion for CDI in patients with IBD presenting with symptoms of a disease flare: institution of appropriate testing and early treatment ensures optimal outcomes.

Prevalence and impact

Initial studies reported CDI to occur infrequently in patients with IBD. However, recent single center reports demonstrated a temporal increase in the frequency of CDI in patients with IBD [3,4]; a finding confirmed by more generalizable studies using large national administrative databases in the United States. Ananthakrishnan et al. demonstrated an increase in CDI complicating IBD hospitalizations between 1998 and 2004 for both UC (24/1000–39/1000) and CD (8/1000–12/1000) [2]. Reports from tertiary centers in Europe from both adult [5] and pediatric IBD [6] cohorts, demonstrated a similar increase in CDI, emphasizing the widespread distribution of the problem.

Clinical Dilemmas in Inflammatory Bowel Disease: New Challenges, Second Edition. Edited by P. Irving, C. Siegel, D. Rampton and F. Shanahan.
© 2011 Blackwell Publishing Ltd. Published 2011 by Blackwell Publishing Ltd.

Risk factors for acquisition of CDI include host and environmental factors. Older age and greater comorbidity are well-recognized risk factors, as are prior antibiotic exposure and healthcare contact. Classically associated with clindamycin use, exposure to any broad-spectrum antibiotic, particularly fluoroquinolones, may increase risk for CDI through disruption of the normal gut flora and subsequent proliferation of *C. difficile*. However, antibiotic use is not essential, as evidenced by recent studies that demonstrated no recent antibiotic use in up to 50% of IBD patients with CDI [3,5]. Immunosuppresion may also be a significant risk factor for CDI: a recent study identified a 2-fold increase in CDI in IBD patients on maintenance immunosuppression (odds ratio (OR) 2.58, 95% confidence interval (CI) 1.28–5.12) [3]. The role of other potential risk factors such as gastric acid suppressive therapy has not been consistently replicated in an IBD population.

The majority of patients with IBD and CDI have colonic involvement [3]; whether underlying disease severity is associated with CDI risk has not been prospectively defined. CDI has also been reported in segments of diverted bowel, ileo-anal pouch, and the small bowel in patients who have had a colectomy.

Presentation and assessment

CDI may present with symptoms that are indistinguishable from an IBD flare. However, the range of presenting symptoms is wide, varying from asymptomatic carriage (reported in up to 8% in an outpatient IBD cohort with mild underlying disease [7]) to diarrhea, abdominal pain, rectal bleeding, and fulminant colitis with toxic megacolon. Fever and leukocytosis with left shift may be seen in those with severe disease. Evaluation with an abdominal X-ray or computed tomography (CT) scan may reveal colonic thickening with dilation in those with fulminant colitis. Colonoscopic evaluation may be useful in defining severity of disease and obtaining samples to rule out cytomegalovirus (CMV) infection; however, colonoscopy as a tool is disappointing in its ability to distinguish between IBD activity and CDI, as these have very similar macroscopic features such as ulceration, friability, granularity, and bleeding. The classic pseudomembranes associated with CDI are rarely seen in patients with underlying IBD [3].

Diagnosis

The diagnosis of CDI is made by culturing the organism from a stool sample or by identifying the toxins in the stool [8]. *C. difficile* in an enterotoxigenic pathogen producing toxins A and B, which lead to spore formation and disruption of the intracellular cytoskeleton. While most infections are caused by strains producing both toxins, a small proportion is caused by strains producing toxin B only (7% of infections) [9]. Thus, it is important to use newer generation enzyme-linked immunosorbent assays (ELISA) tests that detect both toxins. Stool culture is the gold standard but requires additional testing to demonstrate toxicity and has a longer turn-around time. Testing of multiple consecutive stool samples with ELISA for toxin A and B improves sensitivity with an increase in detection rate from 54% with the first sample to 92% with the fourth sample [3] in patients with IBD.

Prognosis

CDI has been shown to have both short- and long-term consequences in patients with IBD. Varying rates of colectomy for CDI have been reported in IBD patients, ranging from 23–45% in tertiary center hospitalized cohorts [3,10]. In addition, it may be associated with longer hospital stays and a 4-fold greater mortality [2]. A higher rate of adverse outcomes extending 1 year out from the initial infection has been reported with higher rates of hospitalizations, surgery, and an increased need for therapy escalation [10,11].

Treatment

There is little evidence to guide treatment of CDI when it complicates IBD, and what follows is derived from reports on management of CDI not associated with UC or CD.

If possible, cessation of the offending antibiotic should be the first step in the management of CDI. Metronidazole in doses of 500 mg orally three times daily for 10–14 days is a good first choice for treatment of mild CDI in which scenario it has efficacy comparable to vancomycin [12]. However, recent studies have highlighted a high failure rate with metronidazole in those with severe disease. Vancomycin, 125–500 mg orally four times daily, is the only FDA-approved agent for the treatment of CDI and has superior efficacy compared to metronidazole in the treatment of severe disease (97% cure rate vs. 76%, $p = 0.02$) [13]. It is our agent of choice in patients with IBD with disease severe enough to require hospitalization. Intravenous vancomycin has no role in the treatment of CDI, though intravenous metronidazole is a good adjunctive therapy to use in patients who are unable to tolerate oral therapy, have ileus or have developed toxic megacolon. Other drugs that have been studied but have limited data supporting their use, particularly in patients with IBD, are probiotics (particularly *Saccharomyces boulardii*), anion-binding resins, teicoplanin, and rifaximin [14]. For treatment of severe disease in people without IBD, intravenous immunoglobulin (IVIG) (150–400 mg/kg, single dose) therapy has demonstrated some success in case reports, as has intracolonic administration of vancomycin and fecal biotherapy. In patients with severe or refractory disease, toxic megacolon or bowel perforation, early surgical consultation and comanagement is essential.

There are still limited data on how to manage concomitant immunosuppression in IBD patients who develop CDI, particularly the hospitalized cohort. Escalation of immunosuppresion in the setting of active CDI should be avoided; sometimes a reduction in corticosteroid dosing may be needed. Ben-Horin and colleagues retrospectively reviewed outcomes in 155 IBD patients hospitalized with CDI and found that use of steroids and immunosuppressive agents worsened the outcome, leading to an increased colectomy rate, compared with antibiotic treatment alone [15]. Whether specific immunosuppressive agents were culprits for worse outcomes, or underlying increased severity of the IBD was the factor leading to colectomy was not answered by this retrospective analysis. The potential for specific IBD medications to lead to CDI was addressed by Schneeweiss and colleagues, who recently used an administrative database from British Columbia, Canada, to assess patterns of infection in >10,000 IBD patients followed over a 5 year time period [16]. Initiation of corticosteroids in IBD patients was associated with a tripling of risk for CDI, while initiation of anti-TNF agents was not. In patients with fulminant colitis, making a distinction between CDI and active severe IBD may be difficult to determine, which may require that both antibiotics against CDI and active immunosuppresion be used either simultaneously or in rapid succession.

Recurrence of CDI may be seen in 15–35% of patients after an initial episode, and more frequently in those with multiple episodes of CDI. In addition to repeating courses of vancomycin and/or metronidazole, a prolonged course of vancomycin with a gradual taper over 6 weeks, a prolonged course of rifaximin, IVIG, and probiotics have all been tried with some success [14]. A thorough analysis of potential environmental sources of reinfection as well as strict instruction on hand-hygiene practices should be undertaken.

Prevention

Environmental exposure and person-to-person transmission is the key mode of acquisition of CDI. *C. difficile* spores are fairly resistant to environmental degradation; a 10% sodium hypochlorite solution has the best efficacy in decreasing environmental spore burden [17]. Hand washing is key in preventing person-to-person transfer. Alcohol-based hand gels do not eradicate *C. difficile* spores; thorough hand-washing with soap-and-water is important before and after contact with patients with suspected CDI [17].

Conclusions

The rise in CDI has had a significant impact on the IBD patient population, particularly patients suffering from IBD colitis. IBD patients are a high-risk group for contracting CDI, and are also at risk for worse clinical outcomes. Identification of the infection is challenging, particularly when one considers the low sensitivity of stool ELISA testing for the presence of toxins A and B. IBD therapy may influence the course of CDI, particularly in hospitalized patients, and attempts to limit corticosteroid use are warranted. Both metronidazole and vancomycin are effective for the treatment of CDI in IBD patients, but hospitalized individuals may benefit from the improved efficacy of vancomycin in the setting of severe illness. The high carriage rates of *C. difficile* in IBD patients and their increased susceptibility to infection, along with defining optimal treatment strategies remain important areas for clinical investigation.

References

1. Bartlett JG, Chang TW, Gurwith M, Gorbach SL, Onderdonk AB. Antibiotic-associated pseudomembranous colitis due to toxin-producing clostridia. *N Engl J Med* 1978; **298**: 531–534.
2. Ananthakrishnan AN, McGinley EL, Binion DG. Excess hospitalisation burden associated with Clostridium difficile in patients with inflammatory bowel disease. *Gut* 2008; **57**: 205–210.
3. Issa M, Vijayapal A, Graham MB, et al. Impact of Clostridium difficile on inflammatory bowel disease. *Clin Gastroenterol Hepatol* 2007; **5**: 345–351.
4. Rodemann JF, Dubberke ER, Reske KA, Seo da H, Stone CD. Incidence of Clostridium difficile infection in inflammatory bowel disease. *Clin Gastroenterol Hepatol* 2007; **5**: 339–344.
5. Bossuyt P, Verhaegen J, Van Assche G, Rutgeerts P, Vermeire S. Increasing incidence of *Clostridium difficile*-assiocated diarrhea in inflammatory bowel disease. *J Crohns colitis* 2009; **3**: 4–7.

6. Pascarella F, Martinelli M, Miele E, Del Pezzo M, Roscetto E, Staiano A. Impact of Clostridium difficile infection on pediatric inflammatory bowel disease. *J Pediatr* 2009; **154**: 854–858.

7. Clayton EM, Rea MC, Shanahan F, et al. The vexed relationship between Clostridium difficile and inflammatory bowel disease: an assessment of carriage in an outpatient setting among patients in remission. *Am J Gastroenterol* 2009; **104**: 1162–1169.

8. Bartlett JG, Gerding DN. Clinical recognition and diagnosis of Clostridium difficile infection. *Clin Infect Dis* 2008; **46**(Suppl. 1): S12–S18.

9. Drudy D, Harnedy N, Fanning S, O'Mahony R, Kyne L. Isolation and characterisation of toxin A-negative, toxin B-positive Clostridium difficile in Dublin, Ireland. *Clin Microbiol Infect* 2007; **13**: 298–304.

10. Jodorkovsky D, Young Y, Abreu MT. Clinical Outcomes of Patients with Ulcerative Colitis and Co-existing Clostridium difficile Infection. *Dig Dis Sci* 2009, **55**(2): 415–420.

11. Chiplunker A, Ananthakrishnan AN, Beaulieu DB, et al. Long-Term Impact of Clostridium difficile On Inflammatory Bowel Disease. *Gastroenterology* 2009; **136**(Suppl. 1): S1145.

12. Gerding DN, Muto CA, Owens RC, Jr. Treatment of Clostridium difficile infection. *Clin Infect Dis* 2008; **46**(Suppl. 1): S32–S42.

13. Zar FA, Bakkanagari SR, Moorthi KM, Davis MB. A comparison of vancomycin and metronidazole for the treatment of Clostridium difficile-associated diarrhea, stratified by disease severity. *Clin Infect Dis* 2007; **45**: 302–307.

14. Issa M, Ananthakrishnan AN, Binion DG. Clostridium difficile and inflammatory bowel disease. *Inflamm Bowel Dis* 2008; **14**: 1432–1442.

15. Ben-Horin S, Margalit M, Bossuyt P, et al. Combination immunomodulator and antibiotic treatment in patients with inflammatory bowel disease and clostridium difficile infection. *Clin Gastroenterol Hepatol* 2009; **7**: 981–987.

16. Schneeweiss S, Korzenik J, Solomon DH, Canning C, Lee J, Bressler B. Infliximab and other immunomodulating drugs in patients with inflammatory bowel disease and the risk of serious bacterial infections. *Aliment Pharmacol Ther* 2009; **30**: 253–264.

17. Gerding DN, Muto CA, Owens RC, Jr. Measures to control and prevent Clostridium difficile infection. *Clin Infect Dis* 2008; **46**(Suppl. 1): S43–S49.

8 Prebiotics and synbiotics: panacea or placebo

James O. Lindsay

Digestive Diseases Clinical Academic Unit, Barts and the London NHS Trust,
The Royal London Hospital, Whitechapel, London, UK

LEARNING POINTS

- The intestinal microbiota has both inflammatory and immunoregulatory potential.

- IBD is associated with alterations in the microbiota.

- Probiotics are living microbes that, when introduced to the gut, are capable of benefiting the host.

- Prebiotics are selectively fermented carbohydrates that induce specific changes to gastrointestinal microbiota, which confer health benefit.

- Synbiotics are a combination of pre- and probiotics.

- There is insufficient clinical trial data to support the use of prebiotics or synbiotics in patients with IBD.

Introduction: the pathogenesis of inflammatory bowel disease (IBD)

Although the exact etiology of IBD has not been established, it clearly involves both genetic and environmental factors resulting in a shift in the normal balance within the mucosal immune system. Regulatory pathways that promote tolerance to luminal antigens may be overcome by proinflammatory responses, thereby resulting in intestinal inflammation (reviewed in [1]). There is evidence from animal models that the intestinal microbiota drives inflammation. Likewise, in patients with IBD, higher concentrations of *bacteroides* and enterobacteria are found in regions of inflamed mucosa; disease activity deteriorates in both Crohn's disease (CD) and pouchitis when the fecal stream is restored to previously defunctioned intestine; and finally, the recently identified genetic associations of IBD highlight intracellular bacterial pattern recognition and autophagy as key players in disease pathogenesis. In contrast, there is also evidence that aspects of the commensal microbiota protect the mucosa from inflammation by decreasing intestinal permeability, increasing epithelial defence mechanisms, and promoting an immunoregulatory acquired immune response (reviewed in [2]). In addition, bacterial fermentation of soluble fiber in the diet results in the release of short chain fatty acids that have proven regulatory impact on the mucosal immune system.

The microbiota in IBD

The appreciation that the intestinal microbiota plays a complex role in both driving inflammation and promoting intestinal homeostasis coupled with advances in molecular microbiology has facilitated identification of differences in the microbial composition of patients with IBD and healthy controls. The characterization of this dysbiosis depends on the technique used and whether attention is focused on the fecal flora, the composition of the mucosa adherent bio-film, or invasion of bacteria into the epithelium [3]. Although this work is ongoing, clear differences have been detected between people with IBD and healthy controls, and people with active and quiescent IBD. For example, reduced levels of *Faecalibacterium prausnitzii* (*F. prausnitzii*) have been seen in patients with active disease, and low levels of this organism in CD ileocecal resection specimens predict subsequent endoscopic disease recurrence [4]. In addition, both *F. prausnitzii* and bifidobacteria species have been shown to have immunoregulatory effects in vitro and in vivo [5,6]. Therefore, there is a

---

Clinical Dilemmas in Inflammatory Bowel Disease: New Challenges, Second Edition. Edited by P. Irving, C. Siegel, D. Rampton and F. Shanahan.
© 2011 Blackwell Publishing Ltd. Published 2011 by Blackwell Publishing Ltd.

clear rationale for therapeutic strategies designed to reverse this dysbiosis, both as a treatment for patients with active disease and as maintenance of remission.

Probiotics in IBD

The majority of clinical trials in this area have investigated the clinical efficacy of probiotics. They include organisms such as lactobacilli, bifidobacteria, enterococci, and yeast species such as *Saccharomyces boulardii* (reviewed in [7,8]). However, with the exception of VSL#3 for primary prevention and maintenance of antibiotic-induced remission in pouchitis, and *Escherichia coli Nissle (E. coli Nissle)* in the maintenance of medically induced remission in mild/moderate ulcerative colitis (UC), most well designed adequately powered clinical trials of probiotic therapy in IBD have not shown benefit [7,8]. This may reflect the differences in the probiotic preparations and technical issues with their delivery to inflamed areas of the intestine. However, it may also reflect the heterogeneity of patients with IBD, in whom the particular genetic, environmental, and microbial drivers for intestinal inflammation are specific to the individual.

Prebiotics and synbiotics: introduction

Prebiotics such as fructooligosaccharides (FOS) and galactooligosaccharides (GOS) are selectively fermented short-chain carbohydrates that promote specific changes in the composition and/or activity of the gastrointestinal microbiota that confer a health benefit. Combinations of probiotics and prebiotics are termed synbiotics. Their theoretical advantage is that any clinical benefit is not reliant on delivery of specific bacterial species to the inflamed intestine as they act to enhance the immunoregulatory potential of an individual's own microbiota [7,8]. Their fermentation releases short-chain fatty acids that also have immunoregulatory potential. FOS of differing chain lengths have been shown to increase fecal and mucosal bifidobacteria and *F. Prausnaitzii* in healthy controls, and studies in animal models have demonstrated clear therapeutic potential in both the prevention and treatment of experimental colitis. Clinical improvements were associated with a reduction in proinflammatory cytokine release, reduced intracellular STAT-2 and NF-κB signaling, reduced expression of homing markers such as MAdCAM 1 and increased release of the immunoregulatory cytokine IL-10 [8] .

Clinical trials in UC

A series of small open label studies have evaluated a prebiotic germinated barley foodstuff and found evidence for therapeutic efficacy in patients with mild to moderately active UC [9]. However, adequately powered placebo-controlled trials of this agent have not been performed and there is debate over its classification as a prebiotic. In a placebo-controlled trial, 19 patients with moderately active colitis were treated with 3 g per day 5-ASA and randomized to receive either 12 g prebiotic FOS/inulin or placebo [10]. All patients experienced a significant reduction in disease activity at 14 days with no difference between the prebiotic and placebo groups. However, patients treated with prebiotic, but not those treated with placebo, experienced a significant reduction in fecal calprotectin at 7 and 14 days. Likewise, a randomized double-blind, double-dummy pilot study in 18 patients with UC has suggested that synbiotics may have a role in reducing inflammation [11]. A combination of FOS/inulin and *Bifidobacterium longum (B. longum)* resulted in reduction in histological and sigmoidoscopy disease scores, although there was no significant benefit on symptom scores. However, mucosal-associated bifidobacteria were increased associated with a decrease in both proinflammatory cytokines and antimicrobial human beta defensins. Although, it is disappointing that the observed alterations in mucosal inflammation in these two trials did not translate into clinically significant benefits, there is clearly a requirement for an adequately powered placebo-controlled trial.

Two small studies have examined the use of prebiotics and synbotics in pouchitis. In the first open label study, ten patients with antibiotic-refractory or antibiotic-dependent pouchitis treated with the synbiotic combination of a lactobacillus and FOS experienced complete clinical and endoscopic remission. The second was a crossover study in 20 patients that demonstrated that inulin was associated with a decrease in histological and endoscopic scores, although no patient had overt clinical pouchitis at enrolment and no change in clinical activity scores was detected [12]. Again, there is a clear mandate for appropriately designed and powered clinical trials.

Clinical trials in CD

Several studies have investigated the role of prebiotics and synbiotics in the maintenance of remission after ileocecal resection for CD and shown no clinical benefit [7, 8,13]. Enrolment to these studies was difficult and it is possible that they were underpowered. A small open label trial of ten patients with active CD treated for 3 weeks with FOS reported a significant reduction in disease activity associated with an increase in fecal bifidobacteria and enhanced lamina propria dendritic cell IL-10 release [14]. This led onto an adequately powered double-blind placebo-controlled trial in patients with moderately active CD on stable medication [15]. In order to minimize the placebo response, patients were required to have biochemical markers of inflammation. After 4 weeks, there was no clinical benefit of FOS compared to placebo in terms of disease activity, quality of life, CRP or fecal calprotectin. In fact, more patients receiving FOS had to withdraw from the study and gastrointestinal side effects were significantly higher in the active compared to the placebo group. Subgroup analyses did not demonstrate clinical benefit in patients dependent on disease duration, location, or genotype. This definitive study demonstrated a lack of clinical benefit for FOS in the treatment of active CD and the higher rate of gastrointestinal side effects, such as flatulence and borborygmi, suggest that patients with active disease should attempt to reduce the prebiotic content of their regular diet.

Conclusions

Interpretation of the current literature on the value of prebiotics and synbiotics in IBD is undermined by insufficient data from well-designed clinical trials. Several small studies have demonstrated a reduction in immunological and biochemical markers of inflammation in both UC and CD, but have not reported an improvement in clinical disease activity scores. The heterogeneity of patients mandates power calculations with appropriate stratification to ensure that a benefit in particular patient subgroups is not missed. It is clear that there is no role for the short-term use of prebiotics to treat active CD. However, the benefit of both prebiotics and synbiotics in active UC and maintenance of remission in both diseases is not clear. Future studies must consider the side effect profile of prebiotics, as symptoms resulting from their fermentation may elevate disease activity indices; therefore, objective markers such as CRP and fecal calprotectin should be measured or endoscopy performed. Finally, attention needs to be paid to the most appropriate timing of prebiotic interventions. A lack of benefit in established disease does not preclude a role in the prevention of disease, either in the postoperative setting or in patients at high risk of developing disease.

References

1. Fiocchi C. Susceptibility genes and overall pathogenesis of inflammatory bowel disease: where do we stand? *Dig Dis* 2009; **27**(3): 226–235.
2. Sartor RB. Microbial influences in inflammatory bowel diseases. *Gastroenterology* 2008; **134**(2): 577–594.
3. Macfarlane GT, Blackett KL, Nakayama T, et al. The gut microbiota in inflammatory bowel disease. *Curr Pharm Des* 2009; **15**(13): 1528–1536.
4. Sokol H, Seksik P, Furet JP, et al. Low counts of Faecalibacterium prausnitzii in colitis microbiota. *Inflamm Bowel Dis* 2009; **15**(8): 1183–1189.
5. Sokol H, Pigneur B, Watterlot L, et al. Faecalibacterium prausnitzii is an anti-inflammatory commensal bacterium identified by gut microbiota analysis of Crohn disease patients. *Proc Natl Acad Sci USA* 2008; **105**(43): 16731–16736.
6. Hart AL, Lammers K, Brigidi P, et al. Modulation of human dendritic cell phenotype and function by probiotic bacteria. *Gut* 2004; **53**: 1602–1609.
7. Hedin C, Whelan K, Lindsay JO. Evidence for the use of probiotics and prebiotics in inflammatory bowel disease: a review of clinical trials. *Proc Nutr Soc* 2007; **66**(3): 307–315.
8. Sartor RB. Therapeutic manipulation of the enteric microflora in inflammatory bowel diseases: antibiotics, probiotics, and prebiotics. *Gastroenterology* 2004; **126**(6): 1620–1633.
9. Kanauchi O, Suga T, Tochihara M, et al. Treatment of ulcerative colitis by feeding with germinated barley foodstuff: first report of a multicenter open control trial. *J Gastroenterol* 2002; **37**(Suppl. 14): 67–72.
10. Casellas F, Borruel N, Torrejón A, et al. Oral oligofructose-enriched inulin supplementation in acute ulcerative colitis is well tolerated and associated with lowered faecal calprotectin. *Aliment Pharmacol Ther* 2007; **25**(9): 1061–1067.
11. Furrie E, Macfarlane S, Kennedy A, et al. Synbiotic therapy (Bifidobacterium longum/ Synergy 1) initiates resolution of inflammation in patients with active ulcerative colitis: a randomised controlled pilot trial. *Gut* 2005; **54**(2): 242–249.
12. Welters CF, Heineman E, Thunnissen FB, et al. Effect of dietary inulin supplementation on inflammation of pouch mucosa in patients with an ileal pouch-anal anastomosis. *Dis Colon Rectum* 2002; **45**(5): 621–627.

13. Chermesh I, Tamir A, Reshef R, et al. Failure of synbiotic 2000 to prevent postoperative recurrence of Crohn's disease. *Dig Dis Sci* 2007; **52**(2): 385–389.

14. Lindsay JO, Whelan K, Stagg AJ, et al. Clinical, microbiological, and immunological effects of fructo-oligosaccharide in patients with Crohn's disease. *Gut* 2006; **55**(3): 348–355.

15. Benjamin JL, Hedin CRH, Koutsoumpas A, et al. A randomised, double-blind, placebo-controlled trial of fructo-oligosaccharides in active Crohn's disease. Gut. 2011 Jan 24. [Epub ahead of print] PMID: 21262918.

9 Worms: light at the end of their burrow

John Leung and Joel V. Weinstock

Division of Gastroenterology, Tufts Medical Center, Boston, MA, USA

LEARNING POINTS

- The exponential increase in IBD incidence is too rapid to be driven by genetic mutation.

- The "IBD hygiene hypothesis" proposes that modern day absence of exposure to intestinal helminths is an important environmental factor contributing to IBD.

- Epidemiological, experimental, and clinical data support the notion that helminths could provide protection against IBD.

- Therapeutic grade helminths have received good manufacturing practice approval as drugs by the United States and European food and drug administrations and are under investigation as potential therapies for IBD and other immunological diseases.

Introduction

Helminthic therapy is a new type of immunotherapy for the treatment of immunological disorders. It involves the administration of a live intestinal helminth or some helminth-associated molecule. Helminths are complex multicellular organisms with a long life span. Colonization of humans with helminths was almost universal until the early twentieth century. Most helminths live symbiotically and coevolved with humans and prehumanoid species over millions of years. Many helminths seem invincible to human defense. They have developed strategies to circumvent our immune responses for their own survival. Modern day absence of exposure to intestinal helminths has been proposed to be an important environmental factor contributing to the development of immunological disor-

ders such as inflammatory bowel disease (IBD). This forms the basis of the IBD hygiene hypothesis and the rationale for the use of helminthic therapy for the treatment of IBD.

Hygiene hypothesis/rational for helminthic therapy

During the past 40 years, there has been a rapid increase in the incidence of immunological disorders such as IBD, type 1 diabetes, multiple sclerosis, and allergic diseases in developed societies, and a similar pattern is emerging in urbanized areas of developing countries [1]. The increase in their incidence is too rapid to be driven solely by genetic factors. Therefore, environmental factors were sought to explain this phenomenon.

In the 1990s, we proposed the "IBD hygiene hypothesis." It states that raising children in extremely hygienic environments negatively affects immune development, and predisposes them to immunological diseases like IBD later in life [2]. Modern hygienic practices have mostly eliminated helminths from industrialized societies. It is widely accepted in the scientific community that appropriate immune development and maturation in mammals relies on interaction with organisms such as helminths. Helminths are worm-like animals that coevolved with our immune systems. Their eradication in the developed countries in the twentieth century and the loss of their capacity to stimulate the regulatory side of our immune systems has resulted in aberrant development of the human immune system rendering us more susceptible to IBD.

Clinical Dilemmas in Inflammatory Bowel Disease: New Challenges, Second Edition. Edited by P. Irving, C. Siegel, D. Rampton and F. Shanahan.
© 2011 Blackwell Publishing Ltd. Published 2011 by Blackwell Publishing Ltd.

The IBD hygiene hypothesis is supported by epidemiological, genetic, animal, and clinical studies. Epidemiological studies show that the frequency of helminth colonization is inversely proportional to the prevalence of IBD and various immunological diseases within a community [2]. Although these studies have not proven a causal relationship, IBD epidemiology supports the postulate that infection with helminths provides protection from IBD. Cases of natural exposure to helminths suppressing ongoing IBD have been reported recently [3]. In addition to epidemiological evidence, the IBD hygiene hypothesis is supported by population genetic analysis. One recent study showed that helminths were the major selective force for the evolution of various interleukins, and some of these helminth-driven interleukin genes predispose individuals to IBD [4]. A third line of evidence comes from animal studies. Protective effects of helminths in immunological disorders have been demonstrated in numerous animal disease models of asthma, type 1 diabetes mellitus, food allergy, experimental autoimmune encephalomyelitis, and IBD [5–7].

Based on the promising findings using helminth infections to treat experimental colitis, we conducted two clinical trials. Both trials suggested that colonization with *Trichuris suis* (*T. suis*) reduces disease activity in Crohn's disease (CD) and ulcerative colitis (UC) [8,9]. *T. suis* is a porcine whipworm closely related to the human whipworm *Trichuris Trichiura* (*T. trichiura*). It is an attractive candidate as a therapeutic organism, since it only transiently colonizes human hosts, does not multiply within or migrate out of the intestine, and it is not known to cause disease. The results of the initial studies were promising. Of the 29 patients with

CD who received *T. suis* ova (2500 ova, every 3 weeks for 24 weeks), 79% responded with significant reduction in symptoms [8]. In a double-blind placebo-controlled trial of 54 patients with an active UC, 43.3% of the patients given *T. suis* ova (2500 ova every 2 weeks for 12 weeks) showed substantial improvement, compared to 16.7% of those given placebo ($p = 0.04$) [9]. Another pilot study led by Dr Croese suggested that another helminth species, *Necator americanus*, was effective for treating CD [10]. In addition to treating IBD, helminthic therapy is currently being studied as a treatment for several other human immunological disorders, including celiac disease, multiple sclerosis, autism, food allergy, and asthma. The pharmaceutical industry is actively studying the potential of these agents to control disease.

Mode of action/mechanisms

IBD is thought to reflect a defect in the regulatory arm of the immune system resulting in failure to control excessive inflammatory responses to luminal contents. Conventional IBD therapies such as glucocorticoids, azathioprine, 6-mercaptopurine (6-MP), methotrexate, and blockers of tumor necrosis factor activity target the disease by crippling the effector arm of the immune system, and thus render patients susceptible to serious infections. In contrast, helminths control aberrant inflammation by restoring the weakened natural regulatory arm of the immune system. Specific immune-modulatory effects of helminthic therapy have recently been characterized (Figure 9.1). They appear to block production of proinflammatory cytokines like IL-17A, IFN-γ, and IL-12/23, while augmenting expression of

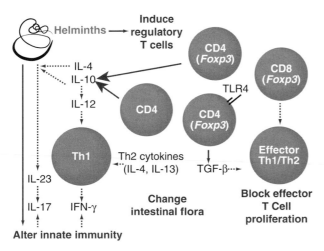

FIGURE 9.1 Helminths suppress aberrant intestinal inflammation by restoring the natural regulatory arm of the immune system [1]. Helminths also induce the production of various subsets of regulatory T cells (e.g., Cd4+ IL-10+ Foxp3+, CD4+ IL-10+, Cd8+ IL-10+ Foxp3+, and CD4+ Foxp3+ TGF-β+ T cells) to block effector T cell proliferation and function [2]. In addition, they modulate innate immunity by altering the function of dendritic cells and/or macrophages to inhibit IFN-γ and IL17 proinflammatory responses [3]. Helminths release factors that alter bacterial flora and indirectly influence mucosal responses. Dotted arrow ($\cdots\blacktriangleright$) indicates inhibition.

regulatory factors such as TGF-β and IL-10, and stimulating various subsets of regulatory T cell [7,11–14]. Helminths also modulate key components of the innate immune system (dendritic cells, alternatively activated macrophages), which helps to control disease [15,16]. A recent study has shown that they alter the composition of the intestinal flora [17], which could have profound effects on mucosal immune reactivity.

Conclusion

Despite an increasing array of medications for IBD, the approved therapies have suboptimal efficacy and are associated with a risk of significant side effects. There remains a large unmet need for better IBD treatments. Helminths and their products hold promise as effective treatments for IBD. They function through a unique and highly physiological process that enhances the regulatory side of the immune system to limit aberrantly strong effector immune function without creating immune deficiency. A clinical grade helminth has achieved GMP approval by the drug regulatory agencies. It is now available for the many clinical trials being conducted in the United States and Europe accessing its safety and efficacy in various immunological diseases. Helminthic therapy may become an attractive alternative to currently available IBD medications given their safety profile, ease of administration, and potential low cost.

References

1. Smits HH, Yazdanbakhsh M. Chronic helminth infections modulate allergen-specific immune responses: Protection against development of allergic disorders? *Ann Med* 2007; **39**(6): 428–439.
2. Weinstock JV, Elliott DE. Helminths and the IBD hygiene hypothesis. *Inflamm Bowel Dis* 2009; **15**(1): 128–133.
3. Büning J, Homann N, von Smolinski D, et al. Helminths as Governors of Inflammatory Bowel Disease. *Gut* 2008; **57**: 1182–1183.
4. Fumagalli M, Pozzoli U, Cagliani R, et al. Parasites represent a major selective force for interleukin genes and shape the genetic predisposition to autoimmune conditions. *J Exp Med* 2009; **206**(6): 1395–1408.
5. Reardon C, Sanchez A, Hogaboam CM, McKay DM. Tapeworm infection reduces epithelial ion transport abnormalities in murine dextran sulfate sodium-induced colitis. *Infect Immun* 2001; **69**(7): 4417–4423.
6. Elliott DE, Setiawan T, Metwali A, Blum A, Urban JF, Weinstock JV. Heligmosomoides polygyrus inhibits established colitis in IL-10-deficient mice. *Eur J Immunol* 2004; **34**(10): 2690–2698.
7. Khan WI, Blennerhasset PA, Varghese AK, et al. Intestinal nematode infection ameliorates experimental colitis in mice. *Infect Immun* 2002; **70**(11): 5931–5937.
8. Summers RW, Elliott DE, Urban JF, Thompson R, Weinstock JV. Trichuris suis therapy in Crohn's disease. *Gut* 2005; **54**(1): 87–90.
9. Summers RW, Elliott DE, Urban JF, Thompson RA, Weinstock JV. Trichuris suis therapy for active ulcerative colitis: a randomized controlled trial. *Gastroenterology* 2005; **128**(4): 825–832.
10. Croese J, O'neil J, Masson J, Cooke S, Melrose W, Pritchard D, et al. A proof of concept study establishing Necator americanus in Crohn's patients and reservoir donors. *Gut* 2006; **55**(1): 136–137.
11. Elliott DE, Metwali A, Leung J, Setiawan T, Blum AM, Ince MN, et al. Colonization with Heligmosomoides polygyrus suppresses mucosal IL-17 production. *J Immunol* 2008; **181**(4): 2414–2419.
12. Elliott DE, Setiawan T, Metwali A, Blum A, Urban JF, Weinstock JV. Heligmosomoides polygyrus inhibits established colitis in IL-10-deficient mice. *Eur J Immunol* 2004; **34**(10): 2690–2698.
13. Setiawan T, Metwali A, Blum AM, et al. Heligmosomoides polygyrus promotes regulatory T-cell cytokine production in the murine normal distal intestine. *Infect. Immun* 2007; **75**(9): 4655–4663.
14. Metwali A, Setiawan T, Blum AM, et al. Induction of CD8+ regulatory T cells in the intestine by Heligmosomoides polygyrus infection. *Am. J. Physiol. Gastrointest. Liver Physiol* 2006; **291**(2): G253–G259.
15. Herbert DR, Hölscher C, Mohrs M, et al. Alternative macrophage activation is essential for survival during schistosomiasis and downmodulates T helper 1 responses and immunopathology. *Immunity* 2004; **20**(5): 623–635.
16. Koyama K. Dendritic cells have a crucial role in the production of cytokines in mesenteric lymph nodes of B10.BR mice infected with Trichuris muris. *Parasitol Res* 2008; **102**(3): 349–356.
17. Walk, ST, Blum, AM, Ewing, S, Weinstock, JV, Young, VB. Alteration of the murine gut microbiota during infection with the parasitic helminth, Heligmosomoides polygyrus. *Inflamm Bowel Dis* 2010. (In press)

10 Do we really need to vaccinate all patients with IBD?

Gauree Gupta and Gil Y. Melmed

Department of Medicine, Cedars Sinai Medical Center and David Geffen School of Medicine at UCLA, Los Angeles, CA, USA

LEARNING POINTS

- Patients with IBD are at increased risk of infection due to underlying immune dysregulation, immunosuppressive therapy, and/or malnutrition.
- Vaccines are underutilized in IBD patients.
- Administer vaccines using standard immunization guidelines.
- Assess vaccination status and risk factors for vaccine-preventable illnesses at the time of initial IBD consultation, including serologic assessments for immunity if indicated.
- Ideally, patients with IBD should be assessed and appropriately immunized before immunosuppressive therapies are needed.
- Avoid live virus vaccines in IBD patients who are immunocompromised.

Patients with inflammatory bowel disease (IBD) are at increased risk of acquiring a vaccine-preventable infection [1]. This increased risk is primarily due to the frequent need for immunosuppressive therapy, and may be further augmented by malnutrition, surgery, and underlying immune dysregulation. Corticosteroids, azathioprine/6-mercaptopurine (6-MP), methotrexate, and antitumor necrosis factor (TNF) alpha therapies are immunosuppressive agents that are often required to control intestinal inflammation and associated complications. Despite specific immunization guidelines for IBD patients published in 2004, vaccines are generally underutilized in IBD patients [2–3]. This may be due to both patient and physician lack of awareness of appropriate indications for vaccination [3].

Studies done in immunosuppressed populations, including IBD, rheumatoid arthritis, and organ transplant recipients, demonstrate that vaccinations are safe and well tolerated, and most patients respond to common vaccines including those against influenza, pneumococcus, and tetanus [4–7]. However, patients on multiple concomitant immunosuppressive agents have diminished serologic responses [8,9]. Vaccinations with non-live vaccines are considered safe. Studies in children and adults with IBD have included subjects who safely received influenza and pneumococcal vaccinations [5–6, 8], although there are case reports of ulcerative colitis (UC) disease flare after vaccination with influenza [10].

In general, all IBD patients should receive standard recommended immunizations as outlined by the Advisory Committee on Immunization Practices (ACIP) of the Center for Disease Control and Prevention (CDC), and the European Crohn's and Colitis Organization (ECCO) [11,12]. Ideally, patients either newly diagnosed with IBD or at their initial IBD consultation should be queried regarding vaccination status, travel history, and risk factors for various infections [1,12]. Where possible, all indicated vaccines (see Table 10.1) should be administered to patients before starting immunosuppressive therapy, in order to maximize the chance of an adequate immune response and allow for administration of live vaccines if needed. However, in cases where patients need to initiate immunosuppressive treatment immediately, these immunizations may need to be postponed.

Clinical Dilemmas in Inflammatory Bowel Disease: New Challenges, Second Edition. Edited by P. Irving, C. Siegel, D. Rampton and F. Shanahan.
© 2011 Blackwell Publishing Ltd. Published 2011 by Blackwell Publishing Ltd.

TABLE 10.1 Vaccine checklist for adults with IBD (>18 years of age)

Vaccine	Initial visit	Follow-up visits
Influenza[a]	Annual vaccination (with killed injected vaccine if immunosuppressed)	Annual vaccination
Pneumococcus	1 dose if not vaccinated within past 5 years	5 years after initial dose
Varicella[b]	2-dose series if no history of varicella confirmed by negative serologies	
Zoster[b]	Single dose for patients age >60	
Measles, Mumps, and Rubella[b]	1 dose if previously unvaccinated and born after 1957	1 dose after age 50 if risk factors present
Hepatitis B Virus	3-dose series if seronegative or with risk factors	Consider checking HBsAb status if immunosuppressed when vaccinated
Diphtheria, Tetanus, and Pertussis	3-dose series if unvaccinated, or 1-time booster with Td	Every 10 years with Td (substitute 1-time dose of Tdap for Td booster)
Meningococcus	1 dose if risk factors present	Consider 1-time revaccination after 5 years if risk factors still present
Human Papilloma Virus	3-dose series for females aged 9–26 years old, consider for all females with IBD, especially if immunosuppressed	

Note: In situations where multiple vaccinations are indicated, clinical judgment of infectious risk should prevail regarding prioritizing the receipt of vaccines. Many non-live vaccines can and should be given on the same day in order to maximize opportunities for vaccination, e.g., influenza and pneumococcal vaccines. Specific vaccine recommendations may vary according to regional guidelines.
[a]Intranasal influenza vaccine is a live virus vaccine. Give inactivated influenza vaccine if patient is immunosuppressed.
[b]Live virus vaccines, generally contraindicated in immunosuppressed patients.

What constitutes immunocompromised status?

Immunocompromised status in children and adults with IBD is defined as treatment with glucocorticoids (prednisone 20 mg/day or equivalent), 6-MP/azathioprine, methotrexate, or biologics, including within 3 months of discontinuing any of these medications [2]. Significant protein-calorie malnutrition, as evidenced by hypoalbuminemia, may also constitute immunocompromised status.

Live virus vaccines should not be given to patients on immunosuppressive medications. In general, it is advised that vaccines be given prior to the initiation of immunosuppressive therapy, or 2–3 months after immunosuppressive therapy is discontinued. To avoid the risk of systemic infection from live virus vaccination, it would be conservative to wait 6 weeks prior to restarting immunosuppressive therapy, although there is very limited data assessing this approach.

Vaccines

Influenza

In the United States, 30,000 people die annually from seasonal influenza, and patients on immunosuppressive medications remain at risk for seasonal and H1N1 influenza. Yearly influenza vaccination is recommended for all patients with IBD. The inactivated trivalent influenza vaccine and inactivated H1N1 vaccine are safe in immunosuppressed recipients, whereas the live attenuated intranasal vaccine is contraindicated. Influenza vaccination is effective in inducing immune responses in children with IBD, but may be less effective among those on anti-TNF therapies. The majority of IBD patients develop protective antibody titers following influenza vaccination, regardless of immunosuppressive medication use. With regard to H1N1 immunization, European studies suggest that vaccination in patients with IBD is safe and effective [13, 14].

Pneumococcus

Pneumococcal vaccination is recommended for children <5 years of age, as well as adults with chronic diseases such as IBD, especially if on immunosuppressive medications. In particular, those with concomitant asthma and other respiratory conditions should receive pneumococcal vaccination. This polysaccharide vaccine is safe in patients receiving immunosuppression. The combination of immunomodulators and anti-TNF therapy is associated with impaired antibody responses in patients with Crohn's disease, but most patients do develop at least partial immunity after vaccination [8].

Hepatitis B virus (HBV)

The 3-dose hepatitis B vaccination series is safe in immunosuppressed patients, and is indicated for all children. ECCO guidelines recommend HBV vaccination in all seronegative patients with IBD, and in general vaccination is advised for those with HBV risk factors, such as intravenous drug use, travel to endemic regions, high-risk sexual behavior, hemodialysis patients, prisoners, and healthcare providers [12].

Diphtheria, tetanus, and pertussis vaccines

Vaccination against tetanus and diphtheria toxoids (Td) is recommended for children, and for adults a Td or Tdap (Td plus pertussis vaccination) booster shot every 10 years is recommended. Td and Tdap are noninfectious, safe, and can be given to all IBD patients as part of routine immunization [11].

Meningococcus

Meningococcal vaccination is recommended for children aged 2–10 years old with risk factors for meningococcal infection, such as travelers to endemic areas, and those with splenic dysfunction or who have had a splenectomy. The vaccine is also recommended for patients aged 11–18 years old, and adults with risk factors, such as college freshmen, military recruits, or travelers to endemic areas. This vaccine is noninfectious, and is considered safe even in immunocompromised patients.

Human papilloma virus (HPV)

The HPV vaccine includes the 4 HPV serotypes most strongly associated with progression to cervical dysplasia and cancer. A 3-dose series is recommended for females aged 9–26 years old, and is considered safe in immunosuppressed patients although studies are lacking. Women with IBD may have a higher risk of HPV and abnormal Pap smears, especially those on immunosuppressive medications [15] (see Chapter 21). Therefore, it may be reasonable to consider vaccination for all immunosuppressed women with IBD.

Varicella (chickenpox) and zoster (shingles)

The varicella vaccine is a live virus vaccine recommended as a 2-dose series in children beginning at 12 months age, and in all healthy persons aged >13 years without evidence of immunity. During the initial history of a patient with IBD, varicella immune status should be assessed by asking about previous varicella infection or immunization, and checking varicella titers if there is doubt about prior exposure. Patients not on immunosuppressive therapy with no history of varicella should receive the vaccine. It remains contraindicated in immunosuppressed patients.

The zoster vaccine, also a live virus vaccine, is indicated for all persons aged >60 years, including those with a history of zoster or varicella. Herpes zoster is one of the most common infections affecting patients with IBD receiving immunosuppression [16], but vaccination is currently contraindicated in immunosuppressed individuals, in particular those receiving anti-TNF therapy. In patients receiving "low dose" immunosuppressive therapy (less than or equal to 20 mg/day prednisone, 3 mg/kg azathioprine, 1.5 mg/kg 6-MP) the degree of immunosuppression is not considered sufficiently immunosuppressive to create vaccine safety concerns [17].

Measles, mumps, and rubella (MMR)

Current guidelines advise a 2-dose MMR immunization series in children aged >1 year. In adults, a 1-time MMR dose is generally indicated for naïve adults who were born during or after 1957. A second MMR dose can be given to adults >50 years of age if risk factors are present [11].

This vaccine contains live attenuated viruses, and is contraindicated in immunocompromised IBD patients.

Other vaccines

Those with risk factors for yellow fever, hepatitis A, polio, rabies, cholera, Japanese encephalitis, or typhoid, including those traveling to endemic areas, should receive standard immunizations. However, since immunocompromised IBD patients should not receive live virus vaccines (e.g., yellow fever), they should be informed of the importance of using other protective measures to reduce the risks of travel. These decisions may be best made in collaboration with an expert from a travel clinic (see Chapter 4).

Conclusion

Our ability to prevent illness through vaccination in IBD patients, especially among those on immunosuppression, is critical in the management of this population. Ideally, vaccinations should be considered at the time of a new IBD diagnosis or consultation. It may be difficult for patients newly diagnosed with a chronic, and often disabling, disease to accept earlier and more frequent immunizations. Helping them understand the benefits of protection against infections that are vaccine-preventable, especially before therapies are begun, is important. In this regard, it may be helpful to explain the rationale for preemptive vaccinations in the context of infectious risks associated with immunosuppressive therapies. Such an approach will bolster patient acceptance and hopefully help to optimize opportunities for preemptive intervention in this high-risk population.

References

1. Toruner M, Loftus EV Jr, Harmsen WS, et al. Risk factors for opportunistic infections in patients with inflammatory bowel disease. *Gastroenterology* 2008; **134**(4): 929–936.

2. Sands BE, Cuffari C, Katz J, et al. Guidelines for immunizations in patients with inflammatory bowel disease. *Inflamm Bowel Dis* 2004; **10**(5) : 677–692.

3. Melmed GY, Ippoliti AF, Papadakis KA, et al. Patients with inflammatory bowel disease are at risk for vaccine-preventable illnesses. *Am J Gastroenterol* 2006; **101**(8): 1834–1840.

4. Moscandrew M, Mahadevan U, Kane S. General health maintenance in IBD. *Inflamm Bowel Dis* 2009; **15**(9): 1399–1409.

5. Mamula P, Markowitz JE, Piccoli DA, Klimov A, Cohen L, Baldassano RN. Immune response to influenza vaccine in pediatric patients with inflammatory bowel disease. *Clin Gastroenterol Hepatol* 2007; **5**(7): 851–856.

6. Lu Y, Jacobson DL, Ashworth LA, et al. Immune response to influenza vaccine in children with inflammatory bowel disease. *Am J Gastroenterol* 2009; **104**(2): 444–453.

7. Chow J, Golan Y. Vaccination of solid-organ transplantation candidates. *Clin Infect Dis* 2009; **49**(10): 1550–1556.

8. Melmed GY, Agarwal N, Frenck RW, et al. Immunosuppression impairs response to pneumococcal polysaccharide vaccination in patients with inflammatory bowel disease. *Am J Gastroenterol* 2010; **105**(1): 148–154.

9. Glück T, Müller-Ladner U. Vaccination in patients with chronic rheumatic or autoimmune diseases. *Clin Infect Dis* 2008; **46**(9): 1459–1465.

10. Fields SW, Baiocco PJ, Korelitz BI. Influenza vaccinations: should they really be encouraged for IBD patients being treated with immunosuppressives? *Inflamm Bowel Dis* 2009; **15**(5): 649–651.

11. Kroger AT, Atkinson WL, Marcuse EK, Pickering LK; Advisory Committee on Immunization Practices (ACIP) Centers for Disease Control and Prevention (CDC). General recommendations on immunization: recommendations of the Advisory Committee on Immunization Practices (ACIP). *MMWR Recomm Rep* 2006; **55**(RR-15): 1–48.

12. Rahier JF, et al. European evidence-based consensus on the prevention, diagnosis and management of opportunistic infections in inflammatory bowel disease. *J of Crohns Colitis* 2009; **3**(2): 47–91.

13. Molnar T, Farkas K, Jankovics I, et al. Appropriate response to influenza A (H1N1) virus vaccination in patients with inflammatory bowel disease on maintenance immunomodulator and/or biological therapy. *Am J Gastroenterol* 2011; **106**:370–372.

14. Rahier JF, Papay P, Salleron J, et al. H1N1 vaccines in a large observational cohort of patients with inflammatory bowel disease treated with immunomodulators and biological therapy. *Gut* 2011; **60**(4):456–462.

15. Kane SV, Khatibi B, Reddy D. Use of immunosuppressants results in a higher incidence of abnormal Pap smears in women with inflammatory bowel disease. *Am J Gastroenterol* 2008; **103**(3): 631–636.

16. Gupta G, Lautenbach E, Lewis JD. Incidence and risk factors for herpes zoster among patients with inflammatory bowel disease. *Clin Gastroenterol Hepatol* 2006; **4**(12): 1483–1490.

17. Harpaz R, Ortega-Sanchez IR, Seward JF; Advisory Committee on Immunization Practices (ACIP) Centers for Disease Control and Prevention (CDC). Prevention of herpes zoster: recommendations of the Advisory Committee on Immunization Practices (ACIP). *MMWR Recomm Rep* 2008; **57**(RR-5): 1–30

PART III:
Investigating IBD

LIBRARY, UNIVERSITY OF CHESTER

JET LIBRARY

JET LIBRARY

Biomarkers in IBD: myth or marvel?

Richard B. Gearry[1,2] and Andrew S. Day[3,4]

[1]Department of Medicine, University of Otago, Dunedin, Otago, New Zealand
[2]Department of Gastroenterology, Christchurch Hospital, Christchurch, New Zealand
[3]Department of Paediatrics, University of Otago, Dunedin, Otago, New Zealand
[4]Paediatric Gastroenterology, Christchurch Hospital, Christchurch, New Zealand

---

LEARNING POINTS

- Classical markers such as erythrocyte sedimentation rate, C-reactive protein, and platelet count are easily measured and provide useful clinical information, but may be poorly specific and sensitive.

- Fecal biomarkers are more specific for gastrointestinal inflammation, useful for distinguishing organic from nonorganic disease and provide prognostic information for patients in clinical remission.

- Serological tests for distinguishing ulcerative colitis and Crohn's disease from indeterminate colitis and for predicting complicated disease promise much but still lack sufficient sensitivity and are not recommended for routine use.

- Future studies should integrate biomarkers with clinical and other patient data to determine which factors are predictive of poor outcomes. Only then should prospective studies of personalized medicine be compared with usual standard of care.

Introduction

The clinical assessment of a patient's symptoms and signs is a physician's primary means of determining inflammatory bowel disease (IBD) activity. While clinical assessment provides valuable insights, it is nonspecific and may reflect noninflammatory processes such as irritable bowel syndrome or small intestinal bacterial overgrowth. The gold standard for the assessment of intestinal inflammation is direct endoscopic visualization of the intestinal mucosa along with histological assessment of mucosal biopsies.

However, endoscopy is invasive, expensive, and exposes the patient to risk. Consequently, performing endoscopy each time a patient is reviewed is not acceptable. Inflammatory biomarkers promise a noninvasive and inexpensive means of determining the degree of intestinal inflammation, but can they deliver on this promise?

Biomarkers are defined by the National Institutes of Health (NIH) as "a characteristic that is objectively measured and evaluated as an indicator of normal biologic processes, pathogenic processes, or pharmacologic responses to a therapeutic intervention." This chapter focuses on classical serological biomarkers, fecal biomarkers, and the emerging serological biomarkers (see Table 11.1).

Classical biomarkers

Nonendoscopic assessment of gut inflammation has traditionally relied on serum markers of inflammation, including erythrocyte sedimentation rate (ESR), C-reactive protein (CRP), orosomucoid, platelets, albumin, and ferritin. The advantages of these tests include easy access to serum, low cost, and prompt measurement. However, disadvantages include relatively poor specificity and sensitivity. CRP appears to be the best of these markers and in one report provided sensitivity of 81% and specificity of 70% in differentiation of children with IBD from those with non-IBD conditions [1]. A prospective study has also shown that CRP concentration at diagnosis correlates with disease extent and risk of colectomy in UC, and the risk of subsequent resection in those with terminal ileal CD [2].

Clinical Dilemmas in Inflammatory Bowel Disease: New Challenges, Second Edition. Edited by P. Irving, C. Siegel, D. Rampton and F. Shanahan.
© 2011 Blackwell Publishing Ltd. Published 2011 by Blackwell Publishing Ltd.

TABLE 11.1 Strengths and weaknesses of biomarkers of gut inflammation

Type of biomarker	Examples	Strengths	Weaknesses
Standard	ESR, CRP, platelets	Inexpensive Widely available	Low specificity Require blood testing
Fecal	Calprotectin, S100A12, lactoferrin	Stool based (noninvasive) High specificity and sensitivity Correlate with inflammation Prediction of future relapse	Not widely available Cost
Serological	ASCA, pANCA, OMP-C, CBir1	Roles in indeterminate colitis Prediction of disease behavior	Diagnostic role not fully defined Require blood testing Not widely available Cost

Note: Fecal and serological biomarkers have augmented the roles of standard serum-based markers of gut inflammation. Examples of each group of biomarkers are provided, along with summaries of strengths and weaknesses for each group.

Fecal biomarkers

Although standard blood tests continue to be widely used, their disadvantages have prompted interest in more specific tests, including fecal assays that more reliably indicate gut inflammation. To date, the most promising disease specific markers are members of the S100 family of calcium-binding proteins and lactoferrin (an iron-binding glycoprotein with antimicrobial properties).

Fecal biomarkers have several clinical roles. Currently, indications include identifying patients with diarrhea who are likely to have an inflammatory cause, differentiating between inflammatory and functional symptoms in IBD patients and predicting the future course of the disease.

In a large prospective study, Tibble and colleagues measured fecal calprotectin in patients presenting with undifferentiated diarrhea to a hospital gastroenterology clinic [3]. These patients were subsequently investigated as usual with the attending doctor blinded to the calprotectin concentration. Those with a calprotectin greater than 10 mg/L were 27.8 times (95% confidence interval [CI], 17.6–43.7; $P < 0.0001$) more likely to have organic disease than a functional cause for their symptoms—calprotectin outperformed both ESR and CRP and may therefore have a role in identifying those newly referred patients who are unlikely to require further invasive investigation.

Fecal markers may also predict future relapse in IBD patients. In one study, patients with calprotectin >50 μg/g had a 13-fold increased risk of relapse, with specificity for relapse in CD of 83% [4]. Costa and colleagues [5] also demonstrated that calprotectin concentration predicted relapse, but only in UC. Further studies have demonstrated that higher calprotectin concentrations are associated with subsequent relapse, including in children [6].

Children are a particularly important population for the use of noninvasive biomarkers. In addition to calprotectin and lactoferrin, fecal S100A12 (Calgranulin C or ENRAGE) has been extensively tested in children and shows a high (97%) sensitivity and specificity [1]. Finally, calprotectin is correlated strongly with mucosal healing, particularly following successful induction of remission of IBD with biologic agents and is now routinely measured in randomized trials of new therapeutic agents.

Emerging serological biomarkers

While the classical and fecal biomarkers described above provide a snapshot of intestinal inflammation, a series of new serological markers against microbial antigens may play roles in diagnosing IBD, distinguishing between CD and UC in those with indeterminate colitis (IC) and indicating long-term prognosis [7]. These antibodies include antineutrophil cytoplasmic antibody with perinuclear staining (pANCA), anti-*Saccharomyces cerevisiae* antibody (ASCA), antibodies against laminaribioside (ALCA), antibodies against chitobioside (ACCA), outer membrane porin C (Omp C), I2 antibody (novel homologue of the bacterial transcription-factor families), and antibody to bacterial flagellin (CBir1).

As with calprotectin, the emerging serological antibodies have been assessed in patients undergoing a standard diagnostic work up for IBD. Most studies have demonstrated high specificity of these tests but limited sensitivity. A combination of antibodies may be more useful, particularly with sequential antibody testing—this approach resulted in a diagnostic accuracy of 84% in a prospectively recruited pediatric cohort [8]. However, the limited sensitivity of these tests for differentiating IBD from non-IBD leaves their role undefined.

While the role of these tests in diagnosing IBD remains unclear, there are more data regarding their ability to differentiate CD from UC. Whereas early studies assessed all patients with IBD, an important prospective study of patients with IC demonstrated that those who were seronegative for ASCA and pANCA were most likely to remain IC, while those positive for either marker were more likely to be reclassified as CD or UC respectively ($p<0.001$) [9]. The addition of Anti-OmpC and I2 did not significantly improve the predictive value of these tests [10], although anti-CBirl may help to further define the uncommon pANCA + CD patients [11].

The most promising role for serum antibody markers may be as part of a suite of biomarkers, which when assessed in conjunction with clinical data, may be able accurately to predict the course of CD, particularly disease behavior and therefore the requirement for more aggressive therapies and surgery. ASCA positivity is associated with an increased risk of complicated (Montreal B2 or B3) disease [12]. Furthermore, the addition of anti-I2 and anti-Omp C to ASCA demonstrated an 8.6-fold (95% CI 4.0–18.9) increased risk of CD patients having either fibrostenotic disease behavior or requiring a small bowel resection for those with all three antibodies compared to those with none [13].

While these studies suggest a promising role for these biomarkers to predict outcome and determine personalized therapy, more comprehensive prospective studies are required that include clinical variables such as elements of disease phenotype, response to previous therapy, cigarette smoking and genotype (particularly *NOD2*). To some extent, this has been achieved in two recently reported studies. A multicenter study prospectively recruited 796 pediatric CD patients at the time of diagnosis and followed them clinically after measuring a wide range of serological and genetic biomarkers and clinical data [14]. Those with ASCA+/CBirl+/OmpC+ status were 9.5-fold more likely to have internal penetrating (Montreal B3) behavior than

those without positive antibodies. A follow-up study of this same cohort using system dynamics analysis modeling reported a wide range of significant risk factors, including female gender, small bowel, or perianal disease, increasing serologic titre, pANCA + (reduced risk), colonic or upper GI tract disease location (reduced risk) in addition to treatment factors such as early corticosteroid use, early immunomodulator (reduced risk), early (reduced risk) or late and early combination immunomodulator and biologic therapy (reduced risk) [15]. Such a model is likely to help to determine therapeutic decisions in IBD management, but similar studies need to be undertaken in adults where the role of different variables is greater (e.g., cigarette smoking) before randomized prospective studies comparing a personalized approach to standard of care are performed.

Conclusions

Two categories of biomarkers may supplement conventional clinical and endoscopic assessment of patients with IBD. First are biomarkers of disease activity, which include CRP, ESR, and platelet count and which have been most usefully complemented by fecal markers such as calprotectin concentrations. Second are biomarkers that are predictive of clinical course and/or of disease subset (UC versus CD versus IC). The latter include combinations of various serum antibodies and, in the future, genetic testing. While these promise much, they have yet to deliver and are not recommended for routine clinical practice.

References

1. Sidler MA, Leach ST, Day AS. Fecal S100A12 and fecal calprotectin as noninvasive markers for inflammatory bowel disease in children. *Inflamm Bowel Dis* 2008; **14**: 359–366.
2. Henriksen M, Jahnsen J, Lygren I, Stray N, Sauar J, Vatn MH, et al. C-reactive protein: a predictive factor and marker of inflammation in inflammatory bowel disease. Results from a prospective population-based study. *Gut* 2008; **57**: 1518–1523.
3. Tibble JA, Sigthorsson G, Foster R, Forgacs I, Bjarnason I. Use of surrogate markers of inflammation and Rome criteria to distinguish organic from nonorganic intestinal disease. *Gastroenterology* 2002; **123**: 450–460.
4. Tibble J, Teahon K, Thjodleifsson B, Roseth A, Sigthorsson G, Bridger S, et al. A simple method for assessing intestinal inflammation in Crohn's disease. *Gut* 2000; **47**: 506–513.

5. Costa F, Mumolo MG, Ceccarelli L, Bellini M, Romano MR, Sterpi C, et al. Calprotectin is a stronger predictive marker of relapse in ulcerative colitis than in Crohn's disease. *Gut* 2005; **54**: 364–368.

6. Walkiewicz D, Werlin SL, Fish D, Scanlon M, Hanaway P, Kugathasan S. Fecal calprotectin is useful in predicting disease relapse in pediatric inflammatory bowel disease. *Inflamm Bowel Dis* 2008; **14**: 669–673.

7. Dubinsky M. What is the role of serological markers in IBD? Pediatric and adult data. *Dig Dis* 2009; **27**: 259–268.

8. Dubinsky MC, Johanson JF, Seidman EG, Ofman JJ. Suspected inflammatory bowel disease—the clinical and economic impact of competing diagnostic strategies. *Am J Gastroenterol* 2002; **97**: 2333–2342.

9. Joossens S, Reinisch W, Vermeire S, Sendid B, Poulain D, Peeters M, et al. The value of serologic markers in indeterminate colitis: a prospective follow-up study. *Gastroenterology.* 2002; **122**: 1242–7.

10. Joossens S, Colombel JF, Landers C, Poulain D, Geboes K, Bossuyt X, et al. Anti-outer membrane of porin C and anti-I2 antibodies in indeterminate colitis. *Gut* 2006; **55**: 1667–1669.

11. Targan SR, Landers CJ, Yang H, Lodes MJ, Cong Y, Papadakis KA, et al. Antibodies to CBir1 flagellin define a unique response that is associated independently with complicated Crohn's disease. *Gastroenterology* 2005; **128**: 2020–2028.

12. Vasiliauskas EA, Kam LY, Karp LC, Gaiennie J, Yang H, Targan SR. Marker antibody expression stratifies Crohn's disease into immunologically homogeneous subgroups with distinct clinical characteristics. *Gut* 2000; **47**: 487–496.

13. Mow WS, Vasiliauskas EA, Lin YC, Fleshner PR, Papadakis KA, Taylor KD, et al. Association of antibody responses to microbial antigens and complications of small bowel Crohn's disease. *Gastroenterology* 2004; **126**: 414–424.

14. Dubinsky MC, Kugathasan S, Mei L, Picornell Y, Nebel J, Wrobel I, et al. Increased immune reactivity predicts aggressive complicating Crohn's disease in children. *Clin Gastroenterol Hepatol* 2008; **6**: 1105–1111.

15. Siegel CA, Siegel LS, Hyams J, Kugathasan S, Markowitz J, Rosh JR, et al. Real-time tool to display the predicted disease course and treatment response for children with Crohn's disease. *Inflamm Bowel Dis* 2011; **17**(1):30–38.

12 Radiation exposure in IBD: how do we minimize the dangers?

Owen J. O'Connor[1], Alan N. Desmond[2], Fergus Shanahan[3], and Michael M. Maher[4]

[1]Department of Radiology, University College Cork, National University of Ireland, Cork, Ireland
[2]Department of Gastroenterology and General Internal Medicine, Cork University Hospital, Wilton, Cork, Ireland
[3]Department of Medicine, Alimentary Pharmabiotic Centre, University College Cork, National University of Ireland, Cork, Ireland
[4]Department of Radiology, Alimentary Pharmabiotic Centre, University College Cork, National University of Ireland, Cork, Ireland

---

LEARNING POINTS

- Radiation exposure in IBD is increasing, particularly in patients with Crohn's disease (CD).

- Computed Tomography (CT) provides valuable diagnostic information but causes most of the radiation exposure in IBD.

- Radiation exposure in IBD can be minimized by careful selection of patients, adopting low-dose radiation protocols for CT, and by deployment of other modalities such as ultrasound and magnetic resonance imaging (MRI).

- While access to MRI and ultrasonography has become widespread, these modalities are unlikely to completely replace CT imaging in the near future.

- Continual audit of CT usage and referrals coupled with improved education and dialogue between clinicians and radiologists is likely to help minimize radiation exposure. This educational process should begin in medical school.

Introduction

The use of diagnostic imaging, including examinations that involve exposure to ionizing radiation, has increased in patients with inflammatory bowel disease (IBD) in recent decades. This can potentially affect patients with Crohn's disease (CD), who are young, often require repeated examinations, already have a disease-related risk of carcinoma and lymphoma, and may receive radiosensitizing drugs and immunomodulatory agents that compound these risks. While the diagnostic information gained from imaging has been hugely beneficial to the management of most patients, clinicians need to familiarize themselves with the relative radiation exposures associated with commonly used diagnostic procedures (Table 12.1), and should maintain a judicious approach to selecting patients for imaging.

Radiation exposure in IBD

Patients with CD receive significantly greater radiation exposure than those with ulcerative colitis (UC) [1]. A study of radiation doses among patients with CD over a 15-year period demonstrated increasing use of imaging with 85% of dose during the final 5 years of the study period being due to CT [2]. Average cumulative effective doses per patient increased from 7.9 mSv to 25 mSv when the first 5-year period was compared with the final 5-year period. Younger patients with more severe disease requiring surgery or steroids were more likely to receive greater radiation exposure. Almost 16% of patients had cumulative effective exposure (>75 mSv) that has been estimated to potentially increase cancer mortality risk by 7%, although controversy remains regarding the nature of the relationship between radiation exposure and actual cancer risk [3].

Clinical Dilemmas in Inflammatory Bowel Disease: New Challenges, Second Edition. Edited by P. Irving, C. Siegel, D. Rampton and F. Shanahan.
© 2011 Blackwell Publishing Ltd. Published 2011 by Blackwell Publishing Ltd.

TABLE 12.1 Summary of radiation exposures associated with imaging procedures [24]

	Study type	Mean effective dose (mSv)	Equivalent number of chest radiographs
Plain film	PA chest radiograph	0.02	1
	Plain film abdomen	0.7	35
	Pelvic radiograph	0.6	30
	Upper GI series	6	300
	Small bowel series	3–5	250
	Barium enema	8	400
CT	Head	2	100
	Thorax	7	350
	CT pulmonary angiogram	15	750
	Abdomen	8	400
	Pelvis	6	300
	Virtual colonoscopy	10	500
Nuclear medicine	Bone scan (^{99m}-Tc-MDP)	6.3	315
Angiography	Coronary angiogram	7	350
MRI		Nil	
Ultrasound		Nil	

It is noteworthy that subgroups of patients with IBD may have an increased risk of small bowel, large bowel, and hepatobiliary carcinoma as well as small bowel lymphoma, depending primarily on the severity and distribution of chronic inflammation, but also influenced perhaps by immune modulation and radiation exposure [4,5].

Radiation exposure and CT

CT directly depicts extraluminal features of IBD that may not be apparent on endoscopy, but increasing use of CT has increased radiation exposure (Figure 12.1) [2,6]. CT has been reported to represent 10% of all studies using ionizing radiation, yet it imparts two-thirds of the overall radiation dose [7]. Mean annual exposures in the general patient population due to ionizing radiation have been estimated to be 0.39 mSv and 0.59 mSv in the United States and the Netherlands, respectively [8,9].

Detrimental effects of X-rays may be either deterministic or stochastic. Deterministic effects become worse with increasing exposure, have thresholds but fortunately rarely occur [10]. The probability of stochastic effects occurring

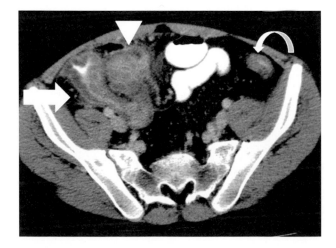

FIGURE 12.1 The value of CT in demonstrating intra- and extraluminal features of CD in a 34-year-old male. There is extensive thickening of the terminal ileum consistent with ileitis and similarly the cecum (arrow) and descending colon are thickened consistent with colitis (curved arrow). In addition, there is an acute inflammatory mass in the right iliac fossa (arrowhead) because of localized perforation, which would be difficult to diagnose endoscopically and may increase risk of complication if colonoscopy were performed.

is variable and has no threshold. Greater exposure increases the likelihood of a stochastic effect, but there is no dose below which there is no possibility of an effect occurring. Such effects include cancer and may occur years following exposure. It is estimated that for every 6000 routine abdominal and head CT examinations performed in children under the age of 15, five cancers directly attributable to ionizing radiation will occur [11].

Approaches to minimizing radiation exposure in CT

Disease-specific low-dose CT is an emerging method of limiting radiation exposures. For example, noncontiguous CT imaging of the thorax with doses as low as for a chest radiograph may be used to minimize pediatric exposure but maximize diagnostic yield [12].

Diagnostic low-dose CT in patients with IBD is particularly challenging. The major effect of exposure reduction at CT is increased image noise, which can impact image resolution, particularly of solid organs such as the liver, spleen, and kidneys. Typically, radiation exposure cannot be reduced to the extent it can in the thorax because the inherent contrast resolution required to resolve soft tissues that have only slightly varying attenuation values can be negatively impacted. CT exposure may be optimized using prepatient collimation, X-ray filters, improved detector geometry, noise-reduction filters, automatic tube current modulation, and iterative reconstruction [13].

CT imaging had traditionally been performed using fixed tube kilovoltage and amperage settings. This meant that larger regions of the body such as the mid-abdomen receive the same exposure as smaller regions such as the pelvis. This inefficient exposure resulted in some regions being over-irradiated (without any benefit in terms of image quality) and others potentially underexposed (with increased image noise and reduced image quality). Image quality in CT, unlike that of conventional radiography, is not reduced by overexposure and the difference between an adequately exposed and an overexposed image is not apparent. Automatic tube current modulation (ATCM) was developed to tailor the amperage of CT to patient size. Tube current is adjusted during the scan depending on X-ray attenuation, tube potential, table speed, pitch, and rotation time so that user-specified noise indices are achieved within each imaged section thereby minimizing exposure [14,15]. This method ensures that thicker regions of the body are imaged using higher tube currents than thinner less attenuating

areas. A reduction in tube-current time product can be achieved in 87% of examinations using ATCM with an average tube-current time product reduction of 32% [15].

Noise reduction filters are software programs applied to reconstructed CT images that reduce image noise on studies performed with reduced tube current. These filters improve the diagnostic quality of low-dose exams producing images, which compare favorably with normal-dose examinations, but like all advances in imaging techniques have some disadvantages including "oversmoothening" of images with potential impact on lesion detection in organs such as the liver [16]. Noise reduction filters can be used with ATCM to improve image quality, while significantly reducing radiation exposure.

Image quality following low-dose CT is affected by the reconstruction algorithm used. CT is normally reconstructed using filtered back projection. Iterative reconstruction is an alternative method of image reconstruction, which is currently being proposed and refined in an effort to improve the diagnostic acceptability of images acquired with reduced radiation exposure. This method is less affected by noisy data (due to reduced radiation) than filtered back projection and has only recently become commercially available for medical imaging.

Alternative imaging strategies for minimizing radiation exposure

CT imaging of IBD is increasingly being complemented or replaced by imaging methods which do not involve exposure to ionizing radiation such as magnetic resonance imaging (MRI) and ultrasound for the purpose of minimizing exposure. MRI represents a realistic alternative to CT and barium studies for certain patients (Table 12.2), and in some respects offers advantages over the other modalities in characterizing CD. Small bowel follow-through has traditionally been performed for the evaluation of small bowel disease in IBD but has an effective exposure of 3–5 mSv [17]. MRI may be used as an alternative to barium studies and CT for examining the small and large bowel. A recent retrospective study demonstrated MR studies performed primarily for small bowel examination to have a sensitivity of 80%, a specificity of 100%, a positive predictive value of 1.0, and a negative predictive value of 0.8 for the detection of colitis compared with colonoscopy [18]. One criticism of MRI is that mucosal detail is inferior to that of small bowel follow-through [19]. A comparison of the

TABLE 12.2 Summary of advantages and disadvantages of IBD-imaging modalities

Modality	Advantages	Disadvantages
Plain film	Inexpensive Fast to perform Easy access	Diagnostic yield very limited for a given radiation dose Sick patients proceed to CT/MRI/ultrasound irrespective of findings
CT	Fast Ease of access Sensitive for both intra- and extraluminal disease Good for imaging critically ill	High radiation dose Usually requires contrast administration
MRI	No Radiation Excellent soft-tissue resolution Requires intravenous contrast less often than CT Excellent for imaging fistula/sinuses	More expensive than CT Less accessible than CT Longer imaging times than CT Associated with claustrophobia Difficult to differentiate air from calculi Incompatible with most ventilator equipment
Ultrasound	No radiation Real-time imaging Excellent for imaging solid organs and fluid-filled structures Excellent for guiding intervention	Poor imaging of intraluminal contents Limited by artifact because of air Body habitus dependent Operator dependent Takes time to learn

sensitivities of CT and MR enterography with that of small bowel follow-through for the detection of Crohn's enteritis has demonstrated comparable results [19]. However, MRI and CT were superior to small bowel follow-through for the detection of extraenteric disease such as fistulae and abscess [19]. Therefore, accurate gastrointestinal imaging using MR with peroral contrast rather than nasojejunal intubation has the potential to safely reduce radiation exposure [19]. MRI may prove particularly useful for the assessment of treatment response, for imaging the terminal ileum and cecum following incomplete colonoscopy and for imaging of nonacute patients. Residual intraluminal air, long examination times, increased cost, and reduced out-of-hours access represent obstacles to the replacement of CT by MRI [6]. In the critically ill patient, MRI, compared with CT, is much more difficult to perform.

Ultrasound provides another alternative to ionizing radiation for the evaluation of intestinal and extraintestinal manifestations of IBD such as gallstones and renal calculi (Table 12.2) [6]. Ultrasound can be used to examine the small and large bowel with sensitivities of and specificities 78–96% and 86–100%, respectively, but is operator-dependent and limited by patient body habitus [6]. Ultra-sound appears best able to examine the terminal ileum and cecum, and can also be used to assess for strictures and fistulae [6].

Improving referral practices

Studies assessing clinicians' knowledge of radiation exposure and associated risks have demonstrated disappointing results with significant underestimation of typical radiation exposures associated with diagnostic imaging studies [20]. In response to the need for greater awareness, the European Council Euratom directive of 1997 recommended that radiation protection incorporating radiation exposure education should be integrated into the curriculum of medical schools [21]. Similar concerns about radiation exposure have precipitated the formation of *Image Gently*, a campaign in the United States aimed at increasing public awareness of radiation exposure in children [22]. The provision of a *radiation diary* to IBD patients has been proposed as a means of increasing awareness regarding radiation exposure among clinicians and patients alike [6]. Experts in the field of radiation dose optimization have advocated color-coding of imaging studies in an effort to identify imaging studies that are associated with exposure to ionizing radiation (red) and those that are not (green) [23]. In the current era of multidisciplinary patient care, collaboration between physicians and radiologists at multidisciplinary conferences, both with regard to the imaging and management of individual patients and the creation of agreed imaging algorithms, is to be encouraged. It may be possible to define clinical indications that justify CT and those where the use of ultrasound or MR is more appropriate. These indications would be used to choose the appropriate imaging modality.

Conclusion

There is increasing awareness of the importance of radiation exposure reduction and optimization in IBD. The optimal strategy for minimizing radiation exposure in IBD has not yet been determined, but requires a multifaceted collaborative approach. The path and pace of the process of exposure minimization will, in part, be determined by educational initiatives and modification of referral practices among clinicians. Radiologists in turn need to integrate low-dose CT imaging protocols into routine practice and encourage the use and development of alternative imaging methods that do not require ionizing radiation such as ultrasound and MRI where feasible.

References

1. Newnham E, Hawkes E, Surender A, James SL, Gearry R, Gibson PR. Quantifying exposure to diagnostic medical radiation in patients with inflammatory bowel disease: are we contributing to malignancy? *Aliment Pharmacol Ther* 2007; **26** (7): 1019–1024.

2. Desmond A, O' Regan K, Curran C, McWiliams S, Fitzgerald T, Maher MM, Shanahan F. Crohn's disease: factors associated with exposure to high levels of diagnostic radiation. *Gut* 2008; **57**: 1524–1529.

3. Cardis E, Vrijheid M, Blattner M, et al. The 15-country collaborative study of cancer risk among radiation workers in the nuclear industry: estimates of radiation-related cancer risks. *Radiat Res* 2007; **167**: 396–416.

4. Bernstein CN, Blanchard JF, Kliewer E, Wajda A. Cancer risk in patients with inflammatory bowel disease: a population-based study. *Cancer* 2001; **91**: 854–862.

5. Jess T, Loftus EV Jr, Velayos FS et al. Risk of intestinal cancer in inflammatory bowel disease: a population-based study from Olmsted county, Minnesota. *Gastroenterology* 2006; **130**: 1039–1046.

6. Herfarth H, Palmer L. Risk of radiation and choice of imaging. *Dig Dis* 2009; **27** (3): 278–284.

7. Mettler FA, Wiest PW, Locken JA, Kelsey CA. CT scanning: patterns of use and dose. *J Radiol Prot* 2000; **20**: 353–359.

8. Harrach RJ, Gallegos GM, Peterson SR. Supplementary notes on radiological disease. Available from: www.llnl.gov/saer/saer03_pdfs/Related_Documents/Radiological_Dose.pdf

9. Brugmans MJ, Buijs WC, Geleijins J, Lembrechts J. Population exposure to diagnostic use of ionizing radiation in the Netherlands. *Health Phys* 2002; **82**: 500–509.

10. Koenig TR, Wolff D, Mettler FA, Wagner LK. Skin injuries from fluoroscopically guided procedures: part 1, characteristics of radiation injury. *AJR Am J Roentgenol* 2001; **177**: 3–11.

11. Brenner D, Elliston C, Hall E, Berdon W. Estimated risks of radiation-induced fatal cancer from pediatric CT. *AJR Am J Roentgenol* 2001; **176** (2): 289–296

12. Takahashi M, Maguire WM, Ashtari M, et al. Low-dose spiral computed tomography of the thorax: comparison with the standard-dose technique. *Invest Radiol* 1998; **33**: 68–73.

13. Kalra MK, Rizzo S, Maher MM, et al. Chest CT performed with z-axis modulation: scanning protocol and radiation dose. *Radiology* 2005; **237**: 303–308.

14. Donnelly LF, Emery KH, Brody AS, et al. Minimising radiation dose for pediatric body applications of single-detector helical CT: strategies at a large children's hospital. *Am J Roentgenol* 2001; **176**: 303–306.

15. Kalra MK, Maher MM, Toth TL, Kamath RS, Halpern EF, Saini S. Comparison of Z-axis automatic tube current modulation technique with fixed tube current CT scanning of abdomen and pelvis. *Radiology* 2004; **232** (2): 347–353.

16. Kalra MK, Wittram C, Maher MM, et al. Can noise reduction filters improve low-radiation-dose chest CT images? Pilot study. *Radiology* 2003; **228**: 257–264.

17. Brenner DJ, Hall EJ. Computed tomography–an increasing source of radiation exposure. *N Engl J Med* 2007; **357** (22): 2277–2284.

18. Cronin CG, Lohan DG, Browne AM, Roche C, Murphy JM. Does MRI with oral contrast medium allow single-study depiction of inflammatory bowel disease enteritis and colitis? *Eur Radiol* 2010; **20** (7): 1667–1674.

19. Lee SS, Kim AY, Yang SK, Chung JW, et al. Crohn disease of the small bowel: comparison of CT enterography, MR enterography, and small-bowel follow-through as diagnostic techniques. *Radiology* 2009; **251** (3): 751–761.

20. Jacob K, Vivian G, Steel JR. X-ray dose training: are we exposed to enough? *Clin Radiol* 2004; **59**: 928–934.

21. Council Directive 97/43/Euratom of 30 June 1997 on health protection of individuals against the dangers of ionizing radiation in relation to medical exposure and repealing Directive 84/466/Euratom. *Official Journal of the European Communities* 1997; **L180**: 0022–0027.

22. Sidhu MK, Goske MJ, Coley BJ, et al. Image gently, step lightly: increasing radiation dose awareness in pediatric interventions through an international social marketing campaign. *J Vasc Interv Radiol* 2009; **20** (9): 1115–1159.

23. Suhova A, Chubuchny V, Picano E. Principle of responsibility in medical imaging. *Ann Ist Super Sanita* 2003; **39** (2): 205–212.

24. Mettler FA, Jr, Huda W, Yoshizumi TT, Mahesh M. Effective doses in radiology and diagnostic nuclear medicine: a catalog. *Radiology* 2008; **48** (1): 254–263.

13 Surveillance colonoscopy in UC: what is the best way to do it?

Matthew D. Rutter

Tees Bowel Cancer Screening Centre, University Hospital of North Tees, Stockton-on-Tees, Cleveland, UK

LEARNING POINTS

- Better patient risk stratification can guide surveillance intensity.
- Severity of inflammation is an important risk factor.
- Most dysplasia is macroscopically detectable with careful inspection.
- Pancolonic dye-spraying enhances dysplasia detection.
- Expert repeat colonoscopy and review of histology should be performed if dysplasia is detected.
- Well-circumscribed dysplastic lesions are often endoscopically resectable.

Introduction

Increased risk

Patients with colitis have a high risk of developing colorectal cancer (CRC). Population-based studies demonstrate that those with ulcerative colitis (UC) or Crohn's colitis have a risk 5–6 times that of the general population[1,2]. Sadly, when cancers do occur, they often occur at a younger age than in the general population, with over a quarter presenting before the age of 40.

Recent studies have shown a reduction in the cancer risk, the most likely explanations being either because of improved control of colonic inflammation or because of the beneficial effect of surveillance programs. Although there have been no randomized controlled trials to demonstrate the efficacy of colitis surveillance, the British Society of Gastroenterology (BSG), American Society for Gastrointestinal Endoscopy (ASGE), American Gastroenterological Association (AGA), Crohn's and Colitis Foundation of America (CCFA), and European Crohn's and Colitis Organisation (ECCO) all recommend colonoscopic surveillance of colitis.

Recently several advances in risk stratification, surveillance technique, and dysplasia management have been made that are likely to improve colitis surveillance efficacy.

Risk stratification

Colitis surveillance effectiveness is contingent on focusing on patients most likely to develop CRC. One of the most important risk factors for colitic cancer is disease extent—a population-based study showed that patients with proctitis had no significantly increased risk, those with left-sided disease had 2.8 times the risk, and those with pancolitis 14.8 times the risk of the general population [1]. As disease extent may change over time, the BSG guideline recommendation is to perform an index screening colonoscopy approximately 10 years after the onset of colitic symptoms, thereafter basing the surveillance strategy on the maximum documented extent of disease to date.

A recently discovered risk factor is disease severity. A case-control study demonstrated that severity of inflammation was independently associated with the risk for colonic neoplasia (odds ratio (OR) 4.7, $p < 0.001$) [3]. Further studies have confirmed this, and this may prove an important discovery, as it is a potentially modifiable risk factor. It is not only current inflammation that increases risk—studies have demonstrated a 2-fold-increased neoplasia risk in patients with postinflammatory polyps, which arise during healing of previous severe colonic ulceration [4].

Clinical Dilemmas in Inflammatory Bowel Disease: New Challenges, Second Edition. Edited by P. Irving, C. Siegel, D. Rampton and F. Shanahan.
© 2011 Blackwell Publishing Ltd. Published 2011 by Blackwell Publishing Ltd.

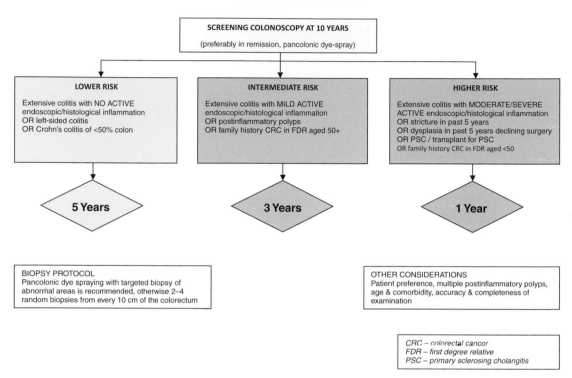

COLITIS SURVEILLANCE AS PROPOSED BY THE BRITISH SOCIETY OF GASTROENTEROLOGY

SCREENING COLONOSCOPY AT 10 YEARS

(preferably in remission, pancolonic dye-spray)

LOWER RISK

Extensive colitis with NO ACTIVE endoscopic/histological inflammation
OR left-sided colitis
OR Crohn's colitis of <50% colon

INTERMEDIATE RISK

Extensive colitis with MILD ACTIVE endoscopic/histological inflammation
OR postinflammatory polyps
OR family history CRC in FDR aged 50+

HIGHER RISK

Extensive colitis with MODERATE/SEVERE ACTIVE endoscopic/histological inflammation
OR stricture in past 5 years
OR dysplasia in past 5 years declining surgery
OR PSC / transplant for PSC
OR family history CRC in FDR aged <50

5 Years

3 Years

1 Year

BIOPSY PROTOCOL
Pancolonic dye spraying with targeted biopsy of abnormal areas is recommended, otherwise 2–4 random biopsies from every 10 cm of the colorectum

OTHER CONSIDERATIONS
Patient preference, multiple postinflammatory polyps, age & comorbidity, accuracy & completeness of examination

CRC – colorectal cancer
FDR – first degree relative
PSC – primary sclerosing cholangitis

FIGURE 13.1 BSG colitis surveillance algorithm [8].

Other known risk factors include duration of disease (1.6% at 10 years, 8.3% at 20 years, and 18.4% at 30 years UC duration) [5], primary sclerosing cholangitis (a 3–5-fold-increased risk) [6], and a family history of sporadic CRC (a 2-fold-increased risk) [7]. Revised BSG guidelines stratify a patient's risk and recommend an appropriate surveillance frequency accordingly (see Figure 13.1) [8]. These guidelines differ from other societies' that still advocate repeating colonoscopy every 1–2 years after 8 years of disease, regardless of the patients' risk factors [9].

Surveillance colonoscopy

Basics of colonoscopy

It is now recognized that with modern endoscopic equipment and techniques, the majority of colitic dysplastic lesions are macroscopically detectable, although the endoscopic appearance can be subtle, varied, and mimicked by inflammatory and postinflammatory changes. Thus, surveillance colonoscopies should ideally be performed during disease remission; however, they should not be delayed unduly as patients with active inflammation have an increased risk of malignancy. An effective bowel preparation regimen is required to ensure optimal mucosal views. Residual fecal debris should be washed and suctioned, and haustral definition and peristalsis suppressed using antispasm drugs such as hyoscine-N-butylbromide or scopolamine. Procedures should be performed by experienced colonoscopists skilled in interpreting colonoscopic appearances. There is clear evidence that the more time that is spent inspecting the mucosa, the greater the dysplasia yield [11,12].

Dysplasia detection

Conventional surveillance strategies advocate taking at least four random biopsies from every 10 cm of colon and rectum based on the now disproved premise that colitis dysplasia is endoscopically invisible. However, compliance with this biopsy schedule is poor and the associated costs high.

Recent prospective controlled trials have consistently demonstrated improved neoplasia detection, if targeted biopsies are taken after pancolonic dye-spraying. In Kiesslich's study using methylene blue, chromoendoscopy detected three times more dysplasia compared with surveillance using random biopsies (32/84 cf. 10/81, $P = 0.003$) [12]. In Rutter's study of back-to-back colonoscopies in 100 patients, no dysplasia was detected from 2904 random biopsies, two visible dysplastic lesions were detected macroscopically, and a further seven lesions were visible only after dye-spraying with indigo carmine [13]. The revised BSG and AGA guidelines advocate pancolonic dye-spraying with targeted biopsy of abnormal areas [8,10]. Details of the dye-spraying technique are published elsewhere [14].

Although there was much hope that narrow-band imaging (NBI) might supersede dye-spraying, a prospective randomized crossover trial concluded that NBI was no better than standard white light endoscopy (WLE) and therefore cannot be recommended for colitis surveillance [15].

Another image-enhancement technique, autofluorescence imaging (AFI), shows some promise. The results of a small prospective randomized crossover trial were in favor of AFI compared to WLE—ten dysplastic lesions were found in the 25 patients undergoing AFI first, subsequent WLE detecting no further lesions, compared to three dysplastic lesions in the 25 patients undergoing WLE first, subsequent AFI detecting three further lesions ($p = 0.036$) [16]. Further confirmatory studies including assessing the technique against pancolonic dye-spraying are required.

Confocal endomicroscopy (CFE) is an exciting technique that produces real-time in vivo images of the cellular structure of the surface and subsurface layers of the mucosa. However, although CFE improves in vivo characterization of lesions, it is not a technology for lesion detection as lesions must be detected before CFE can be employed.

Dysplasia management

Basic principles

If dysplasia is detected at any surveillance colonoscopy, the histological slides should be reviewed by a second expert gastrointestinal pathologist without delay and the surveillance colonoscopy repeated by an expert colonoscopist

using pancolonic dye-spray and, in this specific situation, taking multiple nontargeted biopsies as well. The clinician can then determine whether there is true dysplasia, whether the dysplasia is in a visible lesion or not, and whether there are multiple dysplastic areas.

Macroscopically visible dysplasia

Dysplastic polyps arising within an area of inflammation have been termed dysplasia-associated lesions/masses (DALMs), and early studies showed high cancer incidences in patients with such lesions. However, the definition of a DALM has evolved over time, and recently the term "adenoma-like mass" (ALM) has been used to describe a proportion of such lesions that can be endoscopically resected and appear to carry a lower cancer risk. As there is no clear-cut histological discriminator between these lesions, the management decision rests on whether the dysplastic lesion can be endoscopically resected: if it can be (ensuring that there is no residual dysplasia by taking biopsies from the mucosa surrounding the resected margin), it is usually not necessary to recommend colectomy. However, if the entire dysplastic area cannot be excised, prompt surgery is required irrespective of the grade of dysplasia.

Macroscopically invisible dysplasia

Where endoscopically invisible high-grade dysplasia has been detected, colectomy is recommended because of high rates of synchronous cancer or rapid progression to cancer in 32–42% of patients [18,19]. The diagnosis of low-grade dysplasia (LGD) in flat mucosa is fraught with controversy, with reported rates of progression to advanced neoplasia varying greatly. Most studies have found that between a fifth and a half of patients will develop a more advanced lesion, but some studies report rates of progression as low as 3–10%. The options of either intensified surveillance or colectomy should be discussed with patients, erring towards the latter in the presence of other risk factors or multifocal LGD. It should be noted that these recommendations and the probability of synchronous cancer are based on data from the era of random surveillance biopsies. The risk of progression to cancer has not yet been defined when using enhanced surveillance techniques [19].

Postinflammatory polyps

Patients with postinflammatory polyps have an increased risk of developing colorectal neoplasia [4]. Also, in the presence of multiple postinflammatory polyps the chance of finding subtle mucosal irregularities is low. A full and frank discussion with the patient about this and other management strategies such as prophylactic surgery is necessary.

Conclusion

The recent improvements in risk stratification, surveillance technique, and dysplasia management should improve colitis surveillance efficacy.

References

1. Ekbom A, Helmick C, Zack M, Adami HO. Ulcerative colitis and colorectal cancer. A population-based study. *N Engl J Med* 1990; **323** (18): 1228–1233.
2. Ekbom A, Helmick C, Zack M, Adami HO. Increased risk of large-bowel cancer in Crohn's disease with colonic involvement. *Lancet* 1990; **336**(8711): 357–359.
3. Rutter M, Saunders B, Wilkinson K, et al. Severity of inflammation is a risk factor for colorectal neoplasia in ulcerative colitis. *Gastroenterology* 2004; **126**(2): 451–459.
4. Rutter MD, Saunders BP, Wilkinson KH, et al. Cancer surveillance in longstanding ulcerative colitis: endoscopic appearances help predict cancer risk. *Gut* 2004; **53**(12): 1813–1816.
5. Eaden JA, Abrams KR, Mayberry JF. The risk of colorectal cancer in ulcerative colitis: a meta-analysis. *Gut* 2001; **48**(4): 526–535.
6. Broome U, Lofberg R, Veress B, Eriksson LS. Primary sclerosing cholangitis and ulcerative colitis: evidence for increased neoplastic potential [see comments]. *Hepatology* 1995; **22**(5): 1404–1408.
7. Askling J, Dickman PW, Karlen P, et al. Family History as a risk factor for colorectal cancer in inflammatory bowel disease. *Gastroenterology* 2001; **120**(6): 1356–1362.
8. Cairns S, Scholefield JH, Steele RJ, et al. Guidelines for colorectal cancer screening and surveillance in moderate and high hisk groups (update from 2002). *Gut* 2010; **59**(5): 666–689.
9. Farraye FA, Odze RD, Eaden J, Itzkowitz SH. AGA technical review on the diagnosis and management of colorectal neoplasia in inflammatory bowel disease. *Gastroenterology* 2010; **138**(2): 746–774.
10. Barclay RL, Vicari JJ, Doughty AS, Johanson JF, Greenlaw RL. Colonoscopic withdrawal times and adenoma detection during screening colonoscopy. *N Engl J Med* 2006; **355**(24): 2533–2541.
11. Toruner M, Harewood GC, Loftus EV, Jr, et al. Endoscopic factors in the diagnosis of colorectal dysplasia in chronic inflammatory bowel disease. *Inflamm Bowel Dis* 2005; **11**(5): 428–434.
12. Kiesslich R, Fritsch J, Holtmann M, et al. Methylene blue-aided chromoendoscopy for the detection of intraepithelial neoplasia and colon cancer in ulcerative colitis. *Gastroenterology* 2003; **124**(4): 880–888.
13. Rutter MD, Saunders BP, Schofield G, Forbes A, Price AB, Talbot IC. Pancolonic indigo carmine dye spraying for the detection of dysplasia in ulcerative colitis. *Gut* 2004; **53**(2): 256–260.
14. Rutter M, Bernstein C, Matsumoto T, Kiesslich R, Neurath M. Endoscopic appearance of dysplasia in ulcerative colitis and the role of staining. *Endoscopy* 2004; **36**(12): 1109–1114.
15. Dekker E, van den Broek FJ, Reitsma JB, et al. Narrow-band imaging compared with conventional colonoscopy for the detection of dysplasia in patients with longstanding ulcerative colitis. *Endoscopy* 2007; **39**(3): 216–221.
16. van den Broek FJ, Fockens P, van Eeden S, et al. Endoscopic tri-modal imaging for surveillance in ulcerative colitis: randomised comparison of high-resolution endoscopy and autofluorescence imaging for neoplasia detection; and evaluation of narrow-band imaging for classification of lesions. *Gut* 2008; **57**(8): 1083–1089.
17. Bernstein CN, Shanahan F, Weinstein WM. Are we telling patients the truth about surveillance colonoscopy in ulcerative colitis? [see comments]. [Review] [28 refs]. *Lancet* 1994; **343**(8889): 71–74.
18. Rutter MD, Saunders BP, Wilkinson KH, et al. Thirty-year analysis of a colonoscopic surveillance program for neoplasia in ulcerative colitis. *Gastroenterology* 2006; **130**(4): 1030–1038.
19. Awais D, Siegel CA, Higgins PD. Modelling dysplasia detection in ulcerative colitis: clinical implications of surveillance intensity. *Gut* 2009; **58**(11): 1498–1503.

PART IV:
Medical Therapy

5-ASA

14 New 5-ASAs for ulcerative colitis: a tiny step or giant stride forward?

L. Campbell Levy

Dartmouth Medical School, Section of Gastroenterology and Hepatology, Dartmouth–Hitchcock Medical Center, Lebanon, NH, USA

LEARNING POINTS

- 5-aminosalicylic acid (5-ASA) agents are the mainstay of therapy for mild-to-moderate ulcerative colitis (UC) and have a long track record of safety.

- Efficacy of different oral 5-ASA agents for the treatment of mild-to-moderate UC is similar.

- Sulfasalazine has more side effects than mesalamine-based agents, but should not be discontinued in patients who are tolerating it.

- Optimal dosing of oral 5-ASA for UC remains unclear, although higher doses may be appropriate for refractory disease.

- There is no evidence that newer extended-release mesalamine formulations are more effective for UC.

- Once daily dosing may improve adherence and hence efficacy.

Introduction

Since 5-aminosalicylic acid (5-ASA) was identified as the therapeutically active moiety of sulfasalazine nearly 35 years ago, efforts have been made to evaluate and improve its efficacy as a treatment for inflammatory bowel disease (IBD). In particular, attempts to address the problem of adherence (see Chapter 55) have resulted in the development of longer acting, once-daily mesalamine agents.

Mechanism of action and pharmacology of different formulations

The precise mechanism of mesalamine's anti-inflammatory effects is unknown, but is probably mediated by a local, topical effect impacting on a range of inflammatory processes [1]. Proposed mechanisms include the interruption of lipoxygenase and cyclooxygenase pathways, decreased production of IL-1, IL-2, and tumor necrosis factor (TNF) in the colonic mucosa, and activation of the peroxisome proliferation activated receptor (PPAR-γ) resulting in multiple downstream effects, including decreased transcriptional activity of nuclear factor kappa B.

Commercially available oral 5-ASA formulations include azo-bond prodrugs, such as sulfasalazine, olsalazine, and balsalazide, and a variety of controlled-release and delayed-release forms.

Newer formulations of mesalamine utilize technology that extends their release in the colon. It is argued that this property enables once daily dosing; however, emerging evidence suggests that older preparations of 5-ASA may also be just as effective when taken once daily [2]. Lialda/Mezavant, contains 1.2 g of mesalamine per tablet, and contains a multimatrix (MMX®) system of wax, stearic acid, and cellulose, while Apriso™/Salofalk a 0.375 g capsule, consists of enteric coated granules in a polymer matrix (INTELLICOR™).

Efficacy and safety of aminosalicylates for UC

Many studies have evaluated the efficacy of 5-ASA for UC, some of which were summarized in two Cochrane meta-analyses investigating 5-ASA for induction and maintenance of remission [3,4]. These analyses included over 2100 patients from 21 studies (nine placebo-controlled). Aminosalicylates were superior to placebo for induction

---

Clinical Dilemmas in Inflammatory Bowel Disease: New Challenges, Second Edition. Edited by P. Irving, C. Siegel, D. Rampton and F. Shanahan.
© 2011 Blackwell Publishing Ltd. Published 2011 by Blackwell Publishing Ltd.

of remission (odds ratio (OR) for failing to induce clinical improvement or remission was 0.40, 95% confidence interval (CI) 0.30–0.53) and for maintenance (OR for failing to maintain clinical or endoscopic remission was 0.47, 95% CI 0.36–0.42). Though there was no difference in adverse effects or withdrawal because of side effects, many of the trials in the study excluded patients intolerant to sulfasalazine, thereby incorporating an inherent bias.

While the differences in efficacy between sulfasalazine and other mesalamine agents appear to be minimal, differences in tolerability are more marked. Due to a dose-dependent effect of the sulfapyridine moiety, adverse effects, such as dyspepsia, diarrhea, fever, rash, and headache, occur in up to 50% of patients [5]. Up to 90% of patients who stop sulfasalazine due to adverse side effects will subsequently tolerate mesalamine without difficulty [1]. Serious adverse effects of oral 5-ASAs are idiosyncratic and exceptional and include blood dyscrasias, pancreatitis, and nephrotoxicity.

Optimal dosing

The presumption that higher mucosal concentrations of drug will improve outcomes is appealing. This concept is supported by a dose-response trend observed in the Cochrane analyses [3,4] and by improved outcomes in extensive UC with the addition of topical to oral therapies. However, evidence for higher doses of oral 5-ASA remains inconsistent.

The trio of ASCEND trials and previous dose-finding trials compared different initial doses of mesalamine (see Table 14.1) [6]. In the ASCEND I and II trials, which assessed a standard dose (2.4 g/day) and a higher dose (4.8 g/day) using the 800 mg Asacol® HD formulation, there was no difference in clinical improvement after 6 weeks among patients with mild and moderate colitis (51% versus 56% respectively, $p =$ NS) [7,8]. However, data limited to patients with moderate disease showed a statistically significant benefit of the higher dose (ASCEND I 57% versus 72% respectively, $p = 0.038$ and ASCEND II 59% versus 72% respectively, $p < 0.05$). In the larger ASCEND III study, 2.4 g was again tested against 4.8 g. All of these patients had moderate disease, and now there was no significant difference in the primary endpoint of overall improvement (66% versus 70% respectively, $p =$ NS) [9]. Among secondary endpoints, there was a statistically significant increase for clinical remission with 4.8 g, but no difference in endoscopic improvement. Despite some evidence of improved dose-related outcomes when partial remission or clinical improvement is studied, evidence of superiority for higher doses is lacking when complete remission is used as a primary endpoint. For MMX mesalamine, two Phase 3 induction trials that studied clinical and endoscopic remission at 8 weeks also showed no difference between 2.4 g/day and 4.8 g/day (37.2% and 35.1%, respectively) [10].

However, some data point to subgroups of patients that may benefit from higher doses. Approximately, 60% of patients who failed to achieve remission in the MMX mesalamine Phase 3 studies subsequently responded to 8 more weeks of 4.8 g/day of MMX mesalamine in an extension study [11]. Among patients in ASCEND III with more refractory UC (previously treated with mesalamine, corticosteroids, rectal therapies, or multiple UC therapies), the higher dose was more effective (69.6% versus 58.1%, $p = 0.011$) [9]. Similarly, a subgroup analysis of ASCEND I and II showed a benefit from the higher dose among patients with the same markers of more severe UC [12].

Despite this signal that higher doses of mesalamine may be more effective for more stubborn UC, this hypothesis

TABLE 14.1 Studies evaluating dosing of delayed-release mesalamine for ulcerative colitis (UC)

Study	Primary end point	Duration (weeks)	Mesalamine dose		
			1.6 g	2.4 g	4.8 g
Schroeder et al. [5]	Response	6	18%		50%
Sninsky et al. [6]	Improvement	6	43%	49%	
Kamm et al. [13]	Remission	8		41%	41%
ASCEND I [7]	Overall improvement	6		51%	56%
Moderate subgroup				57%	72%
ASCEND II [8]	Overall improvement	6		59%	72%
ASCEND III [9]	Overall improvement	6		66%	70%

Source: Siegel [6].

has yet to be fully tested. Even with the advent of newer formulations of mesalamine, it remains unknown whether the upper dose limit of 5-ASA has been reached, or whether the limiting step is delivering the drug to the appropriate site of disease.

Efficacy of newer delayed-release formulation

Complex pharmacology, variability of endpoints in the literature, and strong marketing forces confound differences between the newer mesalamine formulations making it difficult for clinicians to discern an advantage of one over another. However, one clear advantage of the newer formulations is a simpler dosing schedule and lighter pill burden. Without head to head trials, there is no evidence of increased efficacy of the newer formulations over the older 5-ASA agents. However, at least for Asacol® HD and Lialda®/Mezavant, efficacy appears to be equivalent. In a double-blinded, placebo-controlled 8-week study of Lialda®/Mezavant (2.4 g and 4.8 g), both doses of Lialda®/Mezavant were superior to placebo in achieving clinical and endoscopic remission (40.5% at 2.4 g, $P = 0.01$; 41.2% at 4.8 g, $P = 0.007$; placebo 22.1%). A reference arm of patients taking Asacol® 2.4 g/day showed a statistically insignificant benefit over placebo (32.6%, $P = 0.124$) [13]. Statistical comparisons directly between Lialda®/Mezavant and Asacol® were not performed

Apriso™/Salofalk was approved for maintenance of remission on the basis of two randomized trials in which patients taking 1.5 g/day mesalamine remained relapse free after 6 months more often than those taking placebo (79% versus 62% respectively, $p < 0.001$) [14]. This formulation has not been approved for the induction of remission of UC in the United States, despite European studies showing benefit in mild-to-moderate UC in two Phase 3 trials [15]. After 8 weeks of either 3 g/day once daily or the same dose 3 times daily, the rates of clinical (69.6% versus 68.8% respectively, $p = $ NS) and endoscopic remission were comparable (70.7% versus 69.8% respectively, $p = $ NS).

Maintaining adherence to therapy is problematic in many chronic conditions, and IBD is no exception. In a recent online survey, approximately 30% of patients with IBD reported missing medications at least weekly [16]. The importance of adherence was underscored by a recent prospective study that showed nonadherence was associated with a 5-fold increased risk of disease activity over a 2-year period (hazard ratio (HR) 5.5, 95% CI 2.3–13) [17]. Multiple factors contribute to nonadherence including age,

gender, marital status, and the nature of the doctor–patient relationship. However, the complexity of drug regimens is undoubtedly also a major contributor. Though simplifying therapies alone will not solve this multifaceted problem, offering once daily dosing and fewer pills is likely to provide an important start to addressing a difficult issue.

Conclusion

Recent advances in the use of aminosalicylates for mild-to-moderate UC have focused on improving drug delivery and optimizing regimens. While newer 5-ASAs have yet to be shown to be more effective than older preparations, they have resulted in more tolerable regimens with lower pill burdens. These improvements are likely to improve adherence. Future studies are needed to teach us which groups of patients will benefit most from higher doses of 5-ASA and how best to deliver the drug.

References

1. Nielsen OH. Sulfasalazine intolerance. A retrospective survey of the reasons for discontinuing treatment with sulfasalazine in patients with chronic inflammatory bowel disease. *Scand J Gastroenterol* 1982; **17**(3): 389–393.
2. Dignass AU, Bokemeyer B, Adamek H, et al. Mesalamine once daily is more effective than twice daily in patients with quiescent ulcerative colitis. *Clin Gastroenterol Hepatol* 2009; **7**(7): 762–769.
3. Sutherland L, Macdonald JK. Oral 5-aminosalicylic acid for maintenance of remission in ulcerative colitis. *Cochrane Database Syst Rev* 2006 (2): CD000544.
4. Sutherland L, Macdonald JK. Oral 5-aminosalicylic acid for induction of remission in ulcerative colitis. *Cochrane Database Syst Rev* 2006 (2): CD000543.
5. Cunliffe RN, Scott BB. Review article: monitoring for drug side-effects in inflammatory bowel disease. *Aliment Pharmacol Ther* 2002; **16**(4): 647–662.
6. Siegel CA. Accidentally ASCENDing into comparative effective research for inflammatory bowel disease. *Gastroenterology* 2009; **137**(6): 1880–1882.
7. Hanauer SB, Sandborn WJ, Dallaire C, et al. Delayed-release oral mesalamine 4.8 g/day (800 mg tablets) compared to 2.4 g/day (400 mg tablets) for the treatment of mildly to moderately active ulcerative colitis: The ASCEND I trial. *Can J Gastroenterol* 2007; **21**(12): 827–834.
8. Hanauer SB, Sandborn WJ, Kornbluth A, et al. Delayed-release oral mesalamine at 4.8 g/day (800 mg tablet)

for the treatment of moderately active ulcerative colitis: the ASCEND II trial. *Am J Gastroenterol* 2005; **100**(11): 2478–2485.

9. Sandborn WJ, Regula J, Feagan BG, et al. Delayed-release oral mesalamine 4.8 g/day (800-mg tablet) is effective for patients with moderately active ulcerative colitis. *Gastroenterology* 2009; **137**(6): 1934–1943.

10. Sandborn WJ, Kamm MA, Lichtenstein GR, Lyne A, Butler T, Joseph RE. MMX Multi Matrix System mesalazine for the induction of remission in patients with mild-to-moderate ulcerative colitis: a combined analysis of two randomized, double-blind, placebo-controlled trials. *Aliment Pharmacol Ther* 2007; **26**(2): 205–215.

11. Kamm MA, Lichtenstein GR, Sandborn WJ, et al. Effect of extended MMX mesalamine therapy for acute, mild-to-moderate ulcerative colitis. *Inflamm Bowel Dis* 2009; **15**(1): 1–8.

12. Hanauer SB, Ramsey D, Sandborn WJ. Efficacy of delayed-release oral mesalamine in patients who received pre-vious ulcerative colitis treatment. *Gastroenterology* 2008; **134**(Suppl. 1): A490.

13. Kamm MA, Sandborn WJ, Gassull M, et al. Once-daily, high-concentration MMX mesalamine in active ulcerative colitis. *Gastroenterology* 2007; **132**(1): 66–75; quiz 432–433.

14. Zakko S, Gordon GL, Murthy UK, et al. Once-daily mesalamine granules effectively maintain remission from ulcerative colitis: data from 2 phase 3 trials. *Gastroenterology* 2009; **136**(Suppl. 1): A521. [Abstract]

15. Kruis W, Kiudelis G, Racz I, et al. Once daily versus three times daily mesalazine granules in active ulcerative colitis: a double-blind, double-dummy, randomised, non-inferiority trial. *Gut* 2009; **58**(2): 233–240.

16. Loftus EV, Jr. A practical perspective on ulcerative colitis: patients' needs from aminosalicylate therapies. *Inflamm Bowel Dis* 2006; **12**(12): 1107–1113.

17. Kane S, Huo D, Aikens J, Hanauer S. Medication nonadherence and the outcomes of patients with quiescent ulcerative colitis. *Am J Med* 2003; **114**(1): 39–43.

15 Do 5-ASAs prevent cancer?

Richard Logan[1,2] and Venkataraman Subramanian[2]

[1]Division of Epidemiology and Public Health, Queens Medical Centre,
Nottingham University Hospitals, Nottingham, UK
[2]Nottingham Digestive Diseases Centre, Queens Medical Centre, Nottingham University Hospitals NHS Trust,
Nottingham, UK

LEARNING POINTS

- The cancer risk in patients with ulcerative colitis (UC) is increased, but recent studies show the cumulative risk to be much lower than previous estimates.

- Colonoscopic surveillance is currently recommended by most professional gastroenterology bodies, but has not been shown to improve survival.

- Regular 5-aminosalicylic acid (5-ASA) use is associated with a halving of cancer risk in observational studies.

- Whether the chemopreventive effect of 5-ASA is due to an anti-inflammatory effect alone is unclear. Other putative mechanisms include antiproliferative and proapoptotic effects, increase in replication fidelity and inhibition of beta-catenin/Wnt signaling pathways.

- Regular use of aspirin or celecoxib may be more effective than 5-ASA, but more data is needed.

Introduction

The fact that people with ulcerative colitis (UC) have an increased risk of colorectal cancer (CRC) looms large in the minds of UC patients and their doctors. CRC in UC occurs at a younger age than in the general population and risk increases with duration of UC. While some have estimated the cumulative risk to be as high as 18% after 30 years of UC, this is not the experience of most clinicians and recent data shows the risk to be much lower [1–3].

Nevertheless, concerns about the cancer risk have led many authorities to advocate colonoscopic surveillance and where necessary prophylactic colectomy. Evidence that this approach is effective is mixed, and the need for repeated colonoscopy is not popular with patients. The possibility of chemoprevention of cancer has obvious appeal. The suggestion that 5-ASAs might have cancer chemopreventive properties as well as being anti-inflammatory was first raised by a case-control study from Sweden, which found that UC patients who had developed CRC reported less sulfasalazine use than UC patients without cancer [4]. The study was limited by only having access to hospital records, but the effect found was large (odds ratio (OR) for sulfasalazine use for >3 months 0.38, 95% confidence interval (CI) 0.20–0.69) suggesting that if this reflected a causal association then cancer risk might be more than halved.

How might 5-ASAs protect against CRC in UC?

If 5-ASAs have chemopreventive properties, are these additional to their anti-inflammatory effects or are any chemopreventive effects simply a reflection of greater control of chronic inflammation [5]? As normal colonic mucosa becomes malignant, there is an increase in enterocyte proliferation rates and a decrease in apoptosis. Intestinal apoptosis and cyclooxygenase-2 (COX-2) expression in the colon appear to be linked, and COX-2 expression is upregulated in colon cancer. 5-ASAs inhibit not only COX-2 but also lipoxygenase activity, leading to intracellular accumulation of the arachidonic acid and eventually an increase in ceramide formation from sphingomyelin, which exerts a strong proapoptotic effect. In patients with colonic polyps, oral 5-ASA (1 g/day) decreased proliferation (by Ki-67 expression) and increased apoptosis (by TUNEL assay) in colorectal mucosa [6]. In vitro studies have also confirmed

Clinical Dilemmas in Inflammatory Bowel Disease: New Challenges, Second Edition. Edited by P. Irving, C. Siegel, D. Rampton and F. Shanahan.
© 2011 Blackwell Publishing Ltd. Published 2011 by Blackwell Publishing Ltd.

that 5-ASAs inhibit growth and enhance apoptosis of cultured CRC cell lines time- and dose-dependently [7]. The formation of aberrant crypt foci (ACF) is considered an intermediate marker for development of CRC, and has been extensively used as a surrogate end point in assessing the chemopreventive effects of drugs in CRC. In a rat model of CRC, 5-ASAs reduced the number of ACFs and tumor number and load, with a concomitant increase in apoptosis and decrease in proliferation [8].

There is also evidence that 5-ASAs may have chemopreventive effects through various non-COX-related mechanisms. 5-ASAs could modulate apoptosis by blocking the transcription factor, nuclear factor kappa B (NFκB) by upregulating or stabilizing its natural inhibitor IκB [9]. NFκB activation is markedly reduced in colonic mucosa after treatment with 5-ASAs. Reactive oxygen species (ROS) are commonly generated during both acute and chronic inflammation and can induce oxidative DNA damage. 5-ASAs are ROS scavengers and can inhibit formation of ROS from leucocytes dose-dependently, thereby inhibiting oxidative DNA damage [10]. Both sporadic and IBD-associated CRC are associated with microsatellite instability, which leads to the accumulation of frameshift mutations. Gasche et al. have shown that 5-ASAs improve replication fidelity in cultured CRC cell lines by reducing frameshift mutations at microsatellites [11]. Although the molecular mechanism by which 5-ASAs inhibit the generation of frameshift mutations is unclear, there is evidence that these drugs slow down DNA replication and cell division allowing cellular mechanisms time to either repair DNA or induce apoptosis. There is also emerging evidence that 5-ASAs activate PPAR-γ, which in turn suppresses tumor formation by interfering with Wnt/β-catenin signaling [12]. PPAR-γ activation has been shown to reduce proliferation and increase apoptosis and suppression of ACF formation.

What is the clinical and observational evidence?

How well does clinical and observational evidence support the use of 5-ASAs for chemoprevention? While this might seem to be a question suitable for a randomized controlled trial, the obstacles to undertaking such a trial are all too obvious. The end point, whether cancer or dysplasia, is rare (so that huge numbers of patients would need to be recruited), the intervention (treatment with 5-ASAs) would

be needed for many years, and perhaps most importantly there would be ethical problems associated with withholding a standard treatment.

Thus, we are reliant on evidence from (nonrandomized) observational studies with their problems of bias and confounding. There have now been over 20 such studies published. These have predominantly been case-control studies in which the cases have either had cancer or developed dysplasia. The controls have often been other current clinic attenders, a potential source of selection bias to the extent that in one study regular clinic attendance was more strongly associated with protection from CRC than was 5-ASA use. Some studies have been nested in administrative databases that have lacked important clinical data, such as extent and duration of UC, and medication use for more than a few years preceding the case's cancer diagnosis. Most studies have involved fewer than 50 cancer cases and have lacked statistical power. 5-ASA exposure has been measured in a variety of ways (ever use versus never use, duration of use, cumulative dose, dose levels, and dose increments) reflecting the data sources used and the difficulty of capturing years of exposure.

A frequently cited systematic review and meta-analysis of the first 9 observational studies, published in 2005, concluded that there was a protective association between 5-ASA use and cancer or cancer and dysplasia with identical odds ratios (OR) (OR 0.51, 95% CI 0.37–0.69) [13]. Meta-analyses of observational studies do not have the strength of randomized trial meta-analyses in which randomization and blinding offer some protection from bias and confounding. As is often true of observational research, studies with more robust methods have tended to be reported later and generally the more recent studies have shown a lesser protective association than seen earlier. An exception to this is the case-control study performed at the Mayo Clinic by Velayos et al. [14]. Not only is this by far the largest case-control study, the methods used were exemplary. In particular, the authors were able to match cases and controls for date of first attendance at Mayo as well as for duration and extent of UC; they used data routinely collected at clinic visits to assess medication use, including that of nonprescribed drugs such as aspirin. Table 15.1 shows the key findings with regard to medication use from this study.

What is notable is that there was no evidence of a dose-response, i.e., a reduction in CRC risk increased with greater duration of 5-ASA use: if present, this would have

TABLE 15.1 Medication use and risk of colorectal cancer (CRC) in ulcerative colitis (UC) from Mayo Clinic case-control study [14]

	CRC cases (n = 188)[a]	Controls (n = 188)	OR[b]	95% CI
Use of 5-ASA for:				
< 1 year	44%	32%	1.0	Reference
1–5 years	20%	25%	0.4	0.2–0.9
6–10 years	18%	21%	0.6	0.3–1.4
>10 years	18%	22%	0.6	0.3–1.3
Corticosteroids for >1 year	21%	26%	0.4	0.2–0.8
Thiopurine use for >1 year	6%	4%	3.0	0.7–14
OTC Aspirin	5%	17%	0.3	0.1–0.8
NSAIDs	3%	11%	0.1	0.03–0.5

[a]All cases had CRC with UC diagnosed more than 2 years earlier.
[b]Multivariate estimates adjusting for family history (FH) of CRC, smoking, primary sclerosing cholangitis, surveillance colonoscopies performed, and presence of pseudopolyps.

strengthened the evidence for a causal relationship. It was also not clear whether the timing of 5-ASA use was critical or whether protection was still evident if 5-ASAs had been used for several years before being discontinued.

Might other drugs be chemopreventive?

If the chemopreventive mechanism of 5-ASAs is the anti-inflammatory activity, then can we expect thiopurines to also be associated with a reduced risk of colon cancer? This has been difficult to assess in studies so far, as until the late 1990s thiopurines were much less frequently used in UC than they are now, and were often only used when colectomy was the alternative. In most of the case-control studies, the numbers taking a thiopurine were small and the OR suggested an increased cancer risk that was not statistically significant. However, a recent French cohort study of almost 20,000 IBD patients found that thiopurine use compared with never use was associated with a 70% reduction in the risk of colonic cancer or high-grade dysplasia [15]. As shown in Table 15.1, in the Mayo study greater than 1 year of corticosteroid use was also associated with a reduced cancer risk, a finding in keeping with an anti-inflammatory mechanism [14].

The evidence that ursodeoxycholic acid (UDCA) has a chemopreventive effect is arguably the most convincing. Secondary bile acids are thought to play a role in CRC development. UDCA reduces colonic concentrations of secondary bile acids and in experimental models reduces

colon carcinogenesis. Four studies have examined the risk of developing CRC or dysplasia in patients with primary sclerosing cholangitis and UC and all have found risk to be lower in those taking UDCA [16]. However, there are no data on use of UDCA in UC in the absence of liver disease and in a trial of UDCA to reduce recurrence of sporadic colorectal adenomas the reduction in recurrence was modest (12%) and not statistically significant [17].

It was notable that in the Mayo study use of aspirin and NSAIDs were also associated with a reduced cancer risk (Table 15.1) [14]. Both aspirin and celecoxib have been clearly shown to be chemopreventive in sporadic CRC, but concerns about side effects have restricted their use to groups with an increased CRC risk because of familial adenomatous polyposis or hereditary nonpolyposis CRC. No other study has directly enquired about aspirin or NSAID use and more data is needed.

Conclusion

Regular 5-ASA use is associated with an approximate halving of the CRC risk in UC patients. As yet the evidence is not sufficient to be confident that this reflects a causal relationship. Similar reductions in risk have been seen with corticosteroids and thiopurines suggesting an anti-inflammatory mechanism. More data is needed on the effects of aspirin and celecoxib that have already been shown to be chemopreventive in other conditions where there is an increased risk of CRC.

References

1. Eaden JA, Abrams KR, Mayberry JF. The risk of colorectal cancer in ulcerative colitis: a meta-analysis. *Gut* 2001; **48**(4): 526–535.

2. Söderlund S, Brandt L, Lapidus A, et al. Decreasing time-trends of colorectal cancer in a large cohort of patients with inflammatory bowel disease. *Gastroenterology* 2009; **136**(5): 1561–1567.

3. Winther KV, Jess T, Langholz E, Munkholm P, Binder V. Long-term risk of cancer in ulcerative colitis: a population-based cohort study from Copenhagen County. *Clin Gastroenterol Hepatol* 2004; **2**(12): 1088–1095.

4. Pinczowski D, Ekbom A, Baron J, Yuen J, Adami HO. Risk factors for colorectal cancer in patients with ulcerative colitis: a case-control study. *Gastroenterology* 1994; **107**(1): 117–120.

5. Itzkowitz S, Hossain S, Matula S, et al. Histologic inflammation is a risk factor for progression to colorectal neoplasia in ulcerative colitis: a cohort study. *Gastroenterology* 2007; **133**(4): 1099–1105.

6. Reinacher-Schick A, Seidensticker F, Petrasch S, et al. Mesalazine changes apoptosis and proliferation in normal mucosa of patients with sporadic polyps of the large bowel. *Endoscopy* 2000; **32**(3): 245–254.

7. Fina D, Franchi L, Caruso R, et al. 5-aminosalicylic acid enhances anchorage-independent colorectal cancer cell death. *Eur J Cancer* 2006; **42**(15): 2609–2616.

8. Brown WA, Skinner SA, Malcontenti-Wilson C, et al. Non-steroidal anti-inflammatory drugs with different cyclooxygenase inhibitory profiles that prevent aberrant crypt foci formation but vary in acute gastrotoxicity in a rat model. *J Gastroenterol Hepatol* 2000; **15**(12): 1386–1392.

9. Kaiser GC, Yan F, Polk DB. Mesalamine blocks tumor necrosis factor growth inhibition and nuclear factor kappaB activation in mouse colonocytes. *Gastroenterology* 1999; **116**(3): 602–609.

10. Allgayer H, Kruis W. Aminosalicylates: potential antineoplastic actions in colon cancer prevention. *Scand J Gastroenterol* 2002; **37**(2): 125–131.

11. Gasche C, Goel A, Natarajan L, Boland CR. Mesalazine improves replication fidelity in cultured colorectal cells. *Cancer Res* 2005; **65**(10): 3993–3997.

12. Lu D, Cottam HB, Corr M, Carson DA. Repression of beta-catenin function in malignant cells by nonsteroidal antiinflammatory drugs. *Proc Natl Acad Sci USA* 2005; **102**(51): 18567–18571.

13. Velayos FS, Terdiman JP, Walsh JM. Effect of 5-aminosalicylate use on colorectal cancer and dysplasia risk: a systematic review and metaanalysis of observational studies. *Am J Gastroenterol* 2005; **100**(6): 1345–1353.

14. Velayos FS, Loftus EV, Jr, Jess T, et al. Predictive and protective factors associated with colorectal cancer in ulcerative colitis: A case-control study. *Gastroenterology* 2006; **130**(7): 1941–1949.

15. Beaugerie L, Seksik P, Bouvier AM, et al. Thiopurine therapy is associated with a three-fold decrease in the incidence of advanced colorectal neoplasia in IBD patients with long-standing extensive colitis: Results from the CESAME Cohort. *Gastroenterology* 2009; **136**(5): A54.

16. Farraye FA, Odze RD, Eaden J, Itzkowitz SH. AGA technical review on the diagnosis and management of colorectal neoplasia in inflammatory bowel disease. *Gastroenterology* 2010; **138**(2): 746–774.

17. Alberts DS, Martínez ME, Hess LM, et al. Phoenix and Tucson Gastroenterologist Networks Phase III trial of ursodeoxycholic acid to prevent colorectal adenoma recurrence. *J Natl Cancer Inst* 2005; **97** : 846–853.

16 Why do we still use 5-ASAs in Crohn's disease?

Stephen B. Hanauer[1], Henit Yanai[1], and Emma Calabrese[2]

[1]Section of Gastroenterology, Hepatology, and Nutrition, University of Chicago Medical Center, Chicago, IL, USA
[2]University of Rome "Tor Vergata," Rome, Italy

LEARNING POINTS

- Sulfasalazine induces remission in mild-to-moderate colonic Crohn's disease (CD) but not isolated small bowel disease.

- Intolerance to sulfasalazine limits its effectiveness.

- Sulfasalazine has not been shown to be effective for maintenance in CD.

- Although mesalamine appears to induce clinical remission in up to 45% of patients with mild-to-moderate CD, recent placebo-controlled trials have not demonstrated statistically significant benefits.

- Most clinical trials evaluating 5-ASAs for maintenance of CD after a medically induced remission have not been properly designed to assess their efficacy in this role

---

Introduction

5-Aminosalicylates (5-ASAs) have been traditionally used to treat mild-to-moderate inflammatory bowel disease (IBD) and in many practices are considered the first line of therapy due to their high tolerability and safety profile. There is sufficient evidence in the literature to support their role in inducing and maintaining remission in ulcerative colitis (UC) [1]. Nevertheless, a number of controversies with regard to the role of 5-ASAs in Crohn's disease (CD) have been generated. In general, in CD, therapeutic recommendations depend on its location (ileal, ileocolonic, colonic, and other), severity, and complications. Therapeutic approaches are individualized according to the symptomatic response and tolerance to the medical intervention.

The first 5-ASA agent used in clinical practice was sulfasalazine, which is composed of sulfapyridine linked by an azo bond to 5-ASA (mesalamine). Sulfasalazine has been associated with a high incidence of side effects and hence is often not well tolerated. Over recent decades, newer oral and topical (rectal) preparations of 5-ASAs lacking the sulfapyridine moiety, which causes most of the adverse effects of sulfasalazine, have been developed.

Role in inducing remission

Although 5-ASA is commonly used in clinical practice for ileal and ileocolonic disease, the most recent American College of Gastroenterology and European Crohn's and Colitis Organization guidelines suggest that this approach is marginally effective as compared with placebo and less effective than corticosteroids for inducing remission [2,3]. Two large placebo-controlled, randomized studies from the 1970s and 1980s have demonstrated minimal benefit of sulfasalazine versus placebo. In these trials, sulfasalazine (3–6 g daily) was compared with placebo and conventional corticosteroids [4,5]. In the national cooperative study, Summers et al. [5] reported that sulfasalazine was superior to placebo but not to prednisone in inducing clinical remission. This advantage was demonstrable only in patients who had disease involving the colon. In a similar European study, Malchow et al. [4] confirmed the superiority of prednisone in inducing remission but identified some benefit with the combination of prednisone and sulfasalazine in a selected group of patients who had only colonic disease and

---

Clinical Dilemmas in Inflammatory Bowel Disease: New Challenges, Second Edition. Edited by P. Irving, C. Siegel, D. Rampton and F. Shanahan.
© 2011 Blackwell Publishing Ltd. Published 2011 by Blackwell Publishing Ltd.

were primarily steroid-naïve. Subsequently, when it became clear that 5-ASA is the active component of sulfasalazine (in UC), newer formulations of 5-ASA devoid of the sulfa moiety were developed [6]. The newer formulations facilitated targeted delivery to the small intestine and/or colon and administration of higher doses of 5-ASA with improved tolerability; this has led to the virtual abandonment of sulfasalazine. However, sulfasalazine has been accepted as an efficacious therapy in rheumatoid arthritis and may still have a role for inducing remission in selected patients with mild colonic CD and, in particular, for patients with associated arthropathy.

In the early 1990s, randomized controlled trials (RCTs) in CD demonstrated efficacy for 5-ASAs in mild ileal, ileocolonic, and colonic diseases [7,8]. Notwithstanding these results, in 2004, a meta-analysis [9] of three RCTs concluded that the Pentasa® formulation, at a dose of 4 g daily, had merely marginal superiority over placebo, defined by a decrease in the Crohn's Disease Activity Index (CDAI) of only 18 points. This small decrement would be of no clinical significance in a primary analysis. Although there is no head-to-head clinical comparison between the newer 5-ASA formulations, experts' opinion and many years of practice support the notion that all newer 5-ASA formulations have more or less the same efficacy and safety profile if delivered to the sites of active disease in equivalent therapeutic doses. Lastly, clinical trials have not been of sufficient size to compare sulfasalazine to 5-ASAs adequately [10]. Despite the fact that placebo-controlled trials have not demonstrated statistically significant benefits, mesalamine has been observed to induce clinical remission in up to 35–45% of patients with mild-to-moderate CD.

Role in maintaining remission

Despite the common use of 5-ASA for maintenance of remission in CD, there is no consistent evidence from well-designed clinical trials to support its use when induction was achieved with medical therapy. Both the national and European cooperative studies failed to demonstrate any benefit for sulfasalazine in maintaining remission in CD [4,5]. Maintenance therapy with sulfasalazine following sulfasalazine induction has never been evaluated in controlled trials. Furthermore, there is an absence of controlled clinical trials following induction therapy with 5-ASAs; there has never been a trial similar to trials with anti-TNF agents where patients who *responded* to mesalamine were ran-

domized to continuation of maintenance therapy compared with a placebo. In contrast, maintenance trials with 5-ASAs for CD have shown conflicting results but were mostly compromised by heterogeneity in the definitions of remission, variability of disease location and severity, variations in inductive therapy, and the different dosing and formulations used. In particular, 5-ASA has not been efficacious at maintaining remissions after induction with conventional corticosteroids [11].

Five meta-analyses have been performed to clarify the usefulness of 5-ASA formulations for the maintenance of CD. Salomon et al. [12] in 1992 evaluated five trials for medical maintenance of remission and concluded that 5-ASAs were ineffective. In contrast, Steinhart et al. [13] in 1994 analyzed 10 trials and concluded that 5-ASAs, but not sulfasalazine, were effective as a maintenance therapy. It should be noted that this meta-analysis analyzed patients with medically and surgically induced remission as a pooled group. A third meta-analysis by Messori et al. [14] in the same year evaluated five clinical trials and also concluded that 5-ASA significantly reduced the relapse frequency at 6, 12, and 24 months. A fourth meta-analysis by Cammà et al. [15] in 1997 found that 5-ASA significantly lowers the relative risk of relapse in patients with surgically induced remission (−13.1%; 95% confidence interval (CI), −21.8–4.5%), but does not lower the relative risk of relapse in patients with medically induced remission (−4.7%; 95% CI, −9.6–2.8%). Finally, the most recent Cochrane meta-analysis by Akobeng and Gardener [16] in 2005, based on six eligible trials, found no evidence indicating that 5-ASA preparations are superior to placebo for maintaining medically induced remission in CD patients at 12 or 24 months. At 12 months, the odds ratio was 1.00 and at 24 months, the odds ratio was 0.98. The current available literature does not provide sufficient evidence to support the use of 5-ASA or sulfasalazine as maintenance therapy in CD.

Role in maintaining remission in postoperative patients

Postoperative maintenance studies have shown conflicting results. There appears to be a modest maintenance benefit for patients with ileal disease treated with more than 3 g/day of 5-ASA [11,15,17]; however, these results are less impressive than the alternatives: thiopurines alone or in combination with antibiotics or infliximab [2].

Role in chemoprevention for colorectal cancer (CRC) prevention

Multiple studies have assessed the utility of 5-ASA in preventing dysplasia and cancer in patients with UC, whereas fewer studies have assessed this endpoint in patients with CD. It is believed that 5-ASAs may have unique chemopreventive properties. Nevertheless, it is still unclear if it is their exclusive property or an effect mediated through improved control of inflammation (see Chapter 15). Information is lacking regarding chemopreventive effects of other therapies compared with that of 5-ASAs [18]. On the basis of this information, it is reasonable to continue prescribing low-dose 5-ASA (1.2 g/day) for patients with colonic CD.

Conclusions

5-ASAs have been used in CD worldwide for several decades. The data for sulfasalazine as an inductive agent in CD is based on evidence from several large trials completed over 30 years ago. If tolerated, sulfasalazine may be used as an inductive agent in mild-to-moderate colonic CD. There have not been adequate studies to demonstrate whether sulfasalazine responders will benefit from continued sulfasalazine maintenance therapy, but sulfasalazine has not maintained steroid-induced remissions. Similarly, while the initial clinical trial data were highly supportive of mesalamine induction therapy for mild—to-moderate CD, the evolution of data has been substantially more controversial. Despite consistent induction benefits compared with placebo, antibiotics, and budesonide, more recent clinical trials have not confirmed benefits compared with placebo therapy.

There is evidence to support a modest effect for 5-ASA in preventing postsurgical recurrence in patients who have had resections for ileal disease; however, information from recent clinical trials support other more efficacious alternatives. The low-cost and high-safety profiles of 5-ASAs are promoting their widespread use in clinical practice. Whether or not 5-ASA provides any chemoprophylactic benefits in CD remains to be demonstrated.

References

1. Sutherland L, MacDonald JK. Oral 5-aminosalicylic acid for induction of remission in ulcerative colitis. *Cochrane Database Syst Rev* 2003; (3): CD000543.

2. Lichtenstein GR, Hanauer SB, Sandborn WJ. Management of Crohn's disease in adults. *Am J Gastroenterol* 2009; **104**(2): 465–483; quiz 464, 484.

3. Travis SP, Stange EF, Lémann M, et al. European evidence based consensus on the diagnosis and management of Crohn's disease: current management. *Gut* 2006; **55**(Suppl 1): i16–i35.

4. Malchow H, Ewe K, Brandes JW, et al. European Cooperative Crohn's Disease Study (ECCDS): results of drug treatment. *Gastroenterology* 1984; **86**(2): 249–266.

5. Summers RW, Switz DM, Sessions JT Jr, et al. National Cooperative Crohn's Disease Study: results of drug treatment. *Gastroenterology* 1979; **77**(4 Pt 2): 847–869.

6. Azad Khan AK, Piris J, Truelove SC. An experiment to determine the active therapeutic moiety of sulphasalazine. *Lancet* 1977; **2**(8044): 892–895.

7. Singleton JW, Hanauer SB, Gitnick GL, et al. Mesalamine capsules for the treatment of active Crohn's disease: results of a 16-week trial. Pentasa Crohn's Disease Study Group. *Gastroenterology* 1993; **104**(5): 1293–1301.

8. Tremaine WJ, Schroeder KW, Harrison JM, et al. A randomized, double-blind, placebo-controlled trial of the oral mesalamine (5-ASA) preparation, Asacol, in the treatment of symptomatic Crohn's colitis and ileocolitis. *J Clin Gastroenterol* 1994; **19**(4): 278–282.

9. Hanauer SB, Stromberg U. Oral Pentasa in the treatment of active Crohn's disease: A meta-analysis of double-blind, placebo-controlled trials. *Clin Gastroenterol Hepatol* 2004; **2**(5): 379–388.

10. Feagan BG. Aminosalicylates for active disease and in the maintenance of remission in Crohn's disease. *Eur J Surg* 1998; **164**(12): 903–909.

11. Modigliani R, Colombel JF, Dupas JL, et al. Mesalamine in Crohn's disease with steroid-induced remission: effect on steroid withdrawal and remission maintenance, Groupe d'Etudes Therapeutiques des Affections Inflammatoires Digestives. *Gastroenterology* 1996; **110**(3): 688–693.

12. Salomon P, Kornbluth A, Aisenberg J, et al. How effective are current drugs for Crohn's disease? A meta-analysis. *J Clin Gastroenterol* 1992; **14**(3): 211–215.

13. Steinhart AH, Hemphill D, Greenberg GR. Sulfasalazine and mesalazine for the maintenance therapy of Crohn's disease: a meta-analysis. *Am J Gastroenterol* 1994; **89**(12): 2116–2124.

14. Messori A, Brignola C, Trallori G, et al. Effectiveness of 5-aminosalicylic acid for maintaining remission in patients with Crohn's disease: a meta-analysis. *Am J Gastroenterol* 1994; **89**(5): 692–698.

15. Camma C, Giunta M, Rosselli M, et al. Mesalamine in the maintenance treatment of Crohn's disease: a meta-analysis adjusted for confounding variables. *Gastroenterology* 1997; **113**(5): 1465–1473.

16. Akobeng AK, Gardener E. Oral 5-aminosalicylic acid for maintenance of medically-induced remission in Crohn's Disease. *Cochrane Database Syst Rev* 2005; (1): CD003715.

17. Lochs H, Mayer M, Fleig WE, et al. Prophylaxis of post-operative relapse in Crohn's disease with mesalamine: European Cooperative Crohn's Disease Study VI. *Gastroenterology* 2000; **118**(2): 264–273.

18. Rubin DT, Cruz-Correa MR, Gasche C, et al. Colorectal cancer prevention in inflammatory bowel disease and the role of 5-aminosalicylic acid: a clinical review and update. *Inflamm Bowel Dis* 2008; **14**(2): 265–274.

Steroids

17 Steroids in Crohn's disease: do the benefits outweigh the dangers?

A. Hillary Steinhart[1,2]

[1]Inflammatory Bowel Disease Centre, Mount Sinai Hospital, University of Toronto, Toronto, ON, Canada
[2]University of Toronto, Toronto, ON, Canada

LEARNING POINTS

- Steroids are highly effective and rapidly improve the symptoms of active Crohn's disease (CD).
- Steroids do not maintain remission when used chronically in CD.
- Steroid dependency occurs in approximately one-third of patients.
- Steroid intolerance and adverse effects are common and may be serious.
- Steroids should be used only for a defined duration and with clear goals.
- The potential role of short courses of steroids as part of a multidrug regimen is still evolving.

Introduction

The glucocorticosteroids (steroids), such as prednisone, prednisolone, methylprednisolone and others, are a class of therapy that is known for its potent anti-inflammatory effect. As a result, steroids are effective treatment for a wide variety of inflammatory disorders irrespective of the underlying pathogenesis. For more than 5 decades, steroids have been the mainstay of medical therapy for the management of active Crohn's disease (CD). In addressing the question of whether the benefits of steroids are worth their risk, it is necessary to define both the benefit and the risk.

Benefits of steroids

The benefits of steroids relate to their significant efficacy and rapidity of action in most forms of CD. In patients with CD who have symptoms that are secondary to intestinal inflammation, treatment with steroids improves symptoms to the point where patients are considered to be in "clinical remission" in 60–93% of patients depending upon the dose, duration of therapy, and definition of remission [1–3]. Responses are observed in patients irrespective of disease location, and in many instances, troublesome extraintestinal manifestations such as arthritis or erythema nodosum will also improve. The rapidity with which they improve symptoms has been another important reason for the widespread use of steroids in the treatment of acute flares of disease activity.

Limitations of therapeutic effects of steroids

Unfortunately, the acute benefits of steroids are not sustained over prolonged periods, and they should, therefore, not be used for maintenance of remission [1–4]. There has also been concern that steroids may alter the natural history of CD and increase the incidence of certain disease-associated complications. As a result, it has been suggested that their use may result in a greater need for surgical management of CD and its complications. Population-based studies from Copenhagen county in Denmark and Olmstead county in Minnesota, USA have both found that approximately 30–35% of patients end up requiring surgery within 1 year of initiation of steroid therapy [5,6]. It is not clear whether the use of steroids is simply a reflection of the treating physician's overall impression of the severity of the CD or whether steroid therapy fundamentally changes

---

Clinical Dilemmas in Inflammatory Bowel Disease: New Challenges, Second Edition. Edited by P. Irving, C. Siegel, D. Rampton and F. Shanahan.
© 2011 Blackwell Publishing Ltd. Published 2011 by Blackwell Publishing Ltd.

the underlying disease process in such a way as to predispose to complications that require surgical management.

One reason for the apparent contrast between the good short-term results seen with steroid therapy and the high rate of disease complications requiring surgery within 1 year of treatment may be the low rate of mucosal healing observed in patients treated with steroids. Despite obtaining clinical remission in 92% of patients, Modigliani and colleagues observed endoscopic healing in only 29% of patients after 7 weeks of prednisolone therapy, 1 mg/kg/day [2]. This suggests that although steroid therapy may reduce inflammation sufficiently to improve symptoms acutely, it does not result in mucosal healing and that this lack of healing, in turn, leads to ongoing intestinal damage and complications.

Adverse effects of steroids

In addition to concerns about long-term efficacy, there have been concerns among physicians and patients about the numerous and well-described side effects and potential complications of steroids. When steroids are used for acute therapy, most patients experience at least one side effect and many experience multiple [7]. Although most side effects resolve with tapering and discontinuation of therapy, they can be extremely troubling to patients and may preclude further use of steroids. For patients who do not experience short-term side effects or who are able to tolerate them, the ongoing or repeated use of steroids can lead to numerous long-term complications such as osteoporosis, cataract formation, impaired wound healing, hypertension, diabetes, buffalo hump, growth delay in children, and adrenal suppression. These short- and long-term side effects and complications need to be considered within the context of the effectiveness of steroids, particularly with the advent of the biologic therapies.

The topically active steroid, budesonide, when given orally as a controlled release formulation, has been shown to be an effective and well-tolerated means of treating symptoms of mild to moderately active ileal and ileocecal CD [8]. However, maintenance therapy with budesonide, although well tolerated, does not appear to improve remission rates over a 1-year period [9].

Studies from Copenhagen county and Olmstead county have shown that roughly one-third of patients treated with steroids for an acute flare of CD will become steroid-dependent over the following year [5,6]. Steroid dependence is a problem on several levels. Firstly, the risk of experiencing adverse effects of therapy increases with higher doses and longer duration of therapy. Secondly, the fact that a patient is dependent on steroids does not necessarily mean that the patient has achieved adequate control of symptoms or mucosal healing. Steroid dependence may simply reflect a steroid dose level below which the symptoms become unmanageable or intolerable. Thirdly, the ongoing use of steroids, even at low dose, may lead to increased risk of complications. In the TREAT registry of over 6000 CD patients, the three factors that were associated with increased risk of serious infection were the severity of the Crohn's disease, the use of narcotics, and the use of steroids. Steroids were the only factor associated with an increased risk of death [10].

Co-administration of immunomodulators with steroids

As a result of the lack of long-term efficacy, the frequent occurrence of steroid dependence, the lack of mucosal healing, and the potential for short- and long-term adverse events associated with steroid therapy, there has been increasing use of antimetabolite immunomodulator therapies whenever steroid therapy is required for management of an acute flare. The use of either of the purine analogs, azathioprine or 6-mercaptopurine, or methotrexate results in improved long-term clinical remission rates and reduced steroid requirements [11,12]. However, the immunomodulator-based, steroid-sparing strategies have not yet been consistently shown to reduce the requirement for surgery. These drugs also have a slow onset of clinical action and, as a result, are not well suited for treatment of acutely ill patients.

Role of anti-TNF therapies

Anti-TNF-based therapies rapidly induce clinical remission and mucosal healing resulting in a reduction in hospitalizations and surgeries for Crohn's disease. Their introduction has clearly changed the way we must think about using steroids. Anti-TNF therapies share with steroids the advantage of being rapidly effective for multiple disease locations and manifestations, but they also have the advantage over steroids of being effective for maintenance therapy with a favorable side effect profile.

The place of steroids in treatment of Crohn's disease

The advent of anti-TNF therapies suggests that steroids may become a historical footnote in the management of Crohn's disease. However, there are still situations where steroids may be the preferred treatment or part of a multidrug regimen. For patients with mild-to-moderately active ileal or ileocecal disease, the use of budesonide is an effective and safe strategy, although the optimal maintenance strategy remains unclear. For patients with moderate-to-severely active CD or CD in other locations, budesonide is not appropriate and the use of systemic steroids or anti-TNF therapy needs to be considered. The anti-TNF therapies are expensive and require the use of injection or infusion for administration. Steroids, although available for intravenous therapy, are also available in inexpensive, orally administered forms that are well absorbed with once daily dosing. Route of administration may be important for some patients, but the cost of anti-TNF therapy may be a more important mitigating factor in treatment decisions. In those instances, the use of a short course of steroids for a predetermined period of time with the introduction of a steroid-sparing strategy may be indicated. However, there needs to be a readiness to move to alternative therapy if steroids, in combination with an immunomodulator, do not achieve the predetermined treatment goals, or if therapy is associated with significant or intolerable side effects.

There is also indirect evidence that steroids may be a part of an effective multidrug treatment regimen that includes an anti-TNF agent. In the COMMIT study, which was designed to determine whether the use of methotrexate increased the rate of steroid-free remission in patients being treated with the anti-TNF agent, infliximab, all patients received steroids for a period of 1 to 6 weeks prior to initiation of infliximab [13]. With this strategy, approximately 80% of patients achieved steroid-free remission, a rate which is higher than that reported in any previous anti-TNF trial. This suggests that the use of a short course of steroids prior to the introduction of anti-TNF therapy may enhance the latter's clinical effectiveness. No endoscopic outcomes were available from that trial and surgical rates have not been reported, but the very high rates of steroid-free remission over a 1-year period warrant further examination of steroids as part of a multidrug or sequential therapeutic regimen.

In conclusion, earlier use of immunomodulator drugs for long-term therapy and the option of biologic agents, such as the anti-TNF-α agents, are changing the way in which steroids are used in patients with CD. However, it must be conceded that the case against steroids is not closed, and that in many countries early use of biologic agents is neither a realistic nor desirable option. In some instances, adverse reactions or loss of efficacy eliminates the option of anti-TNF therapy. For these situations, experienced clinicians can achieve much by attention to detail, continued use of traditional immunosuppressants, and judicious and sparing use of steroids.

References

1. Summers RW, Switz DM, Sessions JT, Jr., et al. National Cooperative Crohn's Disease Study: results of drug treatment. *Gastroenterology* 1979; **77**: 847–869.
2. Modigliani R, Mary JY, Simon JF, et al. Clinical, biological, and endoscopic picture of attacks of Crohn's disease. Evolution on prednisolone. Groupe d'Etude Therapeutique des Affections Inflammatoires Digestives. *Gastroenterology* 1990; **98**: 811–818.
3. Chun A, Chadi RM, Korelitz BI, et al. Intravenous corticotrophin vs. hydrocortisone in the treatment of hospitalized patients with Crohn's disease: a randomized double-blind study and follow-up. *Inflamm Bowel Dis* 1998; **4**(3): 177–181.
4. Steinhart AH, Ewe K, Griffiths AM, Modigliani R, Thomsen OO. Corticosteroids for maintenance of remission in Crohn's disease. *Cochrane Database Syst Rev* 2003; (4): CD000301.
5. Munkholm P, Langholz E, Davidsen M, Binder V. Frequency of glucocorticoid resistance and dependency in Crohn's disease. *Gut* 1994; **35**(3): 360–362.
6. Faubion WA, Jr., Loftus EV, Jr., Harmsen WS, Zinsmeister AR, Sandborn WJ. The natural history of corticosteroid therapy for inflammatory bowel disease: a population-based study. *Gastroenterology* 2001; **121**(2): 255–260.
7. Singleton JW, Law DH, Kelley ML, Jr., Mekhjian HS, Sturdevant RA. National Cooperative Crohn's Disease Study: adverse reactions to study drugs. *Gastroenterology* 1979; **77**: 870–882.
8. Greenberg GR, Feagan BG, Martin F, et al. Oral budesonide for active Crohn's disease. Canadian Inflammatory Bowel Disease Study Group. *N Engl J Med* 1994; **331**(13): 836–841.
9. Greenberg GR, Feagan BG, Martin F, et al. Oral budesonide as maintenance treatment for Crohn's disease: a

placebo-controlled, dose-ranging study. Canadian Inflammatory Bowel Disease Study Group. *Gastroenterology* 1996; **110**(1): 45–51.

10. Lichtenstein GR, Feagan BG, Cohen RD, et al. Serious infections and mortality in association with therapies for Crohn's disease: TREAT registry. *Clin Gastroenterol Hepatol* 2006; **4**(5): 621–630.

11. Markowitz J, Grancher K, Kohn N, Lesser M, Daum F. A multicenter trial of 6-mercaptopurine and prednisone in children with newly diagnosed Crohn's disease. *Gastroenterology* 2000; **119**(4): 895–902.

12. Feagan BG, Fedorak RN, Irvine EJ, et al. A comparison of methotrexate with placebo for the maintenance of remission in Crohn's disease. North American Crohn's Study Group Investigators. *N Engl J Med* 2000; **342**(22): 1627–1632.

13. Feagan BG, McDonald JWD, Panaccione R, et al. A randomized trial of methotrexate in combination with infliximab for the treatment of Crohn's disease. *Gut* 2008; **57**(Suppl II): A66.

Immunomodulators

18 Thioguanine nucleotide measurement: nonadherent, underdosed, shunter, or refractory?

Miles P. Sparrow

Department of Gastroenterology, The Alfred Hospital, Melbourne, VIC, Australia

LEARNING POINTS

- Correctly optimized thiopurine immunomodulators achieve most treatment goals in IBD.

- Measurement of the thiopurine metabolites 6-thioguanine nucleotides (6-TGN) and 6-methylmercaptopurine (6-MMP) helps clarify reasons for nonresponse or adverse events to immunomodulators.

- 6-TGN levels > 235 pmol/8 × 10^8 RBC are associated with clinical response and the risk of myelotoxicity.

- 6-MMP levels > 5700 pmol/8 × 10^8 RBC are associated with toxicity, especially hepatotoxicity.

- Metabolite measurements group nonresponders into four broad groups—nonadherence, underdosing, "thiopurine resistance" (shunters to 6-MMP), and "thiopurine refractoriness." This facilitates dosage optimization or discontinuation of therapy.

- In shunters, low-dose allopurinol in combination with a reduced thiopurine dose optimizes thiopurine metabolism and clinical efficacy.

- Metabolite measurements do not replace the need for regular laboratory monitoring of blood counts and liver function tests.

Introduction

The aims of treatment in inflammatory bowel disease (IBD) are evolving, with the minimum acceptable therapeutic goal being the induction and maintenance of corticosteroid-free remission. Preferably, IBD therapies should lead to a reduction in hospitalizations and surgeries, and ideally to mucosal healing, which, it is hoped, will change the natural history of disease. When correctly used, the thiopurine immunomodulators azathioprine (AZA) and 6-mercaptopurine (6-MP) will achieve these goals in the majority of patients. However, with traditional weight-based dosing of thiopurines, nonresponse rates of up to 40–50% can occur. Accordingly, recent advances in pharmacogenomics and the use of metabolite monitoring have allowed for further optimization and "personalization" of thiopurine dosing, although whether these developments definitely equate to improved clinical outcomes remains to be determined.

Thiopurine metabolism and the role of metabolite monitoring

AZA and 6-MP are inactive prodrugs that require enzymatic conversion to produce active metabolites (Figure 18.1). AZA is nonenzymatically converted to 6-MP, after which three competing enzymatic pathways, including thiopurine methyltransferase (TPMT), metabolize 6-MP to produce the active nucleotide metabolites 6-thioguanine nucleotides (6-TGN) and 6-methylmercaptopurine (6-MMP). TPMT activity has a trimodal distribution with 89% of the population possessing normal or high activity (homozygous high), 11% having intermediate activity (heterozygotes), and 0.3% having negligible enzyme activity and being susceptible to severe myelotoxicity at usual drug dosages [1]. A 6-TGN level of greater than 235 pmol/8 × 10^8 RBC has been

Clinical Dilemmas in Inflammatory Bowel Disease: New Challenges, Second Edition. Edited by P. Irving, C. Siegel, D. Rampton and F. Shanahan.
© 2011 Blackwell Publishing Ltd. Published 2011 by Blackwell Publishing Ltd.

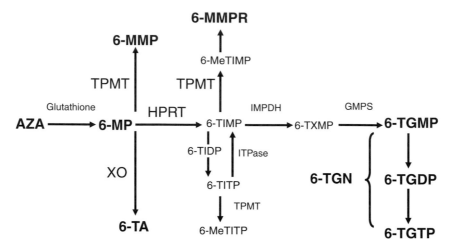

FIGURE 18.1 Thiopurine metabolism. AZA, azathioprine; 6-MP, 6-mercaptopurine; 6-MMP, 6-methylmercaptopurine; 6-MMPR, 6-methylmercaptopurine ribonucleotides; 6-TA, 6-thiouric acid; 6-TGN, 6-thioguanine nucleotides; 6-TGMP, 6-TGDP, 6-TGTP, 6-thioguanine mono-, di-, and triphosphates; 6-TIMP, 6-TIDP, 6-TITP, 6-thioinosine mono, di- and triphosphates; 6-MeTIMP, 6-methyl thioinosine monophosphate; 6-MeTITP, 6-methyl thioinosine triphosphate; 6-TXMP, 6-thioxanthine monophosphate; TPMT, thiopurine methyltransferase; XO, xanthine oxidase; HPRT, hypoxanthine phosphoribosyltransferase; IMPDH, inosine monophosphate dehydrogenase; GMPS, guanosine monophosphate synthetase; ITPase, inosine triphosphatase.

correlated with an increased likelihood of response, while 6-MMP levels greater than 5700 pmol/8×10^8 RBC have been associated with hepatotoxicity in the form of elevated transaminases [2]. Initial studies in metabolite monitoring were small, sometimes retrospective, and produced conflicting results, but more recently well-designed prospective studies and meta-analyses support the association between 6-TGN levels and clinical response [3,4].

Indications for the measurement of thiopurine metabolites

In patients in whom a steroid-free remission is achieved with weight-based dosing of thiopurines, metabolite measurements are unnecessary. However, metabolite measurements are indicated in patients not responding or experiencing adverse events to an adequate weight-based dose

of thiopurine therapy as they help clarify the reasons for nonresponse and guide subsequent dosage optimization. Although stable metabolite levels are measurable 4 weeks after the initiation of thiopurines, most patients should be given a full 3-month trial of therapy before nonresponse is declared and metabolites are indicated. Broadly, metabolite measurements group thiopurine nonresponders into four groups—nonadherence, underdosing, "thiopurine resistant," and "thiopurine refractory," as is outlined in Table 18.1. Of these groups, the two most common, easily surmountable reasons for nonresponse are nonadherence and underdosing.

Nonadherence

Nonadherence is likely when levels of both 6-TGN and 6-MMP are negligible or absent. Nonadherence, as detected solely by metabolite monitoring, has been detected in up to

TABLE 18.1 Metabolite profiles categorizing reasons for treatment failure with thiopurines

6-TGN	6-MMP	Interpretation	Recommendation
↓↓/Absent	↓↓/Absent	Nonadherence	Patient education
↓	↓	Underdosing	Increase thiopurine dose
Therapeutic	<5700	Thiopurine refractory	Change to alternate therapy
↓	↑	"Shunter"	Dose reduction and allopurinol

20% of patients in some studies. Without metabolite measurement, these patients may otherwise have been assumed to be true thiopurine nonresponders [5].

Underdosing

Underdosing of thiopurines is suggested when levels of 6-TGN are subtherapeutic (<235 pmol/8×10^8 RBC) and 6-MMP levels are detectable but less than 5700 pmol/8×10^8 RBC. Subtherapeutic levels can be seen in up to 40–50% of patients who again otherwise may have been incorrectly assumed to be thiopurine nonresponders [6]. Metabolite monitoring can then be used to optimize dose escalation, as shown in a study of 106 steroid-dependent patients (70 Crohn's disease (CD), 36 ulcerative colitis (UC)) in whom steroid-free remission was attained in 72% of patients at 6 months with dose escalation. Furthermore, 86% of patients achieving 6-TGN levels > 250 pmol/8×10^8 RBC achieved remission, compared to no patients with 6-TGN levels below this threshold ($p < 0.01$) [7].

Thiopurine refractory

Patients with therapeutic or high levels of both 6-TGN and 6-MMP and yet having active or steroid-dependent disease are truly "thiopurine refractory," and further thiopurine therapy only exposes the patient to the risk of adverse events—alternative therapeutic agents are needed. This was demonstrated in a study of 55 patients with refractory disease (43 CD, 12 UC) in whom dose escalation with metabolite monitoring was employed. In patients with an initial 6-TGN level of 100–200 pmol/8×10^8 RBC at the commencement of dose escalation, 77% of patients entered steroid-free remission, compared to patients with an initial "therapeutic" 6-TGN level > 400 pmol/8×10^8, in whom no patient entered remission with dose escalation ($p < 0.05$) [8].

Thiopurine resistant

The final group of nonresponders are identified by subtherapeutic levels of 6-TGN due to "shunting" of metabolism to produce high levels of 6-MMP—this pattern of metabolism is seen in up to 15% of patients and is due in part to high intrinsic TPMT activity. This subgroup of patients have previously been considered "thiopurine resistant," but recent studies from several centers have demonstrated that this metabolic pattern can be reversed by the addition of low doses of the xanthine oxidase inhibitor, allopurinol. In an initial study of 20 refractory patients (12 CD, 6 CD, and

2 indeterminate colitis) shunting toward 6-MMP production, 100 mg allopurinol was added and simultaneously the thiopurine dose was reduced to 25–50% of the original dose. This combination produced an increase in 6-TGN levels from 191 pmol/8×10^8 RBC to 400 pmol/8×10^8 RBC ($p < 0.001$) and a striking reduction in 6-MMP levels from 10,604 pmol/8×10^8 RBC to 2000 pmol/8×10^8 RBC ($p < 0.001$). This metabolic switch was accompanied by the clinical benefits expected with effective thiopurine therapy, as measured 3 months after the addition of allopurinol. Disease activity scores fell, with partial Harvey Bradshaw indices decreasing from 4.9 to 1.5 in CD patients ($p = 0.001$) and partial Mayo scores decreasing from 4.1 to 2.9 in UC patients ($p = 0.13$). Steroid-sparing was also achieved with mean prednisolone dosages reducing from 17.6 mg to 1.8 mg daily ($p < 0.001$), and a reversal of the transaminitis, otherwise associated with elevated 6-MMP levels, was seen. Although leukopenia occurred in 5 patients, it was reversible with further thiopurine dose reduction in all patients and without infectious sequelae [9]. Follow-up of this cohort for a mean of 36 months has demonstrated continuing clinical benefits and no evidence of the hepatic complications of nodular regenerative hyperplasia or veno-occlusive disease that have been associated with very high 6-TGN levels seen with 6-thioguanine therapy [10]. These findings have subsequently been replicated in additional single-center studies, but as yet, the mechanism of this favorable metabolic interaction remains unknown.

Clinicians contemplating the use of concomitant allopurinol to optimize thiopurine metabolism in "shunters" must consider the potential risks (leukopenia) and benefits (thiopurine efficacy, steroid-sparing, avoidance of risks and costs of alternative medications) in each individual patient. If this therapeutic maneuver is employed, a low dose of allopurinol (100 mg daily) is recommended in combination with *simultaneous* thiopurine dose reduction—a dose reduction *to* 25–50% of the original immunomodulator dose (i.e., *by* 50–75%) is required. White blood cell counts should be checked weekly for the first 4 weeks after allopurinol is added, then alternate weekly for the next 4 weeks, after which clinicians' routine monitoring intervals can be employed. Therefore, leukopenia can be promptly reversed by further immunomodulator dose reduction. Metabolite measurements should be repeated approximately 4 weeks after the addition of allopurinol to ensure therapeutic levels have been attained. The use of allopurinol to optimize thiopurine efficacy can only be recommended when measurement of metabolites is readily available.

Conclusions

In IBD, as in any lifelong medical disorder, before one therapy is discontinued due to presumed inefficacy, clarification of the reason for nonresponse is important. Metabolite measurements help clarify reasons for nonresponse to thiopurines and may allow for subsequent "therapeutic salvage" via dosage optimization. Just as importantly, metabolite measurements may identify patients who are simply not taking the prescribed drug, or patients who are truly thiopurine refractory and in whom alternative therapies are needed. As thiopurines do not work in every patient, dosage optimization will not always be successful, but, as a minimum, it is recommended that a set of metabolite measurements are drawn in each patient before they are declared a true thiopurine nonresponder.

References

1. Weinshilboum RM, Sladek SL. Mercaptopurine pharmacogenetics: monogenic inheritance of erythrocyte thiopurine methyltransferase activity. *Am J Hum Genet* 1980; **32**(5): 651–662.

2. Dubinsky MC, Lamothe S, Yang HY, et al. Pharmacogenomics and metabolite measurement for 6-mercaptopurine therapy in inflammatory bowel disease. *Gastroenterology* 2000; **118**(4): 705–713.

3. Ansari A, Arenas M, Greenfield SM, et al. Prospective evaluation of the pharmacogenetics of azathioprine in the treatment of inflammatory bowel disease. *Aliment Pharmacol Ther* 2008; **28**(8): 973–983.

4. Osterman MT, Kundu R, Lichtenstein GR, et al. Association of 6-thioguanine nucleotide levels and inflammatory bowel disease activity: a meta-analysis. *Gastroenterology* 2006; **130**(4): 1047–1053.

5. Gearry RB, Barclay ML, Roberts RL, et al. Thiopurine methyltransferase and 6-thioguanine nucleotide measurement: early experience of use in clinical practice. *Intern Med J* 2005; **35**(10): 580–585.

6. Bloomfeld RS, Onken JE. Mercaptopurine metabolite results in clinical gastroenterology practice. *Aliment Pharmacol Ther* 2003; **17**(1): 69–73.

7. Roblin X, Serre-Debeauvais F, Phelip JM, et al. 6-tioguanine monitoring in steroid-dependent patients with inflammatory bowel diseases receiving azathioprine. *Aliment Pharmacol Ther* 2005; **21**(7): 829–839.

8. Roblin X, Peyrin-Biroulet L, Phelip JM, et al. A 6-thioguanine nucleotide threshold level of 400 pmol/8 × 10(8) erythrocytes predicts azathioprine refractoriness in patients with inflammatory bowel disease and normal TPMT activity. *Am J Gastroenterol* 2008; **103**(12): 3115–3122.

9. Sparrow MP, Hande SA, Friedman S, et al. Effect of allopurinol on clinical outcomes in inflammatory bowel disease nonresponders to azathioprine or 6-mercaptopurine. *Clin Gastroenterol Hepatol* 2007; **5**(2): 209–214.

10. Leung Y, Sparrow MP, Schwartz M, Hanauer SB. Long term efficacy and safety of allopurinol and azathioprine or 6-mercaptopurine in patients with inflammatory bowel disease. *J Crohn's Colitis* 2009; **3**(3): 162–167.

19 Thiopurines and the sun: what should be done?

Conal M. Perrett[1], Jane M. McGregor[2,3], and Catherine A. Harwood[2]

[1] University College London Hospitals, London, UK
[2] Centre for Cutaneous Research, Blizard Institute of Cell and Molecular Science, Barts and The London School of Medicine and Dentistry, Queen Mary University of London, London, UK
[3] Barts and the London NHS Trust, London, UK

LEARNING POINTS

- Patients on immunosuppressive drugs, including thiopurines, are at increased risk of skin cancer. Risk factors include age, duration of immunosuppression, skin phototype, and ultraviolet radiation (UVR) exposure.

- Thiopurines are associated with increased skin sensitivity to ultraviolet A (UVA) that constitutes > 90% of incident terrestrial ultraviolet.

- Thiopurine metabolites accumulate in skin DNA and interact with UVA, causing DNA damage that may contribute to skin carcinogenesis.

- Patients receiving thiopurines should be counseled on the importance of photoprotection and self-examination to reduce their skin cancer risk.

- Early detection and prompt referral for treatment of premalignant skin lesions may reduce the incidence of invasive malignancy.

- For patients with extensive premalignancies and/or invasive skin tumors, dose reduction or replacement of thiopurines by alternative agents should be considered on a case-by-case basis.

Introduction

Since their development 50 years ago, the immunosuppressive thiopurines azathioprine (AZA) and 6-mercaptopurine (6-MP) have been used extensively to prevent graft rejection and to treat cancer, autoimmune, and inflammatory diseases. Thiopurines inhibit purine biosynthesis and cause the incorporation of 6-thioguanine (6-TG) nucleotides into DNA [1]. Chronic thiopurine exposure increases the risk of diverse malignancies including non-Hodgkin lymphoma, hepatobiliary carcinoma, and mesenchymal and epithelial cancers [2]. Organ transplant recipients, for whom AZA has long been a component of immunosuppressive regimens, have a 100-fold excess risk of nonmelanoma skin cancer (NMSC). Thiopurine monotherapy for chronic inflammatory disorders, such as inflammatory bowel disease (IBD), is also associated with an excess risk of skin cancer, albeit somewhat lower [3].

Risk factors for skin cancer in these populations include age, duration of immunosuppression, and exposure to ultraviolet radiation (UVR) in sunlight. Immunosuppressive therapy is thought to promote development of invasive malignancy from premalignant skin lesions by reducing tumor surveillance. However, thiopurines, in combination with solar ultraviolet A (UVA) radiation, may also contribute directly to the risk of skin cancer.

What is the evidence that the potential interactions of thiopurines with sunlight increase the risk of cancer? What are the implications for IBD patients receiving thiopurine therapy? Can this risk be managed?

Thiopurines and the sun: what is the risk?

Immunosuppressive therapy increases the risk of skin cancer in transplant patients [4]. In patients with IBD, the elevated skin cancer incidence appears, at least partly, to be due to thiopurines [5].

Clinical Dilemmas in Inflammatory Bowel Disease: New Challenges, Second Edition. Edited by P. Irving, C. Siegel, D. Rampton and F. Shanahan.
© 2011 Blackwell Publishing Ltd. Published 2011 by Blackwell Publishing Ltd.

Organ transplant recipients: a model for thiopurine-associated skin cancer

Skin cancer is the most common malignancy in transplant patients, with a prevalence approaching 70% at 20 years post-transplant [4]. More than 95% are NMSCs (squamous and basal cell carcinomas, SCC and BCC). Compared to age-matched and sex-matched immunocompetent individuals, immunosuppression increases the risk of SCC 65- to 250-fold and of BCC 10-fold. Immunosuppression-related SCCs are frequently multiple and more aggressive than in the general population, with metastatic rates of 5–7% [4,6]. Although rarely fatal, the need for surgical treatment and the consequent risk of facial scarring and disfigurement may cause significant morbidity [4]. The risk of other skin tumors, including melanoma, Kaposi sarcoma, appendageal tumors, and Merkel cell carcinoma, is also increased [4,7,8].

UVR is a causative factor for NMSC in both transplant patients and the general population. Most tumors are more prevalent in regions of high ambient solar radiation, have a predilection for sun-exposed sites such as the face and hands, and are more common in those with fair skin phototype (burns easily and tans with difficulty) and a history of chronic UV exposure and sunburn [6]. Other risk factors include older age at transplantation, duration of thiopurine exposure, and the presence of premalignant actinic keratoses [9].

IBD and skin cancer

Several series have reported the occurrence of skin cancers in IBD patients using thiopurines [10,11]. A prospective study of 1634 immunosuppressed nontransplant patients, 20% of whom had IBD—most (68%) receiving AZA—found an excess of SCC [12]. A population-based cohort study of 4776 IBD patients found a 5.5-fold increase in SCC in Crohn's disease (CD) [13]. An increased relative risk of 1.4 (CI 1.0–1.9) was reported in a Danish cohort of 5546 patients with ulcerative colitis (UC) [14] and an excess SCC standardized incidence ratio of 1.92 (CI 1.46–2.47) amongst 21,788 CD patients [15]. A recent retrospective analysis of 26,403 patients with CD and 26,974 with UC showed a 60% excess risk of NMSC [5]; use of any immunosuppressant was associated with an adjusted odds ratio (OR) of 3.28 (CI 2.62–4.10) and use of thiopurines with an OR of 3.56 (CI 2.81–4.50), rising to 4.27 (CI 3.08–5.92) for persistent (>365 days) use. In comparison, there were lower but still significantly elevated adjusted ORs of 2.07 (CI 1.28–3.33) for recent biologic use in patients with CD

and 2.18 (OR 1.07–4.46) for persistent biologic use. A further recent study suggested that ongoing use of thiopurines was associated with an OR of developing NMSC of 7.3 (CI 2.7–19.8) whilst previous exposure was associated with an OR of 5.1 (CI 1.7–15.3) The absolute risk of developing NMSC, however, was low at 0.59 (CI 0.25–1.16) per 10,000 patient-years in people taking thiopurines aged under 50 [16].

Not all studies have confirmed this association. Both Fraser et al. [17] and Connell et al. [18] found no increase in skin cancer in 626 and 755 IBD patients on thiopurines, respectively. Some tumor registry-based series have also failed to detect an increased risk, possibly in part because of poor reporting of NMSC. In addition, studies focusing on cancer mortality may obscure a real increase in skin cancer-related morbidity [19].

The smaller excess risk of NMSC associated with thiopurines in patients with IBD compared with transplant patients probably reflects the way thiopurines are used in this disease. Thiopurines are frequently used as monotherapy in IBD in contrast to a two- or three-drug regimen to prevent graft rejection, with an overall higher immunosuppressive burden. Some of the other immunosuppressants in transplant patients also have carcinogenic properties, for example, calcineurin inhibitors [20,21]. In addition, thiopurine exposure in transplant patients is continuous and often lifelong, whereas the majority of IBD patients are treated intermittently, for shorter periods.

Molecular mechanisms of thiopurine-associated skin cancer

The pathogenesis of thiopurine-related skin cancer is probably multifactorial; reduced immune surveillance, UVR, oncogenic viruses, and host genetic factors may each play a role. In addition, thiopurines may be mutagenic, either directly or via an interaction with UVR.

The parallels between malignancy in transplant patients and patients with HIV/AIDS highlight the importance of *immunosuppression* per se with consequent reduced tumor surveillance as a contributor to increased cancer risk [2]. *UVR* is mutagenic; ultraviolet B (UVB; 290–320 nm), comprising <1% of terrestrial solar radiation, is directly mutagenic through the formation of DNA lesions such as pyrimidine dimers, while UVA (320–400 nm), comprising > 95% of solar radiation, is indirectly mutagenic via the generation of reactive oxygen species. In addition, UVR is immunosuppressive and may increase skin cancer risk by

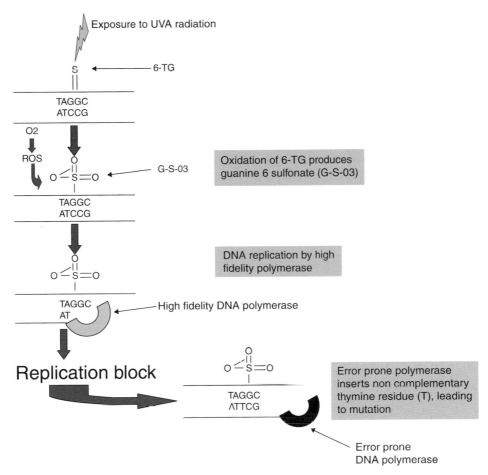

FIGURE 19.1 Generation of mutagenic oxidative DNA damage by the interaction of 6-TG and UVA: 6-TG, a metabolite of AZA, is incorporated into the DNA of skin cells of patients receiving AZA. UVA photoactivates 6-TG to produce guanine-6-sulfonate (G-S-O3). DNA strands separate and a high fidelity DNA polymerase attempts to synthesise a new strand. However, G-S-O3 is a powerful block to high fidelity replicative DNA polymerases, resulting in recruitment of low fidelity error prone polymerases which facilitate the insertion of a non-complementary residue leading to mutations (25).

locally reducing tumor surveillance. Immunosuppression-associated malignancies are usually due to known or suspected *oncogenic viruses* [2], which, in the skin, include Kaposi sarcoma, post-transplant lymphoproliferative disorder, and possibly Merkel cell carcinoma [22]. Although human papillomaviruses are likely suspects, a causative association with SCC remains unproven [23].

Direct thiopurine mutagenicity
UV-dependent
AZA enhances UV-induced skin carcinogenesis in mice [24,25]. It also increases the UVA (but not UVB) sensitivity of skin [26,27] by permitting the substitution of

DNA by 6-TG [1,28]. Normal DNA does not absorb UVA, whereas DNA 6-TG absorbs maximally at 342 nm [26]. The absorbed UVA energy is transferred to molecular oxygen to generate reactive oxygen species that damage DNA and proteins. The oxidized DNA bases block DNA replication and transcription—consistent with the enhanced skin UVA sensitivity—and some are potentially mutagenic (Figure 19.1) [26].

UV-independent
The cytotoxicity of thiopurines requires an intact DNA mismatch repair (MMR) system [28], and chronic thiopurine exposure provides a selective pressure that favors

the proliferation of MMR-deficient cells. Since these cells have an increased rate of spontaneous mutation, the time taken for their transformation to malignancy is short. Sebaceous carcinomas—rare appendageal skin tumors characteristic of the MMR-deficient Muir–Torre syndrome—are more common in thiopurine-exposed individuals in whom acquired deficiencies of MMR proteins have been demonstrated [7].

Two in vivo studies also suggest that thiopurines may be directly mutagenic. Analysis of the *PTCH* gene in BCCs from thiopurine-treated patients suggested a possible signature mutation consistent with the potential mutagenicity of DNA 6-TG [29]. Nguyen et al. [30] reported a similar mutational signature in the *HPRT* gene of peripheral T lymphocytes of thiopurine-treated patients with IBD. The frequency of mutation was related to the duration and total dose of thiopurine treatment. Since the same mutational signature is present in *PTCH* from BCCs arising on non-sun-exposed skin of patients on a thiopurine [29] and in T lymphocytes of IBD patients, these findings are consistent with direct and UVA-independent mutagenicity mediated by DNA 6-TG.

What should be done?

Advice aimed at preventing or reducing the impact of skin cancer in patients with IBD should take into account the pathogenetic mechanisms discussed above. Strategies should include assessment and advice on individual risk, education on photoprotection and self-surveillance, and rapid referral to dermatologists for management of suspicious skin lesions.

1. **Risk assessment:** Patients receiving thiopurines should be counseled on the increased risk of skin cancer, particularly those with risk factors including fair skin type, high previous chronic sun exposure and sunburn, evidence of photodamage, older age, and prolonged thiopurine exposure.
2. **Photoprotection:** Advice should be routinely provided before starting treatment. This includes avoidance of sunburn, intentional tanning, use of artificial tanning devices, and unnecessary sun exposure, especially between 11 am and 3 pm in spring through to autumn. Sunscreens with broad-spectrum UVB and UVA protection should be recommended year round as UVA is present as the main component of UVR throughout the year. Additional measures include use of broad-

brimmed hats, sunglasses, and protective clothing. To minimize the subsequent risk of vitamin D deficiency, vitamin D levels should be monitored and supplemented where necessary.
3. **Self-skin examination:** Patients should be counseled on regular self-skin examination and advised to seek early treatment for any new or suspicious skin lesions. A full skin examination as part of clinical examination prior to starting thiopurines is an opportunity to detect photodamage and (pre) malignant lesions.
4. **Clinical surveillance:** The high risk of skin cancers in transplant patients has prompted many centers to set up dedicated skin cancer surveillance clinics, a key recommendation in the 2006 UK NICE Improving Outcomes Guidance for Melanoma and Other Skin Cancers. Clinicians managing patients with IBD should be alert to the possibility of skin cancer, and rapid access to a dermatology service should be assured.
5. **Thiopurine withdrawal:** For patients developing widespread or multiple premalignancies and invasive skin tumors, dose reduction or replacement of thiopurines by alternative agents should be considered on a case-by-case basis.

Conclusions

Thiopurines are effective treatment for many patients with IBD, but skin cancer is a potential risk, especially in those with high previous UV exposure on long-term therapy. Recognition and assessment of the potential risk by healthcare providers, together with appropriate counseling, monitoring, and, where suspicious skin lesions arise, rapid referral to dermatology clinics, should help reduce the occurrence and impact of these skin cancers in the future.

Acknowledgements

We are extremely grateful to Dr Peter Karran (Mammalian DNA Repair Group, Clare Hall Laboratories, Cancer Research UK) for initiating our interest in thiopurines and skin cancer. We thank both Dr Karran and Dr Natalie Attard for critically reviewing this chapter.

References

1. Karran P, Attard A. Thiopurines in current medical practice: molecular mechanisms and contributions to therapy-related cancer. *Nat Rev Cancer* 2008; **8**(1): 24–36. Review.

2. Gruhlich AE, van Leeuwen MT, Falster MO, Vajdic CM. Incidence of cancers in people with HIV/AIDS compared with immunosupresssed transplant recipients: a meta analysis. *Lancet* 2007; **370**: 59–67.

3. IARC Monographs on the Evaluation of Carcinogenic Risk to Humans: Azathioprine (446-86-6) 1987a; **6**(Suppl. 7): 293.

4. Euvrard S, Kanitakis J, Claudy A. Skin cancers after organ transplantation. *N Engl J Med* 2003; **348**: 1681–1691.

5. Long MD, Herfarth HH, Pipkin C, et al. Increased risk for non-melanoma skin cancer in patients with inflammatory bowel disease. *Clin Gastroenterol Hepatol* 2010 Jan 15. [Epub ahead of print]

6. Harwood CA, Proby CM, McGregor JM, et al. Clinicopathological features of skin cancer in organ transplant recipients: a retrospective case-control series. *J Am Acad Dermatol* 2006; **54**: 290–300.

7. Harwood CA, McGregor JM, Swale VJ, et al. High frequency and diversity of cutaneous appendageal tumours in organ transplant recipients. *J Am Acad Dermatol* 2003; **48**: 401–408.

8. Matin RN, Mesher D, Proby CM, et al. Skin Care in Organ Transplant Patients, Europe (SCOPE) group. Melanoma in organ transplant recipients: clinicopathological features and outcome in 100 cases. *Am J Transplant* 2008; **8**(9): 1891–1900.

9. Bouwes Bavinck JN, Euvrard S, Naldi L, et al. Keratotic skin lesions and other risk factors are associated with skin cancer in organ-transplant recipients: a case-control study in The Netherlands, United Kingdom, Germany, France and Italy. *J Invest Dermatol* 2007; **127**(7): 1647–1656.

10. Austin AS, Spiller RC. Inflammatory bowel disease, azathioprine and skin cancer: case report and literature review. *Eur J Gastroenterol Hepatol* 2001; **13**: 193–194.

11. Marshall V. Premalignant and malignant skin tumours in immunosuppressed patients. *Transplantation* 1974; **17**: 272–275.

12. Kinlen LJ. Incidence of cancer in rheumatoid arthritis and other disorders after immunosuppressive treatment. *Am J Med* 1985; **78**: 44–49.

13. Ekbom A, Helmick C, Zack M, Adami HO. Extracolonic malignancies in inflammatory bowel disease. *Cancer* 1991; **67**: 2015–2019.

14. Mellemkjaer L, Olsen JH, Frisch M, et al. Cancer in patients with ulcerative colitis. *Int J Cancer* 1995; **60**(3): 330–333.

15. Hemminki K, Li X, Sundquist J, Sundquist K. Cancer risks in Crohn disease patients. *Ann Oncol* 2009; **20**(3): 574–580.

16. Peyrin-Biroulet I, Khosrotehrani K, Carrat F et al. *J Crohn's Colitis* 2011; **5**, S9.

17. Fraser AG, Orchard TR, Robinson EM, Jewell DP. Long-term risk of malignancy after treatment of inflammatory bowel disease with azathioprine. *Alimentary Pharmacology & Therapeutics* 2002; **16**(7): 1225–1232.

18. Connell WR, Kamm MA, Dickson M, et al. Long-term neoplasia risk after azathioprine treatment in inflammatory bowel disease. *Lancet* 1994; **343**: 1249–1252j.

19. McGregor JM, Perrett CM, Harwood CA. What about therapy-related cancer morbidity? *Br Med J Rapid Responses* 2009. [Online rapid response to Kempen JH, Daniel E, Dunn JP et al. Overall and cancer related mortality among patients with ocular inflammation treated with immunosuppressive drugs: retrospective cohort study. *BMJ* 2009; **339**: b2480.]

20. Hojo M, Morimoto T, Maluccio M, et al. Cyclosporine induces cancer progression by a cell-autonomous mechanism. *Nature* 1999; **397**: 530–534.

21. Yarosh DB, Pena AV, Nay SL, et al. Calcineurin inhibitors decrease DNA repair and apoptosis in human keratinocytes following ultraviolet B irradiation. *J Invest Dermatol* 2005; **125**: 1020–1025.

22. Feng H, Shuda M, Chang Y, Moore PS. Clonal integration of a polyomavirus in human Merkel cell carcinoma. *Science* 2008; **319**(5866): 1096–1100.

23. Harwood CA, Proby CM. Human papillomaviruses and non melanoma skin cancer. *Curr Opin Infect Dis* 2002; **15**(2): 101–114.

24. Reeve VE, Greenoak GE, Gallagher CH, et al. Effect of immunosuppressive agents and sunscreens on UV carcinogenesis in the hairless mouse. *Aust J Exp Med Sci* 1985; **63**: 655–665.

25. Kelly GE, Meikle W, Sheil AG. Effects of immunosuppressive therapy on the induction of skin tumours by ultraviolet irradiation in hairless mice. *Transplantation* 1987; **44**: 429–434.

26. O'Donovan P, Perrett CM, Zhang X, et al. Azathioprine and UVA light generate mutagenic oxidative DNA damage. *Science* 2005; **309**: 1871–1874.

27. Perrett CM, Walker SL, O'Donovan P, et al. Azathioprine photosensitises human skin to UV-A radiation. *Br J Dermatol* 2008; **159**: 198–204.

28. Swann PF, Waters TR, Moulton DC, et al. Role of postreplicative DNA mismatch repair in the cytotoxic action of thioguanine. *Science* 1996; **273**: 1109–1111.

29. Harwood CA, Attard NR, O'Donovan P, et al. PTCH mutations in basal cell carcinomas from azathioprine-treated organ transplant recipients. *Br J Cancer* 2008; **99**(8): 1276–1284.

30. Nguyen T, Vacek PM, O'Neill P, et al. Mutagenicity and potential carcinogenicity of thiopurine treatment in patients with inflammatory bowel disease. *Cancer Res* 2009; **69**(17): 7004–7012. Epub 2009 Aug 25.

20 Do thiopurines worsen risk and prognosis of cervical neoplasia?

Melissa A. Smith[1] and Jeremy D. Sanderson[1,2]

[1]Department of Gastroenterology, St Thomas' Hospital, Guy's and St. Thomas' NHS Foundation Trust, London, UK
[2]Nutritional Sciences Research, Kings College London, London, UK

LEARNING POINTS

- Immunosuppression, and thiopurines in particular, increase the risk of developing malignancy.

- Cervical cancer is caused by the human papilloma virus (HPV) 16 and 18 and, therefore, higher rates would be expected in immunosuppressed patients.

- Initial reports that cervical dysplasia and cancer may be more common in patients with IBD even in the absence of immunosuppression have not been substantiated.

- Several studies have failed to show a significant association between the use of azathioprine in IBD and the occurrence of cervical cancer, although most showed a trend towards a higher incidence.

- The impact of azathioprine on the prognosis of cervical cancer in IBD is not known.

Introduction

Azathioprine (AZA), 6-mercaptopurine (6-MP), and 6-thioguanine make up the group of drugs known as thiopurines. In the treatment of inflammatory bowel disease (IBD), AZA and 6-MP are first-line immunomodulatory agents used to induce and maintain clinical remission, heal fistulae, and minimize exposure to steroid treatment. While generally safe and well tolerated, the development of malignancy as a late complication of thiopurine use in IBD is of concern.

One in ten cancers diagnosed in women worldwide is a cervical cancer, with the highest incidence being seen in southern Africa and Central America where it is the commonest cancer in women. In the Western world, cervical cancer is the 12th most common cancer in women, but is a particular concern as it often affects young women, with a peak incidence in women in their 30s. Significant healthcare resources are expended on screening for cervical cancer and more recently in vaccinating against the causative human papilloma virus (HPV) serotypes 16 and 18 with which most cases are associated.

It has been proposed that there is an association between IBD itself and the development of cervical neoplasia. Initial reports from relatively small cohorts suggested that while an excess of cancers could not be detected, there was an increase in cervical dysplasia in the IBD population [1,2]. However, recent findings dispute this [3–5], and a large Canadian population-based database [6] recently reported no excess cervical cancer risk in ulcerative colitis (UC) and attributed a small excess in Crohn's disease (CD) to oral contraceptive use.

Thiopurines and cancer risk

It is widely accepted that immunosuppression is a risk factor for the development of tumors. Evidence from HIV and post-transplant cohorts demonstrates that immunosuppression is associated with a huge excess of cancers with an infectious etiology, including cervical cancer. The CD4 count acts as a strong predictor of death due to all malignancies in the HIV-positive population, and the degree of immunosuppression achieved post-transplant determines an individual's overall risk of cancer. Since approximately 99% of cervical cancers are related to HPV infection, immunosuppression could theoretically increase the risk of individuals with IBD developing cervical cancer.

Clinical Dilemmas in Inflammatory Bowel Disease: New Challenges, Second Edition. Edited by P. Irving, C. Siegel, D. Rampton and F. Shanahan.
© 2011 Blackwell Publishing Ltd. Published 2011 by Blackwell Publishing Ltd.

However, any increase in incidence associated simply with the effects of immunosuppression will be common to all treatments in this category and are unavoidable in the current management of IBD.

However, there are various ways in which thiopurines might specifically contribute to carcinogenesis (see also Chapter 19). Incorporation of "rogue" thiopurine nucleotides into DNA promotes DNA damage in a variety of ways, promoting mutagenesis. Clinical evidence implicates thiopurines in carcinogenesis. Individuals with IBD treated with thiopurines have higher rates of somatic mutations in circulating white cells than thiopurine-naïve patients, [7] an effect which was found to be proportional to dose and duration of AZA treatment, and which formed a specific thiopurine "signature" [7]. Specific cytogenetic abnormalities have been shown to occur in practice in some malignancies occurring in patients on AZA treatment [8,9], and risk of malignancy has been linked (in a variety of disease backgrounds) to the total dose of AZA received, thiopurine metabolite levels, and thiopurine methyltransferase mutations. Comparing different post-transplant immunosuppression regimes has also implicated thiopurines as being particularly associated with development of malignancy, although this finding has not been universal.

The risk of cervical cancer in thiopurine-treated IBD

In the IBD literature, there are limited data on the effect of thiopurines on the occurrence of cervical cancer. There are many case reports of cervical cancer occurring during AZA treatment, but these tell us nothing about the relative risk of developing cervical neoplasia during AZA treatment.

A recent study (abstract only) suggested that treatment duration with AZA could be a risk factor [4]. A study looking at the long-term risk of all malignancies in IBD patients treated with AZA found an observed incidence of two cervical cancers in a population of 755 patients where 0.5 cases would have been predicted [10]. Hutfless et al. found, in a cohort of 1165 patients with IBD and 12,124 controls, an odds ratio (OR) of 3.45 (0.82–14.45) for development of cervical cancer on any immunomodulator [11]. However, in none of these three studies was a statistically significantly increased risk of cervical neoplasia in association with immunomodulator use detected.

The large Canadian cohort cited above [6] did not detect a link between *single agent* AZA/6-MP and cervical dysplasia or cancer, but this subgroup was very small, containing only 13 patients from an original study cohort of nearly 248,000 women. On the other hand, those patients who had cashed prescriptions for both steroids and an immunomodulatory agent within the 5-year study period were at an increased risk of cervical cancer (OR 1.41, 95% confidence interval (CI) 1.09–1.81) [6]. In keeping with this, there is evidence from the transplant literature that rates of cervical neoplasia are increased in those on multiple immunosuppressive agents. In a large case-control study from Scotland, immunomodulation did not confer an increased risk of cervical dysplasia and neither did use of oral contraceptives. However, smoking was associated with increased risk [5].

When it does occur, there appears to be a short lag time between commencement of immunosuppression and development of cervical cancer. One study noted that changes associated with HPV infection began to appear on smear results from 18 months after transplantation, occurring at a mean interval of 42 months; the mean interval to development of neoplasia was 47 months [12].

The prognosis of cervical cancer in thiopurine-treated IBD

There is very little data in the literature on the impact of treatment with AZA on the prognosis of cancers in general and none specific to cervical cancer or to patients with IBD. In the context of renal transplants, combined treatment with AZA and a calcineurin inhibitor has been associated with locally advanced prostatic cancer at presentation and with more aggressive behavior in skin cancers. There are also case reports of sarcoma and lymphoma that completely resolved simply in response to stopping AZA treatment. How this relates to cervical cancer in the IBD patient group is unclear.

AZA in patients with a history of cervical cancer

For patients with a previously diagnosed and treated cervical cancer, caution should always be exercised when prescribing immunosuppression. That being said, in the renal transplant setting, cervical cancer is considered low risk for recurrence on immunosuppression, and it is

TABLE 20.1 Overview of the risk of cervical cancer on thiopurine treatment

Reference	Context	Patient numbers	Significantly increased risk?	OR	95% CI
Connell [10]	Tertiary hospital	755 patients	No $p = 0.09$	4 AZA only	Not given
Hutfless [11]	Tertiary hospital	1165 patients 12,124 controls	No	3.45 All immunomodulators	0.82–18.45
Singh [6]	Population-based	19,692 abnormal smears 57,898 controls	No	1.1 All immunomodulators	0.76–1.59
Lees [5]	Tertiary hospital	411 patients	No $p = 0.54$	1.3 Thiopurine only	0.61–2.78

considered safe to start immunomodulators after an individual has been "cancer-free" for 1 year [13].

Conclusion

Therefore, despite legitimate concerns and several findings that suggest that thiopurines could increase the risk of cervical neoplasia in our patients, the available evidence would suggest that the risk is not statistically different to that in the general population. Indeed, we can advise our patients that although there is a theoretically increased risk of cervical cancer in people using thiopurines, this does not seem to have been borne out in clinical practice.

Minimizing risks

There are various things that our patients can do to minimize their risk of contracting cervical cancer. Sexual promiscuity, smoking, and oral contraceptive use are all risk factors that can be addressed. Barrier contraception does not totally prevent transmission of HPV, which can be transferred from skin to skin, but is partially protective and, of course, prevents the spread of other sexually transmitted diseases, particularly chlamydia, which encourage the development of HPV infection. Adherence to cervical cancer screening programs should be encouraged since the evidence suggests that current rates of adherence are suboptimal [14]. Renal transplant guidelines, for example, recommend annual cervical smears for those on immunosuppression [15]. Uptake of HPV vaccination, where relevant, should also be encouraged. Thiopurines should be stopped immediately if cervical cancer develops during treatment (Table 20.1).

References

1. Bhatia J, Bratcher J, Korelitz B, et al. Abnormalities of uterine cervix in women with inflammatory bowel disease. *World J Gastroenterol* 2006; **12**(38): 6167–6171.
2. Kane S, Khatibi B, Reddy D. Higher incidence of abnormal Pap smears in women with inflammatory bowel disease. *Am J Gastroenterol* 2008; **103**(3): 631–636.
3. Lees C, Critchley J, Chee N, et al. Cervical dysplasia and IBD: no effect of disease status or immnosuppressants on analysis of 2199 smear records. *Gastroenterology* 2008; **134**(4): A143.
4. Lyles T, Oster R, Gutierrez A. Prevalence of abnormal PAP smears in patients with IBD om immune modulator therapy. *Gastroenterology* 2008; **134**(4): A143.
5. Lees CW, Critchley J, Chee N, et al. Lack of association between cervical dysplasia and IBD: a large case-control study. *Inflamm Bowel Dis* 2009; **15**(11): 1621–1629.
6. Singh H, Demers AA, Nugent Z, et al. Risk of cervical abnormalities in women with inflammatory bowel disease: a population-based nested case-control study. *Gastroenterology* 2009; **136**(2): 451–458.
7. Nguyen T, Vacek PM, O'Neill P, et al. Mutagenicity and potential carcinogenicity of thiopurine treatment in patients with inflammatory bowel disease. *Cancer Res* 2009; **69**(17): 7004–7012.
8. Arnold JA, Ranson SA, Abdalla SH. Azathioprine-associated acute myeloid leukaemia with trilineage dysplasia and complex karyotype: a case report and review of the literature. *Clin Lab Haematol* 1999; **21**(4): 289–292.
9. Harwood CA, Attard NR, O'Donovan P, et al. PTCH mutations in basal cell carcinomas from azathioprine-treated organ transplant recipients. *Br J Cancer* 2008; **99**(8): 1276–1284.
10. Connell WR, Kamm MA, Dickson M, et al. Long-term neoplasia risk after azathioprine treatment in inflammatory bowel disease. *Lancet* 1994; **343**(8908): 1249–1252.

11. Hutfless S, Fireman B, Kane S, et al. Screening differences and risk of cervical cancer in inflammatory bowel disease. *Aliment Pharmacol Ther* 2008; **28**(5): 598–605.

12. Halpert R, Fruchter RG, Sedlis A, et al. Human papillomavirus and lower genital neoplasia in renal transplant patients. *Obstet Gynecol* 1986; **68**(2): 251–258.

13. Kalble T, Lucan M, Nicita G, et al. EAU guidelines on renal transplantation. *Eur Urol* 2005; **47**(2): 156–166.

14. Long MD, Porter CQ, Sandler RS, et al. Suboptimal rates of cervical testing among women with inflammatory bowel disease. *Clin Gastroenterol Hepatol* 2009; **7**(5): 549–553.

15. EBPG Expert Group on Renal Transplantation. European best practice guidelines for renal transplantation. Section IV: Long-term management of the transplant recipient. IV.6 Cancer after renal transplantation. *Nephrol Dial Transplant* 2002; **17**(Suppl 4): 1–67.

21 Optimizing use of methotrexate

Anna Foley[1] and Peter R. Gibson[1,2]

[1] Department of Gastroenterology and Hepatology, Box Hill Hospital, Box Hill, VIC, Australia
[2] Eastern Health Clinical School, Monash University, Box Hill, VIC, Australia

LEARNING POINTS

- Methotrexate (MTX) is an alternative to thiopurines for the induction and maintenance of remission in Crohn's disease. Some evidence suggests that it is effective for ulcerative colitis as well.

- Parenteral administration is preferred as oral bioavailability is variable.

- Higher induction doses (25 mg/week) are more efficacious than lower doses, but dose reduction should be considered in renal impairment and in long-term maintenance.

- Adequate folate supplementation is essential in preventing and managing side effects.

- Vigilance should be applied to preventing and treating infection, but cessation of therapy is seldom necessary.

- MTX should be avoided in women of childbearing age who are not using contraception. Evidence regarding its safety in men fathering children is lacking.

Introduction

A significant proportion of patients with inflammatory bowel disease (IBD) are refractory to or intolerant of thiopurines. Thus, alternative immunomodulators are sorely needed. Methotrexate (MTX) is effective in IBD but, like thiopurines, needs to be used appropriately to achieve the best outcomes. Optimal use is facilitated by understanding the pharmacology, efficacy, and adverse effects.

Lessons from pharmacology of methotrexate [1,2]

The highly variable bioavailability of oral MTX (between 20% and 80%) has significant implications for its clinical use. Reports of successful MTX use have usually been associated with parenteral administration, following which >95% of the drug will be delivered to the target tissue. Excretion is principally renal such that care should be taken with dosing in patients with renal dysfunction. Recommendations from high-dose MTX therapy should probably be applied to low-dose therapy. Thus, the dose should be reduced by 50% if the creatinine clearance is 10–50 mL/min and its use avoided if below 10 mL/min [3]. The value of MTX metabolites as a guide to dosing has not yet been established.

MTX is a folate analog and a reversible competitive inhibitor of dihydrofolate reductase. As such, it interferes with DNA synthesis resulting in antitumor activity. At low doses, apoptosis of activated T cells is one potential mechanism for immunomodulatory effects. However, MTX also modulates cytokine networks by mechanisms not exclusively related to folate metabolism. MTX accumulates intracellularly and irreversibly affects activated lymphocytes. This is the basis of the slow onset of its immunomodulatory action, but, as a result, allows for weekly administration. Maximal effect occurs in 3–6 months but activity is usually evident within weeks.

In long-term use, drug tolerability and chronic toxicity probably relate to accumulation of MTX in tissues and the depletion of endogenous folate, the latter leading to

Clinical Dilemmas in Inflammatory Bowel Disease: New Challenges, Second Edition. Edited by P. Irving, C. Siegel, D. Rampton and F. Shanahan.
© 2011 Blackwell Publishing Ltd. Published 2011 by Blackwell Publishing Ltd.

increased adenosine production and hyperhomocysteine-mia. This is the basis for concurrent folate therapy, as discussed below.

Efficacy in IBD

While MTX can induce remission, its major role is as a maintenance therapy in IBD. In Crohn's disease, randomized controlled studies of intramuscular MTX (25 mg/week) demonstrate remission rates of about 40% [4,5] and maintenance of remission in up to 65% [6,7] of responding patients. Case series support response rates of above 50% [8,9]. Subcutaneous administration appears equivalent to intramuscular and is far better tolerated [10]. In contrast, controlled studies using lower dose oral MTX failed to show benefit over placebo [4]. Clinical experience in ulcerative colitis mimics that in Crohn's disease [8,9], but evidence of efficacy depends upon reports from large case series since the only controlled studies used low oral doses (10–12.5 mg/week) that showed no benefit over placebo [11].

One of the roles for thiopurines has been to support infliximab (and possibly adalimumab), both to improve primary efficacy and to reduce immunogenicity. The benefit of MTX and anti-TNF therapy as early combination therapy has been well established in rheumatoid arthritis [12]. However, the evidence base for a similar role in IBD is limited. Its effect in reducing levels of antibodies to infliximab has been reported to be equivalent to thiopurines [13]. There is little information on the appropriate dose or the magnitude of its effect.

Thus, MTX should be regarded as an alternative to thiopurines. As a second-line immunomodulator, MTX shows response rates in patients with thiopurine resistance that are comparable to those with thiopurine intolerance [9]. The case for using MTX before thiopurines includes a possibly lower rate of primary intolerance, the convenience of weekly administration, and apparently lower risk of lymphoma (extrapolating from the rheumatological experience [13]), but the convenience of oral dosing, the clinical value of metabolite testing, safety in pregnancy, and, most importantly, the greater evidence base for efficacy and mucosal healing would favor thiopurines as the primary immunomodulator.

Adverse effects

MTX has a range of adverse effects from nuisance to serious and potentially life-threatening, and the likelihood that MTX therapy will be discontinued due to side effects varies from 10% to 30%. Their primary prevention, early detection, and effective management are key elements in optimizing use of MTX.

The most common side effects of low-dose MTX are nausea, gastrointestinal upset, and fatigue. These are part of the acute toxicity of MTX and often occur within a day or two of a dose of MTX. However, they may become more prominent with time, leading to late cessation of therapy. Strategies to address these side effects include dividing the weekly dose and ensuring intracellular folate depletion is corrected. A weekly 5-mg dose of folate is ineffective in improving nausea, but folate 1 mg/day, or folinic acid given the day after the MTX, reduce nausea by up to 50% [15]. Currently, there is no evidence that folate repletion reduces the efficacy of MTX [15,16].

Trivial elevation of aminotransferases is common within the first two weeks of commencing MTX and usually resolves spontaneously. However, it may persist or develop at any time during therapy. It often responds to dose reduction and seldom leads to discontinuation of the drug; resolution should be seen within one month of discontinuation. There are few data regarding the risks of continuing therapy without dose reduction despite elevated aminotransferases. Current practice is to monitor liver function tests every three months and to reduce the dose if they become abnormal. Folate supplementation reduces the risk of abnormal liver function tests [16,17].

The development of hepatic fibrosis is more concerning, and studies in patients with psoriasis suggest it is related to total cumulative dose (>1.5 g). However, this has not been reflected in the IBD population who appear to have a much lower incidence of hepatic fibrosis despite cumulative doses higher than 1.5 g [18]. Liver biopsy is now only recommended based on clinical suspicion and persistently abnormal liver function test, not cumulative dose. Liver function tests are a poor indicator of the development of fibrosis, and other noninvasive markers, such as hepatic elastography, may become useful. The risk of hepatic fibrosis appears to be associated with other conditions that cause liver problems, especially obesity, diabetes, alcohol, and viral hepatitis [15]. These factors are relative contraindications to MTX and should be considered prior to its initiation.

Pneumonitis and pulmonary fibrosis occur in 2% of the rheumatoid population but are extremely rare in patients with IBD [19]. A chest X-ray prior to commencement is recommended in rheumatoid arthritis [20], but no recommendations for or against have been made in patients with IBD.

Macrocytosis is common and probably reflects reduced endogenous folate and perhaps hyperhomocysteinemia. While macrocytosis is generally considered of no consequence, its presence may reflect inadequate folate supplementation. Myelosuppression is less common but risks include high dose MTX, renal impairment, and folate deficiency. Three-monthly monitoring is required with dose reduction for neutropenia.

Like all immunomodulating drugs, MTX use must be considered as increasing the risk of malignancy, notably lymphoma. However, such an association is poorly established in the rheumatoid population [13], and there are no data in patients with IBD. Hepatosplenic T-cell lymphoma has not been reported with MTX.

Most data regarding infection risk are extrapolated from rheumatoid patients where the risk of common infections such as those affecting the respiratory tract and skin must be considered increased, although by how much has not been quantified [21]. The risk of shingles is clearly increased. Opportunistic infections, though reported, seem to be rare unless MTX is used concurrently with corticosteroids or TNF antagonists. The slow offset of action of MTX (weeks) lags well behind the resolution of the vast majority of acute common infections. Stopping the drug will have little effect on the infection but leaves the patient vulnerable to increased disease activity. Thus, the temptation to stop MTX should be resisted in most cases. As for any immunomodulatory drug, attention to prevention of infection by, for example, vaccination (see Chapter 10) and vigilance in at-risk situations is warranted. MTX interacts with some commonly used medications, so careful review of concomitant medications is essential (see Chapter 33).

There is documented embryotoxicity and teratogenicity related to MTX use and it should be avoided in women contemplating pregnancy. All women of childbearing potential should be counseled about adequate contraception. In men, there is no evidence to suggest adverse pregnancy outcomes with MTX [22], although reversible oligospermia has been reported [23]. However, in some countries, including the United Kingdom, avoidance of MTX is recommended in men wanting to father children.

Conclusions (Table 21.1)

The success of MTX as a long-term therapy in patients with IBD is dependent upon its optimal application. This

TABLE 21.1 Guide to the optimal use of methotrexate in patients with inflammatory bowel disease

Before therapy	Hematology, creatinine, liver function tests Chest X-ray[a] Screen for liver diseases Minimize ethanol intake Immunize against vaccine-preventable disease
How to initiate	Dose: Aim for 25 mg weekly Route of administration: Subcutaneous Instruction on self-administration and handling of cytotoxic agents Blood monitoring: 2-weekly liver function tests, hematology
Long-term therapy	Dose may be reduced (e.g., to 15 mg weekly) Safety monitoring mandatory: 3-monthly liver function tests, hematology Folate supplementation essential
When it is not working	Are the symptoms being generated by inflammation? Is the dose sufficient? Is the best route of administration being used? Is compliance an issue?
When it is not tolerated	Are the side effects really due to the methotrexate? Is the dose too high? Is the route of administration the best for the patient? Can the dose be divided? Is folate supplementation adequate?

[a]Recommended for patients with rheumatoid arthritis.

includes attention to indication, dose, mode of administration, and safety. The risk of side effects can be minimized by appropriate screening of patients prior to its initiation, monitoring in the long term, and ensuring adequate folate supplementation.

References

1. Grim J, Chladek J, Martinkova J. Pharmacokinetics and pharmacodynamics of methotrexate in non-neoplastic diseases. *Clin Pharmacokinet* 2003; **42**: 139–151.
2. van Dieren J, Kuipers E, Samsom J, et al. Revisiting the immunomodulators, tacrolimus, methotrexate and mycophenolate mofetil: their mechanisms of action and role in the treatment of IBD. *Inflamm Bowel Dis* 2006; **12**: 311–327.

3. Aronoff GR, Bennett WM, Berns JS, et al. *Drug Prescribing in Renal Failure: Dosing Guidelines in Adults and Children*, 5th Ed. Philadelphia, PA: Am Col of Physicians; 2007, p 101.

4. Alfadhi AA, McDonald JW, Feagan BG. Methotrexate for the induction of remission in refractory Crohn's disease. *Cochrane Database Syst Rev* 2005; (1): CD003459.

5. Feagan BG, Rochon J, Fedorak RN, et al. Methotrexate for the treatment of Crohn's disease. *New Engl J Med* 1995; **332**: 292–297.

6. Chong RY, Hanauer SB, Cohen RD. Efficacy of parenteral methotrexate in refractory Crohn's disease. *Aliment Pharmacol Ther* 2001; **15**: 35–44.

7. Feagan BG, Fedorak RN, Irvine EJ, et al. A comparison of methotrexate with placebo for the maintenance of remission of Crohn's disease. North American Crohn's Study Group Investigators. *New Engl J Med* 2000; **342**: 1627–1632.

8. Fraser A, Morton D, McGovern D, et al. The efficacy of methotrexate for maintaining remission in inflammatory bowel disease. *Alim Pharmacol Ther* 2002; **16**: 693–697.

9. Nathan D, Iser J, Gibson P. A single centre experience of methotrexate in the treatment of Crohn's disease and ulcerative colitis: a case for subcutaneous administration. *J Gastroenterol Hepatol* 2008; **23**: 954–958.

10. Brooks PM, Spruill WJ, Parish RC, et al. Pharmacokinetics of methotrexate administered by intramuscular and subcutaneous injections in patients with rheumatoid arthritis. *Arthritis Rheum* 1990; **33**: 91–97.

11. Chande N, MacDonald JK, McDonald JW. Methotrexate for induction of remission in ulcerative colitis. *The Cochrane Library* 2009; (3).

12. Goekoop-Ruiterman YP, de Vries-Bouwstra JK, Allaart CF, et al. Clinical and radiographic outcomes of four different treatment strategies in patients with early rheumatoid arthritis (the BeST study): A randomised controlled trial. *Arthritis Rheum* 2005; **52**: 3381–3390.

13. Salliot C, van der Heijde D. Long term safety of methotrexate monotherapy in patients with rheumatoid arthritis: a systemic literature research. *Ann Rheum Dis* 2009; **68**: 1100–1104.

14. Vermeire S, van Assche G, Baert F, et al. Effectiveness of concomitant immunosuppressive therapy in suppressing the formation of antibodies to infliximab in Crohn's disease. *Gut* 2007; **56**: 1226–1231.

15. Visser K, Katchamart W, Loza E, et al. Multinational evidence based recommendations for the use of methotrexate in rheumatic disorders with a focus on rheumatoid arthritis: integrating a systematic literature research and expert opinion of a broad international panel of rheumatologists in the 3E Initiative. *Ann Rheum Dis* 2009; **68**: 1086–1093.

16. Van Ede A, Laan R, Rood M, et al. Effect of folic or folinic acid supplementation on the toxicitiy and efficacy of methotrexate in rheumatoid arthritis. *Arthritis Rheum* 2001; **44**: 1515–1524.

17. Prey S, Paul C. Effect of folic or folinic acid supplementation on methotrexate-associated safety and efficacy in inflammatory disease: a systematic review *Br J Dermatol* 2009; **160**: 622–628.

18. Te HS, Schiano TD, Kuan SF, et al. Hepatic effects of long-term methotrexate use in the treatment of inflammatory bowel disease *Am J Gastroenterol* 2000; **95**: 3150–3156.

19. Siegel CA. Review article: practical management of inflammatory bowel disease patients taking immunomodulators. *Aliment Pharmacol Ther* 2005; **22**: 1–16.

20. Anonymous. American College of Rheumatology Ad Hoc Committee on Clinical Guidelines. Guidelines for monitoring drug therapy in rheumatoid arthritis. *Arthritis Rheum* 1996; **39**: 723–731.

21. McLean-Tooke A, Aldridge C, Waugh S, et al. Methotrexate, rheumatoid arthritis and infection risk – what is the evidence? *Rheumatology* 2009; **48**: 867–871.

22. Lamboglia F, D'Inca R, Bertomoro P, et al. Patient with severe Crohn's disease became a father whilst on methotrexate and infliximab therapy. *Inflamm Bowel Dis* 2009; **15**: 648–649.

23. Sussman A, Leonard J. Psoriasis, methotrexate and oligospermia. *Arch Dermatol* 1980; **116**: 215–217.

22 Which calcineurin inhibitor and when?

A. Barney Hawthorne

Department of Medicine, University Hospital of Wales, Cardiff, UK

LEARNING POINTS

- Both cyclosporine and tacrolimus induce remission in corticosteroid-refractory ulcerative colitis, with more controlled data available for cyclosporine.

- The best intravenous (IV) cyclosporine dose is 2 mg/kg/day.

- Oral tacrolimus absorption is slightly faster and more predictable than oral cyclosporine, making IV tacrolimus unnecessary.

- Trough levels are more reliable as a measure of appropriate dosing for tacrolimus than for cyclosporine

- The side effect profiles of the two drugs are similar but not identical.

Introduction

The calcineurin inhibitors cyclosporine and tacrolimus are potent inhibitors of T cell activation, without significant myelosuppressive properties. They are widely used in transplantation and autoimmune disease. In IBD, cyclosporine has gradually gained a place as a salvage treatment for severe or refractory ulcerative colitis (UC). It is not used often in Crohn's disease (CD), as it is only effective at high doses, and TNF inhibitors are more suitable second-line immunosuppressive therapies. Recently, a small number of studies have evaluated tacrolimus in UC. Now the clinician is faced with a choice of using either calcineurin inhibitor, or anti-TNF drugs in UC patients who are failing therapy, and who wish to avoid surgery. As is so often the case, these decisions are hampered by the lack of head-to-head comparisons of these agents in clinical trials.

Cyclosporine in UC

The initial randomized study [1] used a 4-mg/kg/day intravenous (IV) dose in 20 patients failing 7 days IV corticosteroids. Nine of 11 (87%) on cyclosporine responded versus none on placebo. Another small study randomized 29 patients with severe UC to the same high IV dose versus methylprednisolone 40 mg daily with similar response rates of 64% and 53% respectively at day 7 or 8 [2]. The same authors went on to show (in a larger study of 73 patients) that 2 mg/kg/day was as effective as 4 mg/kg/day with response rates at 14 days of 86% and 84%, respectively [3]. Once response is achieved, patients are converted to twice daily oral doses (5–6 mg/kg/day is equivalent to 2 mg/kg/day IV). No randomized controlled trials using initial oral cyclosporine have been performed, but a large number of case series have shown comparable early response rates of about 80% [4]. The optimal trough level is not evidence-based, but should probably match those for transplantation (150–250 ng/mL in induction of remission and 100–200 ng/mL after remission is achieved). The longer term outcomes are best when cyclosporine is used as a bridging therapy to maintenance thiopurines, with 40–50% remaining colectomy-free at 2 years [4].

Tacrolimus in UC

There are less data on tacrolimus in UC, with only one randomized controlled trial. This study [5] evaluated efficacy

---

Clinical Dilemmas in Inflammatory Bowel Disease: New Challenges, Second Edition. Edited by P. Irving, C. Siegel, D. Rampton and F. Shanahan.
© 2011 Blackwell Publishing Ltd. Published 2011 by Blackwell Publishing Ltd.

in 60 hospitalized patients with moderate-to-severe UC who had failed at least 30 mg of prednisolone for 2 weeks. They were randomized to three groups for 2 weeks of either placebo, low-dose tacrolimus (target trough level 5–10 ng/mL), or high-dose tacrolimus (target trough level of 10–15 ng/mL). Although both active treatment groups started on 0.05 mg/kg/day split into twice daily dosing, the final dose at 2 weeks was 0.14 and 0.2 mg/kg in the low- and high-dose groups, respectively. It took 7–8 days to achieve the target trough levels. At 2 weeks, 10% responded in the placebo group, versus 68% in the high-dose group ($p < 0.001$), but only 38% in the low-dose group ($p = $ NS). Patients were then given open-label tacrolimus for a further 10 weeks, with a pooled response rate of 55% and remission rate of 29% at 12 weeks. It is important to note that no patients had colectomy during the short period of observation in this trial. This trial confirms that oral tacrolimus is effective in UC, with a target trough level of 10–15 ng/mL, and a short-term response rate, which is comparable to cyclosporine. Optimal trough levels for maintenance of remission are not evidence-based, but should probably be lower (5–10 ng/mL). There are no other randomized trials of tacrolimus, but several case series show that oral tacrolimus is as effective as IV tacrolimus with comparable outcomes to cyclosporine: 78–90% early response rates, and 50–62% long-term colectomy-free survival [6–8].

Pharmacology

Both cyclosporine and tacrolimus have extremely variable pharmacokinetics, and a narrow therapeutic index, making blood-level monitoring essential. Cyclosporine microemulsion has a better absorption than the earlier oil-based formulations, but is still somewhat dependent on bile, which is not the case for tacrolimus. Cyclosporine absorption is improved when taken with a fatty meal, whereas tacrolimus absorption is reduced. Peak plasma levels after oral ingestion occur at 1–8 hours for cyclosporine, 0.5–6 hours for tacrolimus. Much of the variability in bioavailability of both drugs relates to their metabolism by the CYP3A4 member of the cytochrome P450 superfamily, present mainly in liver, but also in kidney and gut mucosa, and subject to endogenous and exogenous inhibition. Intestinal P-glycoprotein (controlled by *MDR-1* gene) also contributes to variability in absorption. The elimination half-life of cyclosporine is 19 hours, and of tacrolimus 9–12 hours, and both are bile-excreted. Tacrolimus trough levels correlate better with area under the time/concentration curve than do trough levels for cyclosporine [9].

Toxicity

Side effects of calcineurin inhibitors are less problematic in autoimmune disease therapy than in transplant therapy, mainly because they are dose-dependent, and improve with dose reduction or cessation (often not an easy option after transplantation). There are less data available for tacrolimus than for cyclosporine. The range of toxicities is shown in Table 22.1. Renal impairment is multifactorial with calcineurin inhibitors and occurs with both cyclosporine and tacrolimus. In a randomized trial of immunosuppressive regimens in renal transplantation, low-dose tacrolimus caused less renal impairment than low-dose cyclosporine with better allograft survival [10]. Hypertension occurs with both drugs, and is best treated with calcium-channel blockers, which increase renal blood flow (note that diltiazem increases drug levels by reducing metabolism, allowing lower doses to be used). Tacrolimus causes less gum hypertrophy and hirsutism, and is less likely to precipitate gout, whereas cyclosporine is less likely to cause tremor, other neurological effects, glucose intolerance, and gastrointestinal effects. Seizures are only a problem with very high-drug levels, but more likely with IV cyclosporine if cholesterol levels are low, or seizure threshold is reduced by calcineurin-inhibitor induced hypomagnesemia. Potent immunosuppressive therapy carries increased risk of toxicity in the elderly or those with significant comorbidity, and this must be factored into any decision to start a calcineurin inhibitor. Drug interactions are numerous (see Chapter 38), and grapefruit juice can increase levels significantly. The increased infection risk applies to both drugs, and if triple therapy (calcineurin inhibitor, thiopurine, and corticosteroids) is used, cotrimoxazole should be coprescribed. (Without corticosteroids, the pneumocystis pneumonia risk is lower).

When to start a calcineurin inhibitor

The Cochrane library highlights the lack of controlled trial data for both cyclosporine [11] and tacrolimus [12], yet there is no doubt that both these drugs induce remission in active UC. There are two situations where they have a role. In severe corticosteroid-refractory UC in hospitalized patients, these drugs will spare about three quarters of

System	Toxicity	Comparison
Renal	Acute	Equal
	Chronic	C > T[a]
Hypertension		Equal
Neurological	Tremor	
	Headache	T > C
	Seizures	
	Encephalopathy	
Metabolic	Glucose intolerance	T > C
	Increased bone turnover	C > T
	Hyperuricemia	C > T
	Hyperkaliemia	Equal
	Hypomagnesemia	Equal
Infection		Equal
Malignancy		Equal
Dermatological	Gingival hyperplasia, hirsutism	C > T
Gastrointestinal	Anorexia	
	Nausea and vomiting	T > C
	Diarrhea	
	Abdominal discomfort	

TABLE 22.1 Comparative toxicity of calcineurin inhibitors

C, cyclosporine; T, tacrolimus; T > C, toxicity more widely reported for tacrolimus than cyclosporine; C > T, toxicity more widely reported for cyclosporine than tacrolimus.
[a]Data from one renal transplant study show low-dose tacrolimus has less nephrotoxicity, without loss of immunosuppressive efficacy, than low-dose cyclosporine.

patients from colectomy during that admission (and about half will not need colectomy over the next 2–3 years). The timing of intervention is unclear, but it is likely that prolonging ineffective IV corticosteroids, then adding a calcineurin inhibitor will increase the risk of adverse events significantly. There is good evidence that failure to respond to 3 days of IV corticosteroids is predictive of colectomy without further drug intervention [13], so this should guide timing of therapy. The Ho index [14](based on bowel frequency, colonic dilatation, and albumin level) is a good predictor of response to cyclosporine and avoidance of colectomy [15]. The best long-term outcomes are achieved with addition of long-term thiopurine maintenance therapy, so that the cyclosporine or tacrolimus can be stopped after 3–6 months. Thiopurines should be started as soon as possible, to allow for slow onset of action. Once a good response is achieved to cyclosporine or tacrolimus, corticosteroids should be tapered rapidly over a week, to avoid unnecessary triple therapy.

The second scenario is in chronic active UC refractory to conventional immunosuppressive therapy in the clinic setting. Here there are no controlled data, but oral cyclosporine and tacrolimus clearly are treatment options. The diffi-culty is deciding the duration of therapy. Observational studies show tacrolimus is safe over a year or more, with most patients off corticosteroids, but outcomes after stopping are unclear. Patients need to be helped to make an informed choice between risks of longer term cyclosporine or tacrolimus therapy (renal impairment, neoplasia, and infection) and colectomy.

The alternative drug to consider in these situations is a TNF inhibitor (see Chapter 32). There is an urgent need for head-to-head comparisons looking at short- and long-term outcomes (both colectomy-sparing and toxicity) for these two therapy groups.

Conclusions

Calcineurin inhibitors are an effective salvage therapy in corticosteroid-refractory UC. The choice of cyclosporine or tacrolimus is subjective. In hospitalized patients, where IV therapy is convenient, the larger evidence base favors IV cyclosporine, converting to oral in responders. In the outpatient setting, or where oral therapy is necessary, tacrolimus can be used. The pharmacokinetics of tacrolimus make it slightly easier to use, and the side effect profile perhaps favors tacrolimus, particularly where therapy is likely to be prolonged beyond 3–6 months. However, both drugs remain difficult to use and monitor, particularly in view of drug interactions, toxicity, and the need for close monitoring. As with any drug therapy for UC, the patient must always be aware of the option for colectomy, which is likely to have significantly lower risk of serious harm, but at the expense of stoma or pouch, with their attendant impact on quality of life.

References

1. Lichtiger S, Present DH, Kornbluth A, et al. Cyclosporine in severe ulcerative colitis refractory to steroid therapy. *N Engl J Med* 1994; **330**(26): 1841–1845.

2. D'Haens G, Lemmens L, Geboes K, et al. Intravenous cyclosporine versus intravenous corticosteroids as single therapy for severe attacks of ulcerative colitis. *Gastroenterology* 2001; **120**(6): 1323–1329.

3. Van Assche G, D'Haens G, Noman M, et al. Randomized, double-blind comparison of 4 mg/kg versus 2 mg/kg intravenous cyclosporine in severe ulcerative colitis. *Gastroenterology* 2003; **125**(4): 1025–1031.

4. Durai D, Hawthorne AB. Review article: how and when to use ciclosporin in ulcerative colitis. *Aliment Pharmacol Ther* 2005; **22**(10): 907–916.

5. Ogata H, Matsui T, Nakamura M, et al. A randomised dose finding study of oral tacrolimus (FK506) therapy in refractory ulcerative colitis. [see comment] [erratum appears in *Gut* 2006; **55**(11):1684. Note: dosage error in abstract]. *Gut* 2006; **55**(9): 1255–1262.

6. Fellermann K, Tanko Z, Herrlinger KR, et al. Response of refractory colitis to intravenous or oral tacrolimus (FK506). *Inflamm Bowel Dis* 2002; **8**(5): 317–324.

7. Yamamoto S, Nakase H, Mikami S, et al. Long-term effect of tacrolimus therapy in patients with refractory ulcerative colitis. *Aliment Pharmacol Ther* 2008; **28**(5): 589–597.

8. Baumgart DC, Wiedenmann B, Dignass AU. Rescue therapy with tacrolimus is effective in patients with severe and refractory inflammatory bowel disease. *Aliment Pharmacol Ther* 2003; **17**(10): 1273–1281.

9. Kapturczak MH, Meier-Kriesche HU, Kaplan B. Pharmacology of calcineurin antagonists. *Transplant Proc* 2004; **36**(Suppl. 2): 25S–32S.

10. Ekberg H, Tedesco-Silva H, Demirbas A, et al. Reduced exposure to calcineurin inhibitors in renal transplantation. [see comment]. *N Engl J Med* 2007; **357**(25): 2562–2575.

11. Shibolet O, Regushevskaya E, Brezis M, Soares-Weiser K. Cyclosporine A for induction of remission in severe ulcerative colitis. *Cochrane Database Syst Rev* 2005(1): CD004277.

12. Baumgart DC, Macdonald JK, Feagan B. Tacrolimus (FK506) for induction of remission in refractory ulcerative colitis. *Cochrane Database Syst Rev* 2008(3): CD007216.

13. Travis SP, Farrant JM, Ricketts C, et al. Predicting outcome in severe ulcerative colitis. *Gut* 1996; **38**(6): 905–910.

14. Ho GT, Mowat C, Goddard CJ, et al. Predicting the outcome of severe ulcerative colitis: development of a novel risk score to aid early selection of patients for second-line medical therapy or surgery. *Aliment Pharmacol Ther* 2004; **19**(10): 1079–1087.

15. Aceituno M, Garcia-Planella E, Heredia C, et al. Steroid-refractory ulcerative colitis: predictive factors of response to cyclosporine and validation in an independent cohort. *Inflamm Bowel Dis* 2008; **14**(3): 347–352.

Biologics

23 Are all anti-TNF agents the same?

Jennifer L. Jones

Departments of Medicine and Community Health Sciences and Epidemiology, University of Saskatchewan, Royal University Hospital, Saskatoon, SK, Canada

LEARNING POINTS

- There are three antitumor necrosis factor (anti-TNF) antibodies currently used to treat IBD—infliximab, adalimumab, and certolizumab, the latter being available in only a few countries.

- It is unclear if one drug is significantly better than the others and large randomized head-to-head trials are unlikely to be performed to answer this question.

- Therefore, the choice of which drug to use is driven by a number of factors, including availability, cost, route of administration, dosing regimen, immunogenicity, and patient preference

Introduction

The past decade has borne witness to a rapid expansion in the development of biological agents targeting tumor necrosis factor (TNF). They have proven highly effective for the treatment of various chronic inflammatory conditions, including IBD. Despite the fact that most of the biological agents available for the treatment of IBD belong to the same class, antitumor necrosis factor (anti-TNF), some important differences exist with respect to the structure, mechanism of action, pharmacokinetic properties, and efficacy between these agents.

Structure and function

The structures of the TNF antagonists infliximab (IFX), etanercept, adalimumab (ADA), and certolizumab pegol (CERTO) are represented in Figure 23.1. All agents, except

for etanercept, are monoclonal antibodies (mAbs) or fragments of mAbs [1]. IFX and ADA are full length IgG mAbs, whereas CERTO is a monovalent Fab1 antibody fragment covalently linked to polyethylene glycol (PEG) [1]. TNF-antagonist mAbs also differ in their IgG isotopes. All of the anti-TNF agents, with the exception of CERTO, are structurally similar in that they all contain an IgG1 Fc region and are, therefore, capable of antibody-dependent cell-mediated toxicity (ADCC) and complement-dependent cytotoxicity (CDC) [1]. These molecules also have the potential to mediate killing of cells expressing membrane-bound TNF-α (mTNFα) [1]. CERTO lacks the Fc region and is, therefore, not capable of mediating these effects (see Figure 23.1) [2].

Etanercept is a fusion protein composed of the Fc portion of IgG1 and the extracellular domain of the TNF receptor [1]. Despite the overall success of development programs of anti-TNF molecules, initial clinical trials of etanercept in Crohn's disease (CD) were negative [3]. This has led to speculation as to how various structural and mechanistic differences including specificity, neutralization potency, reverse signaling, apoptosis, Fc receptor interactions, and cytotoxicity may have played a role.

Golimumab, another fully human IgG1 anti-TNF antibody is currently undergoing Phase III trials in ulcerative colitis (UC).

Pharmacokinetic properties

All of the TNF antagonists differ in their dosing regimens, pharmacokinetic properties, and immunogenicity (see

Clinical Dilemmas in Inflammatory Bowel Disease: New Challenges, Second Edition. Edited by P. Irving, C. Siegel, D. Rampton and F. Shanahan.
© 2011 Blackwell Publishing Ltd. Published 2011 by Blackwell Publishing Ltd.

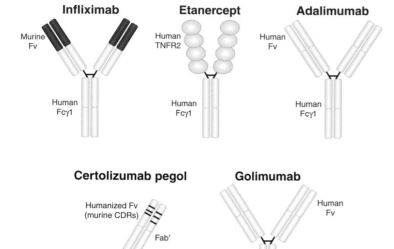

FIGURE 23.1 Simplified diagrams of the molecular structures of 4 TNF antagonists. (Reprinted from [1] with permission from Elsevier.)

Figure 23.2) [4,5]. IFX, which is administered by intravenous (IV) infusion at 5 mg/kg every 8 weeks, reaches high initial serum concentrations that are 13–40-fold greater than the peak concentrations of ADA or etanercept at steady state [5]. The half-life of IFX ($t_{1/2}$) has been estimated to be between 8–10 days. ADA, given as 40 mg subcutaneously every other week, produces steady-state trough serum concentrations of 4–8 μg/mL, which is 3–7 times greater than the clinically effective serum concentrations [1]. This suggests that the mean steady-state serum concentrations of ADA are within the therapeutic window. The $t_{1/2}$ of ADA has been estimated to be between 10–20 days [1]. CERTO,

administered at 100, 200, or 400 mg every 4 weeks, has a plasma $t_{1/2}$ of approximately 14 days [1,6].

Immunogenicity

Clinical consequences of immunogenicity of TNF antagonists include acquired drug resistance and infusion or injection site reactions. Anti-drug antibodies can form multivalent complexes with the target drug, leading to rapid clearance and inactivation of the drug [1]. Strategies to deal with this include dose escalation or the addition of concomitant immunosuppressive therapy to reduce

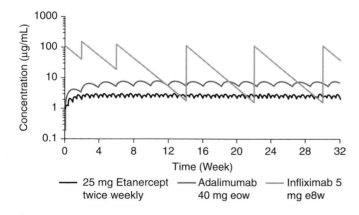

FIGURE 23.2 A pharmacokinetics simulation of serum concentrations of infliximab, etanercept, and adalimumab at steady state in patients with RA treated with each drug at doses and schedules shown. (Reprinted from [1] with permission from Elsevier.)

antibody formation [7–10]. Studies of the immunogenicity of protein-based drugs have suggested that chimeric antibodies are generally more immunogenic than humanized or human antibodies [11]. However, comparisons of the immunogenic potential of the anti-TNF agents are difficult, largely because of differences in the sensitivity of the assays designed to detect anti-drug antibodies, as well as the interference in the assays of the drug itself [9].

Clinical efficacy

Anti-TNF agents, except for etanercept, have proven themselves efficacious for the induction and maintenance of clinical response and remission in patients with CD.

Infliximab

The initial multicenter, prospective, double-blind, placebo-controlled clinical trial by Targan and colleagues studied IFX administered as a single dose of 5, 10, or 20 mg/kg, then followed patients for clinical response out to week 12. Week 4 nonresponders were given an additional open-label dose at 10 mg/kg, then followed for an additional 12 weeks. Eighty-one percent of subjects given the drug at 5 mg/kg responded at week 4, while 33% went into remission compared to 4% of subjects receiving placebo [12].

ACCENT I demonstrated the efficacy of IFX as a maintenance agent [13]. This Phase III multicenter trial examined maintenance of response in subjects with moderate-to-severe CD who had initially responded to a single 5-mg/kg induction dose of IFX. Patients were assigned to one of three treatment arms: (1) placebo at weeks 2, 6, and every 8 weeks until week 46, (2) IFX 5 mg/kg at week 2, 6, and every 8 weeks until week 46, or (3) IFX 5 mg/kg at weeks 2, 6, and then 10 mg/kg every 8 weeks until week 46. 335 of the enrolled 573 patients (58%) responded to treatment at week 2. At week 30, 21% of patients in the placebo group were in remission compared to 39% in the 5-mg/kg group, and 45% in the 10-mg/kg group [13,14]. IFX maintenance therapy has also been shown to be associated with a reduced need for surgery, hospitalizations and procedures, and with improved health-related quality of life [14,15].

IFX is also effective for fistulizing CD. ACCENT II was a double-blind, placebo-controlled study in which efficacy for closure of fistulae, the majority of which were perianal, was evaluated. Thirty-six percent of subjects who initially responded had maintained a complete response to IFX (defined as the absence of draining fistulae) at 54 weeks

(versus 19% in the placebo group) [15]. Finally, IFX has also been shown in subgroup analysis to result in mucosal healing [16].

Adalimumab

CLASSIC I was the first double-blind, placebo-controlled trial of ADA as induction therapy for patients with moderately to severely active CD [17]. 80/40 mg and 160/80 mg dosing regimens were compared to placebo. Both ADA intervention groups were superior to placebo [17]. The CHARM study evaluated the efficacy of adalimumab maintenance therapy after induction therapy [18]. This study demonstrated that initial responders had a 36% remission rate at weeks 26 and 56 for those maintained on 40 mg subcutaneously every other week in comparison to 12% for placebo ($p < 0.001$) [18]. CHARM also evaluated fistula closure as a secondary end point and 33% of initial responders experienced complete closure of their fistula [18]. Ninety percent of those patients with fistula closure at the end of CHARM had maintained fistula closure at the end of a second year of therapy. Lastly, ADA has been shown to be efficacious in those patients who had initially responded to, but then subsequently lost response or tolerance to IFX in the GAIN trial (21% receiving ADA 160/80 mg versus 7% in placebo) [19].

Certolizumab

The Pegylated Antibody Fragment Evaluation in CD Safety and Efficacy (PRECiSE 1) study evaluated the efficacy of CERTO as an induction agent with a primary end point of response at week 6 and 26 [6]. Twenty-two percent of subjects receiving therapy versus 12% receiving placebo achieved a clinical response. Remission rates were not significantly different between groups. In the PRECiSE 2 trial, the primary end point was clinical response at week 26 in patients with an elevated CRP. Of the initial responders at week 6, 62% of patients maintained their response at week 26 versus 34% of those receiving placebo ($p < 0.001$) [20]. A prospective study evaluating the steroid-sparing effects of CERTO is currently underway.

Conclusions

Questions remain as to whether one anti-TNF agent is more efficacious than another, and it is unlikely that adequately powered randomized head-to-head controlled trials will be performed to address this issue, given the extremely large sample size that would be required to answer such a question. For now, issues pertaining to dosing regimen, route of administration, immunogenicity, and patient preference appear to be the major considerations when deciding which agent to use as first- and second-line anti-TNF therapy. In some parts of the world, choice may be affected by the cost and availability of the different drugs and, for a proportion of patients, issues around adherence may also enter into the equation.

References

1. Tracey D, Klareskog L, Sasso EH, Salfeld JG, Tak PP. Tumor necrosis factor antagonist mechanisms of action: a comprehensive review. *Pharmacol Ther* 2008; **117**(2): 244–279.

2. Bourne T, Fossati G, Nesbitt A. A PEGylated Fab' fragment against tumor necrosis factor for the treatment of Crohn disease: exploring a new mechanism of action. *BioDrugs* 2008; **22**(5): 331–337.

3. Sandborn WJ, Hanauer SB, Katz S, et al. Etanercept for active Crohn's disease: a randomized, double-blind, placebo-controlled trial. *Gastroenterology* 2001; **121**(5): 1088–1094.

4. Furst DE, Wallis R, Broder M, Beenhouwer DO. Tumor necrosis factor antagonists: different kinetics and/or mechanisms of action may explain differences in the risk for developing granulomatous infection. *Semin Arthritis Rheum* 2006; **36**(3): 159–167.

5. Nestorov I. Clinical pharmacokinetics of TNF antagonists: how do they differ? *Semin Arthritis Rheum* 2005; **34**(5Suppl.1): 12–18.

6. Schreiber S, Rutgeerts P, Fedorak RN, et al. A randomized, placebo-controlled trial of certolizumab pegol (CDP870) for treatment of Crohn's disease. *Gastroenterology* 2005; **129**(3): 807–818.

7. Baert F, Noman M, Vermeire S, et al. Influence of immunogenicity on the long-term efficacy of infliximab in Crohn's disease. *N Engl J Med* 2003; **348**(7): 601–608.

8. van der Laken CJ, Voskuyl AE, et al. Imaging and serum analysis of immune complex formation of radiolabelled infliximab and anti-infliximab in responders and non-responders to therapy for rheumatoid arthritis. *Ann Rheum Dis* 2007; **66**(2): 253–256.

9. Bendtzen K, Geborek P, Svenson M, Larsson L, Kapetanovic MC, Saxne T. Individualized monitoring of drug bioavailability and immunogenicity in rheumatoid arthritis patients treated with the tumor necrosis factor alpha inhibitor infliximab. *Arthritis Rheum* 2006; **54**(12): 3782–3789.

10. Wolbink GJ, Vis M, Lems W, et al. Development of anti-infliximab antibodies and relationship to clinical response in patients with rheumatoid arthritis. *Arthritis Rheum* 2006; **54**(3): 711–715.

11. Hwang WY, Foote J. Immunogenicity of engineered antibodies. *Methods* 2005; **36**(1): 3–10.

12. Targan SR, Hanauer SB, van Deventer SJ, et al. A short-term study of chimeric monoclonal antibody cA2 to tumor necrosis factor alpha for Crohn's disease. Crohn's Disease cA2 Study Group. *N Engl J Med* 1997; **337**(15): 1029–1035.

13. Hanauer SB, Feagan BG, Lichtenstein GR, et al. Maintenance infliximab for Crohn's disease: the ACCENT I randomised trial. *Lancet* 2002; **359**(9317): 1541–1549.

14. Lichtenstein GR, Yan S, Bala M, Blank M, Sands BE. Infliximab maintenance treatment reduces hospitalizations, surgeries, and procedures in fistulizing Crohn's disease. *Gastroenterology* 2005; **128**(4): 862–869.

15. Sands BE, Anderson FH, Bernstein CN, et al. Infliximab maintenance therapy for fistulizing Crohn's disease. *N Engl J Med* 2004; **350**(9): 876–885.

16. Sandborn WJ. Mucosal healing in inflammatory bowel disease. *Rev Gastroenterol Disord* 2008; **8**(4): 271–272.

17. Hanauer SB, Sandborn WJ, Rutgeerts P, et al. Human anti-tumor necrosis factor monoclonal antibody (adalimumab) in Crohn's disease: the CLASSIC-I trial. *Gastroenterology* 2006; **130**(2): 323–333; quiz 591.

18. Colombel JF, Sandborn WJ, Rutgeerts P, et al. Adalimumab for maintenance of clinical response and remission in patients with Crohn's disease: the CHARM trial. *Gastroenterology* 2007; **132**(1): 52–65.

19. Sandborn WJ, Rutgeerts P, Enns R, et al. Adalimumab induction therapy for Crohn disease previously treated with infliximab: a randomized trial. *Ann Intern Med* 2007; **146**(12): 829–838.

20. Schreiber S, Khaliq-Kareemi M, Lawrance IC, et al. Maintenance therapy with certolizumab pegol for Crohn's disease. *N Engl J Med* 2007; **357**(3): 239–250.

24 One drug or two: do patients on biologics need concurrent immunomodulation?

Glen A. Doherty[1,2] and Adam S. Cheifetz[2]

[1]Centre for Colorectal Disease, St Vincent's University Hospital/University College Dublin, Dublin, Ireland
[2]Center for Inflammatory Bowel Disease, Division of Gastroenterology, Beth Israel Deaconess Medical Center and Harvard Medical School, Boston, MA, USA

LEARNING POINTS

- Concomitant use of an immunomodulator reduces the risk of immunogenicity in patients on episodic ("on demand") antitumor necrosis factor (anti-TNF) therapy, but this does not appear as important when therapy is given on a scheduled basis.

- Data from the SONIC trial suggest that combined use of infliximab and azathioprine in immunomodulator-naive Crohn's disease (CD) is more effective over 1 year than either agent alone.

- There is uncertainty about whether long-term outcomes in CD are altered by the use of concomitant immunomodulation.

- There are no large prospective trials of combination therapy in ulcerative colitis.

- Combining an anti-TNF agent with an immunomodulator may enhance the risk of infection and lymphoma.

- The decision to use a concurrent immunomodulator with anti-TNF therapy should be based on analysis of risks and benefits in each patient.

Introduction

Treatment with antitumor necrosis factor (anti-TNF) compounds has proven to be effective for induction and maintenance treatment of moderate-to-severe Crohn's disease (CD) and ulcerative colitis (UC). Three anti-TNF agents have been approved for use in CD in the United States: (1) infliximab (IFX), (2) adalimumab, and (3) certolizumab pegol. For the moment, only IFX has been approved for use in UC. When IFX was first introduced, concomitant immunomodulator therapy (typically with azathioprine (AZA) or 6-mercaptopurine (6-MP) was generally prescribed, principally with the rationale of reducing immunogenicity. When anti-TNF therapy is given "on demand," there is evidence that the addition of an immunomodulator decreases immunogenicity and prolongs response. There are less data that concomitant immunomodulation reduces immunogenicity when anti-TNFs are given on a scheduled basis, which is now considered standard of care. Over time, concerns have emerged about the safety of combination therapy, particularly the risks of infection and lymphoma. Recent data suggesting an advantage to combination treatment in biologic and immunomodulator naïve patients with CD has now generated significant uncertainty in this area. The risks and benefits of combination therapy are currently a source of considerable debate.

Efficacy of combination therapy

Early studies suggested that combination therapy reduces the immunogenicity of infliximab and decreases the formation of neutralizing antibodies (antibodies to infliximab, ATI) that are associated with an increased risk of infusion reactions and shorter duration of response to therapy [1]. This phenomenon appears most marked in patients receiving episodic therapy. However, anti-TNF drugs are now typically administered on a scheduled basis (e.g., every 8 weeks for infliximab), which enhances the long-term efficacy of biologic therapy and is associated with lower incidence

---

Clinical Dilemmas in Inflammatory Bowel Disease: New Challenges, Second Edition. Edited by P. Irving, C. Siegel, D. Rampton and F. Shanahan.
© 2011 Blackwell Publishing Ltd. Published 2011 by Blackwell Publishing Ltd.

of ATI formation [2]. This has called into question whether there is really any enhanced therapeutic effect when immunomodulation is given concurrently with scheduled anti-TNF treatment. A randomized controlled trial (RCT) of the impact of withdrawing concomitant immunosuppressives in CD patients receiving scheduled IFX did not show any clear benefit of continuing combination therapy beyond 6 months [3]. This study is often cited to justify the use of single agent anti-TNF treatment; however, it was significantly underpowered to find a difference in the main outcome and thus should be interpreted with caution.

However, post hoc analysis of data from large RCTs of anti-TNF agents would also seem to support the notion that monotherapy and combination therapy are equivalent. A combined analysis of outcomes across the ACCENT and ACT trials (four RCTs of IFX with 1383 patients randomized in total) did not show enhanced efficacy in the 40% of patients receiving concomitant immunomodulators [4]. Similarly, there is no evidence of improved responses with the other anti-TNF agents, adalimumab, or certolizumab pegol, in CD patients receiving concomitant immunomodulators [5,6], although immunomodulator therapy may prolong time to dose escalation for patients receiving adalimumab [7].

A number of larger RCTs were designed in order to specifically address the question of whether combined treatment confers any advantage in the era of scheduled maintenance anti-TNF therapy. The results have reignited debate on this subject. The COMMIT (Combination of Maintenance Methotrexate-Infliximab Trial) study of combination therapy failed to show an advantage for the use of concomitant MTX 25 mg weekly by subcutaneous injection [8]. Notably, all patients had received prednisone to induce remission and sustained remission rates were high with approximately 70% in both groups maintaining steroid-free remission to week 50 ($p = 0.63$).

The results of combined therapy with azathioprine in immunomodulator/biologic naïve CD appear different. The recent prospective data from SONIC (Study of Immunomodulators in Naïve patients with Crohn's disease) suggest that outcomes are improved up to 1 year with the combination of IFX and AZA versus either agent alone [9]. Steroid-free remission rates at week 26 were 30% (50/170) with AZA monotherapy, 44% (75/169) with IFX alone, and 57% (96/169) with combination therapy ($p < 0.001$ IFX + AZA versus AZA, $p = 0.006$ IFX alone versus AZA alone, $p = 0.022$ IFX + AZA versus IFX alone). Cor-

responding rates at week 50 were 28% (AZA monotherapy), 40% (IFX alone), and 56% (combination AZA/IFX). Endoscopic mucosal healing was also more frequent with combined therapy. It is worth noting certain limitations of the study, notably that AZA dosing was weight-based without metabolite monitoring, and that individuals with intermediate thiopurine methyltransferase (TPMT) activity were excluded; these individuals often achieve the highest 6-thioguanine (6-TG) levels on treatment, and so the effect of immunomodulator monotherapy may be underestimated. While a beneficial effect may be observed with combination therapy up to 1 year, there are data to suggest that there may be diminishing returns in the longer term [10]. The question of how long patients should remain on combination therapy remains unanswered for the moment.

Toxicity of combination therapy

While the results of the SONIC trial appear definitive, there remains reluctance on the part of many clinicians to adopt routine use of combination therapy in all patients, particularly in those naïve to immunomodulator and biologic therapy because of concerns about toxicity.

Infection

There has been concern from an early stage about the infection risk associated with anti-TNF, particularly serious infection with opportunistic pathogens, mycobacteria, and fungi. Such risks have promoted a cautious approach, which logically must be all the greater when two potent approaches to immune modulation are combined. Indeed, data have emerged highlighting enhanced risk of opportunistic infection with the combination of two or more immunosuppressant strategies [11]. This case-control study examined 100 IBD patients with opportunistic infection and highlighted increased infection risk individually with glucocorticoids, AZA/6-MP, and IFX. In multivariate analysis, while the use of any one of these agents enhanced infection risk with an odds ratio (OR) of 2.9 (95% confidence interval (CI) 1.5–5.3), use of two or more drugs yielded an OR of 14.5 (95% CI, 4.9–43), suggesting an effect that is at best additive, at worst synergistic. However, the majority of these infections were associated with the addition of corticosteroids and not the combination of IFX and AZA/6-MP. Furthermore, in both the SONIC and COMMIT trials the rates of serious infections were equal across the IFX monotherapy and combination therapy groups. Accordingly, it is still

TABLE 24.1 Summary of patient characteristics with the potential to influence a decision to use concomitant immunosuppression in a patient with Crohn's disease (CD)

Patient factors favoring use of combined therapy	Patient factors against use of combined therapy
Young age at disease onset	Young male
Requirement for steroid use at onset	Benign disease phenotype
Perianal disease/Rectal involvement	Limited disease
Extensive disease	Elderly with multiple comorbidities
Penetrating disease	Family history of lymphoma/leukemia
Early surgery/Multiple prior resections	Negative serology panel
Positive/high-titer serology panel	

unclear whether combination therapy increases the rate of serious infections.

Lymphoma

There is also concern about lymphoma risk with combination therapy. Concerns have particularly focused on the risk of hepatosplenic T-cell lymphoma (HSTCL), a rare form of lymphoma seen almost exclusively in young men receiving combination therapy and which is associated with a very poor prognosis [12]. While HSTCL may be exceptionally rare, enhanced risk of other forms of lymphoma may also be an issue. A recent meta-analysis has noted an increased risk of non-Hodgkin's lymphoma (NHL) in patients receiving anti-TNF therapy compared to the general population. Most were receiving combination therapy, and while the risk was not significantly different from that of patients receiving immunomodulator therapy alone, the relatively small number of cases ($n = 13$) may have made it difficult to detect any difference [13].

Conclusion

An individualized rather than a universal approach to the use of combination therapy probably constitutes the optimal strategy. Most of the useful data comes from patients with CD, and the role (if any) for combined immunosuppression in UC is unclear. Some individuals may be at increased risk of harm with combination therapy; young men in particular seem at increased risk of HSTCL when combination therapy is employed. It is also possible that older patients with comorbid illnesses may also be at increased risk of adverse events.

Conversely, some patients have an aggressive disease course and probably do best with early aggressive therapy in terms of limiting the risk of surgery and long-term disability. Patient characteristics with the potential to influence the threshold for use of a concomitant immunomodulator in CD are shown in Table 24.1. Clinical parameters associated with an aggressive CD phenotype have been identified—young age of onset, requiring prednisone at first flare, perianal disease, and smoking [14]. CD patients with extensive disease are at greater risk of losing significant length of bowel if surgery is necessary, and patients who have had surgery early in the course of their disease or have required multiple previous resections generally require a more aggressive approach to treatment. Early combined immunosuppression may be an advantageous approach in such individuals, and there is evidence to suggest that early aggressive therapy may improve outcomes [15]. However, better risk-stratification tools are required, and it is possible that serum markers, such as serology to microbial antigens, may help in selecting patients at high risk for progression and conversely in selecting low-risk patients in whom combination treatment may be not be justifiable. It would also be useful to identify biomarkers to select individuals at risk of adverse outcomes (particularly serious adverse outcomes such as infection and HSTCL). Future prospective studies would do well to address such issues of patient selection, with a view to greater individualization of therapeutic strategies in IBD. The more information we have in terms of this risk/benefit ratio, the better the decisions we can arrive at in partnership with our patients.

References

1. Baert F, Noman M, Vermeire S, et al. Influence of immunogenicity on the long-term efficacy of infliximab in Crohn's disease. *N Engl J Med* 2003; **348**(7): 601–608.
2. Rutgeerts P, Feagan BG, Lichtenstein GR, et al. Comparison of scheduled and episodic treatment strategies of infliximab in Crohn's disease. *Gastroenterology* 2004; **126**(2): 402–413.

3. Van Assche G, Magdelaine-Beuzelin C, D'Haens G, et al. Withdrawal of immunosuppression in Crohn's disease treated with scheduled infliximab maintenance: a randomized trial. *Gastroenterology* 2008; **134**(7): 1861–1868.

4. Lichtenstein GR, Diamond RH, Wagner CL, et al. Clinical trial: benefits and risks of immunomodulators and maintenance infliximab for IBD-subgroup analyses across four randomized trials. Aliment Pharmacol *Ther* 2009; **30**(3): 210–226.

5. Colombel JF, Sandborn WJ, Rutgeerts P, et al. Adalimumab for maintenance of clinical response and remission in patients with Crohn's disease: the CHARM trial. *Gastroenterology* 2007; **132**(1): 52–65.

6. Schreiber S, Khaliq-Kareemi M, Lawrance IC, et al. Maintenance therapy with certolizumab pegol for Crohn's disease. *N Engl J Med* 2007; **357**(3): 239–250.

7. Karmiris K, Paintaud G, Noman M, et al. Influence of trough serum levels and immunogenicity on long-term outcome of adalimumab therapy in Crohn's disease. *Gastroenterology* 2009; **137**(5): 1628–1640.

8. Feagan BG. A randomized trial of methotrexate in combination with infliximab for the treatment of Crohn's disease. *Gastroenterology* 2008; **134**(5): 294–296. (Abstract only).

9. Sandborn WJ. One year data from the Sonic Study: a randomized, double-blind trial comparing infliximab and infliximab plus azathioprine to azathioprine in patients with Crohn's disease naive to immunomodulators and biologic therapy. *Gastroenterology* 2009; **136**(5 Supp. 1): A116. (Abstract only).

10. Moss AC, Kim KJ, Fernandez-Becker N, Cury D, Cheifetz AS. Impact of concomitant immunomodulator use on long-term outcomes in patients receiving scheduled maintenance infliximab. *Dig Dis Sci* 2010; **55**(5): 1413–1420.

11. Toruner M, Loftus EV, Jr, Harmsen WS, et al. Risk factors for opportunistic infections in patients with inflammatory bowel disease. *Gastroenterology* 2008; **134**(4): 929–936.

12. Rosh JR, Gross T, Mamula P, Griffiths A, Hyams J. Hepatosplenic T-cell lymphoma in adolescents and young adults with Crohn's disease: a cautionary tale? *Inflamm Bowel Dis* 2007; **13**(8): 1024–1030.

13. Siegel CA, Marden SM, Persing SM, Larson RJ, Sands BE. Risk of lymphoma associated with combination anti-tumor necrosis factor and immunomodulator therapy for the treatment of Crohn's disease: a meta-analysis. *Clin Gastroenterol Hepatol* 2009; **7**(8): 874–881.

14. Beaugerie L, Seksik P, Nion-Larmurier I, Gendre JP, Cosnes J. Predictors of Crohn's disease. *Gastroenterology* 2006; **130**(3): 650–656.

15. D'Haens G, Baert F, van Assche G, et al. Early combined immunosuppression or conventional management in patients with newly diagnosed Crohn's disease: an open randomised trial. *Lancet* 2008; **371**(9613): 660–667.

25 How do we identify patients needing early aggressive therapy and what should we use?

Marc Ferrante and Séverine Vermeire

Department of Gastroenterology, University Hospital Gasthuisberg, Leuven, Belgium

LEARNING POINTS

- A subset of Crohn's disease patients might benefit from early aggressive therapy with immunomodulatory and biological drugs.

- Clinical predictors of poor outcome include young age at diagnosis, extensive small bowel disease, perianal disease, and the need for corticosteroids at diagnosis.

- Although some serologic and genetic predictors of disease progression have been identified, data are not ready to be implemented in daily clinical practice.

- Unless they have perianal disease, therapy with biological agents should be restricted to patients with clear signs of inflammation (increased C-reactive protein and/or endoscopic lesions).

- Combination therapy with a biological and an immunomodulator seems superior to either therapy alone.

Introduction

Recent clinical trials in Crohn's disease (CD) clearly illustrate that treatment with biological agents early in the disease course results in higher steroid-free remission rates and higher mucosal healing rates [1,2]. However, not all patients are good candidates for such a strategy as immunomodulators, and biological agents are not free from adverse events, including opportunistic infections and lymphomas. Therefore, predictors of complicated disease behavior are needed to help select those patients who will benefit most from early aggressive therapy.

Clinical factors identifying complicated disease

A number of clinical risk factors for complicated disease have been described. Beaugerie et al. defined a young age at diagnosis (< 40 years), the presence of perianal disease and the requirement for steroids at diagnosis as risk factors for a subsequent 5-year disabling course of CD [3]. This observation was partially confirmed by Loly et al., who identified ileocolonic involvement as another predictive factor of a disabling disease course [4]. Using another definition, these authors also demonstrated that stricturing behavior and weight loss at diagnosis were both predictive of a severe disease course. In a population-based cohort from New Zealand, perianal involvement at diagnosis was confirmed not only as predictive of complicated disease behavior but also of more rapid progression of CD [5].

Other clinical features that point towards more severe disease with a potential bad outcome include extensive small bowel involvement, deep ulcers at endoscopy, and the presence of growth failure in children. Unfortunately, in all studies, definitions for complicated, severe, and disabling CD vary, for example, from the need for two courses of steroids to formation of an ileostomy. Given the limitations of clinical factors in identifying patients at risk of a complicated disease course and in determining their likely response to treatment, serological and genetic markers have been explored as alternative predictors.

Clinical Dilemmas in Inflammatory Bowel Disease: New Challenges, Second Edition. Edited by P. Irving, C. Siegel, D. Rampton and F. Shanahan.
© 2011 Blackwell Publishing Ltd. Published 2011 by Blackwell Publishing Ltd.

Biomarkers for predicting complicated disease

In the past 20 years, several serologic markers have been associated with IBDs and CD in particular. These markers are antibodies directed against bacterial antigens, including anti-*Saccharomyces cerevisiae* antibodies (ASCA), anti-laminarobioside carbohydrate antibodies (ALCA), anti-laminarin carbohydrate antibodies (anti-L), anti-chitobioside carbohydrate antibodies (ACCA), anti-chitin carbohydrate antibody (anti-C), anti-mannobioside carbohydrate antibodies (AMCA), anti-outer membrane protein C of *Escherichia coli* antibodies (anti-OmpC), anti-*Pseudomonas fluorescens* antibodies (anti-I2), and anti-flagellin antibodies (CBir1). In ulcerative colitis (UC) a strong antibody response is found against neutrophil antigens (pANCA).

Although these serologic markers were originally investigated as a diagnostic tool, their clinical value may turn out to be their association with a complicated disease course and the need for abdominal surgery [6–10]. However, a conditio sine qua non before pronouncing on the predictive value of these markers is the stability of antibody responses over time. The observed increased antibody responses in CD patients with longer disease duration in a large Belgian cohort highlight the importance of prospective longitudinal studies [8]. Up to now, only one relatively small pediatric longitudinal study has reported a relation between the presence and titre of antibodies (ASCA, anti-OmpC, anti-I2, anti-CBir1) at a time when no fistula or strictures were clinically apparent and the subsequent development of complicated disease behavior during a median follow-up of 18 months [10] . We clearly need larger prospective trials to conclude on the predictive role of these serological markers.

Genetic markers of complicated disease

Compared to serologic factors, genetic factors are more appealing for risk stratification, since they are present long before the onset of the disease and before any environmental factor plays a role. In contrast to serologic factors, genetic factors remain stable over time and are unaffected by disease flares. Moreover, as several studies have correlated microbial seroreactivity with genetic mutations in pattern recognition receptors [11,12], genetic markers might well prove superior to antibodies for use in daily clinical practice. The presence of NOD2 variants has been associated with a shorter time to onset of stricturing disease as well as the need for surgery [13]. With the identification of several other susceptibility genes through genome-wide association scanning, the research on genetic markers and their role in disease progression has recently gained more attention. In a large Dutch cohort, Weersma et al. not only described a higher odds ratio (OR) for CD susceptibility with an increasing number of risk alleles and genotypes (NOD2, IBD5, DLG5, ATG16L1, IL23R), but also a more severe disease, a greater need for surgery and a younger age at onset [14]. Henckaerts et al. reported a higher risk of stricturing behavior in patient who were homozygous for the rs1363670 G-allele in *AK097548* gene located near the *IL-12B* gene and encoding for a hypothetical protein [15]. Furthermore, this GG genotype was associated with a shorter time to development of strictures, especially in patients with ileal involvement. In the same cohort, male patients carrying at least one rs12704036 T-allele in a gene desert had the shortest time to development of non-perianal fistula. Presence of a C-allele at the CDKAL1 rs6908425 SNP and absence of NOD2 variants were both independently associated with development of perianal fistula, particularly in smokers with colonic involvement. Of course, these retrospective cohort data need confirmation and the causal variants in these genes still need to be determined. Furthermore, genetic markers will probably never fully explain or predict evolution of disease because of the incomplete penetrance of phenotypes, the rather low absolute risk in the general population, and the role of environmental factors in shaping the disease. Accordingly, it is clear that genetic markers will need to be integrated with other molecular markers, clinical data, and environmental triggers.

What should we use in patients identified as requiring early aggressive therapy?

As indicated above, we need predictors not only of disease progression, but also of response to a more aggressive therapeutic strategy. The SONIC study has demonstrated the superiority of combination therapy with infliximab and azathioprine to azathioprine alone, and to infliximab alone, not only for induction and maintenance of remission, but also for achieving mucosal healing [2]. The importance of mucosal healing for the long-term outcome of patients was further illustrated by the 4-year follow-up data of the step-up and top-down study. In this study, Baert et al demonstrated that patients with mucosal healing at year 2 (observed more frequently in the patients randomized to top-down therapy with anti-TNF and azathioprine) more often remained in clinical remission and off steroids, in the following 2 years [16]. Therefore, if we do start early aggressive therapy with, for example, infliximab, combination therapy with azathioprine and the biological seems superior to either agent alone [2]. The benefit of combination therapy with adalimumab has not yet been explored.

The SONIC trial also clearly illustrated that biological therapy should be reserved for patients with active inflammation, who have either an elevated CRP level at baseline or clear signs of inflammation on imaging studies [2]. In patients without a raised CRP and with absence of endoscopic lesions, the steroid-free remission rates and mucosal healing rates were almost identical between the treatment groups.

Conclusion

In conclusion, clinical predictors of poor outcome in CD have been identified. Patients younger than 40 years at diagnosis, with extensive small bowel disease or perianal disease and needing corticosteroids at diagnosis have a significant risk of complicated disease behavior and will benefit from early aggressive therapy. The search for molecular markers to define and predict disease outcome in common diseases has moved forward rapidly with the help of modern technologies. However, we are not ready to implement this part of molecular research clinically, as many questions remain unanswered. Nevertheless, this research should be encouraged since our ultimate goal is to have at our disposal an individual molecular profile of the patient around the time of diagnosis (based on serum, DNA, tissue) that will allow us to choose the most appropriate management in terms of therapy, intensity of follow-up, and frequency of investigations.

References

1. D'Haens G, Baert F, Van Assche G, et al. Early combined immunosuppression or conventional management in patients with newly diagnosed Crohn's disease: an open randomised trial. *Lancet* 2008; **371**: 660–667.
2. Colombel JF, Sandborn WJ, Reinisch W, et al. Infliximab, azathioprine or combination therapy for Crohn's disease. *N Engl J Med* 2010; **362**: 1383–1395.
3. Beaugerie L, Seksik P, Nion-Larmurier I, Gendre JP, Cosnes J Predictors of Crohn's disease. *Gastroenterology* 2006; **130**: 650–656.
4. Loly C, Belaiche J, Louis E Predictors of severe Crohn's disease. *Scand J Gastroenterol* 2008; **43**: 948–954.
5. Tarrant KM, Barclay ML, Frampton CM, Gearry RB Perianal disease predicts changes in Crohn's disease phenotype-results of a population-based study of inflammatory bowel disease phenotype. *Am J Gastroenterol* 2008; **103**: 3082–3093.
6. Mow WS, Vasiliauskas EA, Lin YC, et al. Association of antibody responses to microbial antigens and complications of small bowel Crohn's disease. *Gastroenterology* 2004; **126**: 414–424.
7. Targan SR, Landers CJ, Yang H, et al. Antibodies to CBir1 flagellin define a unique response that is associated independently with complicated Crohn's disease. *Gastroenterology* 2005; **128**: 2020–2028.
8. Ferrante M, Henckaerts L, Joossens M, et al. New serological markers in inflammatory bowel disease are associated with complicated disease behaviour. *Gut* 2007, **56**: 1394–1403.
9. Seow CH, Stempak JM, Xu W, et al. Novel anti-glycan antibodies related to inflammatory bowel disease diagnosis and phenotype. *Am J Gastroenterol* 2009; **104**: 1426–1434.
10. Dubinsky MC, Lin YC, Dutridge D, et al. Serum immune responses predict rapid disease progression among children with Crohn's disease: immune responses predict disease progression. *Am J Gastroenterol* 2006; **101**: 360–367.
11. Devlin SM, Yang HY, Ippoliti A, et al. NOD2 variants and antibody response to microbial antigens in Crohn's disease patients and their unaffected relatives. *Gastroenterology* 2007; **132**: 576–586.
12. Henckaerts LC, Pierik M, Joossens M, Ferrante M, Rutgeerts PJ, Vermeire S: Mutations in pattern recognition receptor genes modulate seroreactivity to microbial antigens in patients with inflammatory bowel disease. *Gut* 2007; **56**: 1536–1542.
13. Alvarez-Lobos M, Arostegui JI, Sans M, et al. Crohn's disease patients carrying Nod2/CARD15 gene variants have an increased and early need for first surgery due to stricturing disease and higher rate of surgical recurrence. *Ann Surg* 2005; **242**: 693–700.
14. Weersma RK, Stokkers PC, van Bodegraven AA, et al. Molecular prediction of disease risk and severity in a large Dutch Crohn's disease cohort. *Gut* 2009; **58**: 388–395.
15. Henckaerts L, Van Steen K, Verstreken I, et al. Genetic risk profiling and prediction of disease course in Crohn's disease patients. *Clin Gastroenterol Hepatol* 2009; **7**: 972–980.
16. Baert F, Moortgat L, Van Assche G, et al. Mucosal healing predicts sustained clinical remission in patients with early-stage Crohn's disease. *Gastroenterology* 2010; **138**: 463–468.

26 What is the role of biologics in UC?

Joanna K. Law and Brian Bressler

Division of Gastroenterology, University of British Columbia, Vancouver, BC, Canada

> **LEARNING POINTS**
>
> - Antitumor necrosis factor-alpha (anti-TNF-α) agents are the only biologic therapy with high quality evidence supporting their use in ulcerative colitis (UC).
>
> - There is increasing evidence for the use of anti-TNF-α therapy in the treatment of moderate-to-severe UC in the outpatient setting.
>
> - When used as a rescue therapy, infliximab is probably most effective when used early in the nonfulminant patient.
>
> - The evidence for combined immunosuppresion is limited in UC.

Introduction

The severity of ulcerative colitis (UC) varies with some patients requiring only 5-aminosalicylates to maintain remission, while others may have disease resistant to corticosteroids and/or immunomodulators. Patients who fail these therapies have traditionally needed surgery, but emerging evidence suggests that appropriate introduction of other therapies, such as anti-TNF agents, may reduce the need for hospitalization and for surgery in patients with moderate-to-severe UC.

When to initiate a biologic for UC

Outpatient setting

Many patients with mild-to-moderate UC will not require steroids or immunomodulators, but high-risk patients refractory to these treatments may benefit from infliximab to avoid further steroid use, hospitalization, and colectomy. Standard outpatient therapy for active UC generally begins with 5-aminosalicylates followed by oral corticosteroids if needed. Steroid response rate at 30 days is 80% [1], but at 1 year 25% of patients become corticosteroid-dependent and 30% require alternative medical therapy or surgery [2]. Approximately 15% of patients with UC will experience a severe episode requiring hospitalization and intravenous (IV) corticosteroids [3].

In the large ACT 1 and ACT 2 studies, patients with moderate-to-severe active UC were randomized to receive either infliximab or placebo. Approximately 55% of patients had extensive disease, while the remainder had left-sided disease. Seventy-two percent of patients were receiving 5-aminosalicylates, 56% were receiving corticosteroids, and 46% were receiving immunosuppressants at baseline. These studies demonstrated that patients treated with infliximab at weeks 0, 2, and 6 and every 8 weeks thereafter at either 5 mg/kg or 10 mg/kg were more likely to have a clinical response at week 30 than those receiving placebo (62% versus 36%)[4]. Eight out of 79 patients (10%) discontinued steroids in the placebo group versus 31/143 (22%) in the treatment arm. At 54 weeks, 7/79 (9%) remained steroid-free in the placebo group compared to 30/143 (21%) in the combined treatment arms. Furthermore, these studies demonstrated higher rates of mucosal healing (Mayo subscore of 0 or 1 that allows for mild friability on endoscopy) in the treatment arms at weeks 8 and 30 in ACT 1 and ACT 2 and at week 54 in ACT 1, when compared to placebo. They also demonstrated the efficacy and safety of an induction

Clinical Dilemmas in Inflammatory Bowel Disease: New Challenges, Second Edition. Edited by P. Irving, C. Siegel, D. Rampton and F. Shanahan.
© 2011 Blackwell Publishing Ltd. Published 2011 by Blackwell Publishing Ltd.

regimen of three doses and regular maintenance of infliximab 5 mg/kg for patients with moderate-to-severe UC in the outpatient setting for 54 weeks. Both hospitalizations and colectomy (17% placebo versus 10% treatment) rates were significantly reduced in the group of patients receiving infliximab [5].

In patients failing outpatient oral corticosteroid therapy, the next step is generally hospitalization for IV steroids, cyclosporine, or surgery. In one long-term follow-up of 121 patients with refractory UC, who would have otherwise required hospitalization for IV steroids, outpatient treatment with infliximab was initiated. The authors demonstrated that two-thirds of these patients had an initial clinical response with 68% of those responding and demonstrating a sustained clinical response [6]. Seventeen percent of these patients went on to colectomy—the absence of short-term clinical response, baseline C-reactive protein (CRP) level $\geq$5mg/L and previous treatment with IV corticosteroids and/or cyclosporine were all independent predictors of colectomy.

Hospitalized patients

Various small studies have looked at infliximab for hospitalized patients. One randomized placebo-controlled study of 45 patients failing IV steroid compared treatment with infliximab or placebo on days 4 through 8 of admission [7]. The study found a significant difference in colectomy rates, with 29% in the infliximab group compared with 67% in the placebo group undergoing surgery by 70 days. However, in patients with the most severe disease, there was no difference in colectomy rates.

Proposed use of infliximab for the hospitalized severe UC patient

Previous literature has identified simple predictors of patients who will respond poorly to IV corticosteroid therapy [8]. Based on these parameters, the decision to escalate therapy should be made as early as day 3 of treatment. Traditionally, the only options for these patients have been cyclosporine or colectomy. The role of rescue therapy with infliximab in this situation is gaining interest, but it is becoming evident that its role is primarily in the patient with UC that is not fulminant. In one study presented in abstract form, patients were randomized to intravenous cyclosporin (2mg/kg/d) or infliximab if they had failed intravenous steroids for acute severe hospitalized ulcerative colitis [20]. In this intention to treat analysis, 111

patients were randomized and rates of treatment failure were 60% and 54% for cylcosporin and infliximab, respectively (p = 0.49) with response rate at 7 days of 84% and 86% (p = 0/75) with 10 patients in the cyclosporin (18%) and 13 in the infliximab (23%) group required colectomy. The authors concluded that cyclosporin is not more effective that infliximab in severe ulcerative colitis to achieve short term remission or avoid urgent colectomy.

Which drug(s) to initiate

Combined immunosuppression? (see Chapter 26)

The role of combined immunosuppressive therapy when using biologic therapy has two potential benefits that may lead not only to additive but also synergistic effects. First, the immunomodulator has its own efficacy in treating UC. Second, when combination therapy is used formation of anti-TNF antibodies is reduced, which influences trough levels of biologics. The presence of infliximab when trough levels are determined has recently been shown to be a predictor of clinical remission [9]. The UC SUCCESS trial, presented at the 2011 European Crohn's and Colitis Organization meeting, randomized 231 patients with moderate-severe UC failing corticosteroids to one of three treatment arms: azathioprine + placebo; infliximab + placebo; or infliximab + azathioprine. At week 16, patients in the combination therapy group were more likely to have achieved steroid-free remission compared to monotherapy while response and mucosal healing were more likely in the infliximab-treated arms [18]. Since combined immunosuppression has been shown to increase the risk of infectious complications (odds ratio (OR) 2.7, confidence interval (CI) 1.1–6.7)[10] albeit largely driven by the use of corticosteroids rather than the combined use of immunomodulators and anti-TNF. This study [18] suggests that there is an increase in hepatobiliary events in the azathioprine arm (16.46% vs 3.85% and 6.25% in the IFX and IFX + AZA groups, respectively).

Which biologic?

The ACT 1 and ACT 2 studies demonstrate that infliximab is effective and safe when used to induce and maintain remission in patients with UC. The role of short-term infliximab as a bridge to azathioprine therapy or sequential therapy (i.e., cyclosporine then infliximab or vice versa) is unknown, although one small study demonstrated a modest response but significant adverse events including one death suggested that the risks of this strategy outweighs the benefits [11]. At the time of publication, seven randomized controlled trials (RCTs) have looked at the efficacy of infliximab in patients with moderate-to-severe UC, but no trials have yet been published on other anti-TNF agents [12]. The results of a Phase 3 multicenter, randomized, placebo-controlled study comparing the efficacy and safety of two dosing regimens for induction of remission with adalimumab in patients with moderately to severely active UC was recently presented in abstract form. The primary end point of clinical remission at week 8 demonstrated that adalimumab 160/80 was more effective (18.5%) compared to placebo (9.2%, $p = 0.031$) [13]. Efficacy and safety of adalimumab for induction and maintenance of clinical remission in patients with moderate-to-severe UC was presented at the 2011 Digestive Diseases Meeting. 248 patients received adalimumab in an intention to treat (ITT) study and when compared to placebo, adalimumab was more likely to induce remission at weeks 8 and 52 (16.5% and 17.3% vs 9.3% and 8.5%)[19]. There were no new safety concerns than those previously published. In a Phase 2 multicenter study, a humanized antiadhesion molecule to alpha4 beta7 integrin used in patients with active UC was more likely to induce remission than placebo (33% versus 14%) [14].

The use of biologics around the time of surgery

Perioperative use (see Chapter 43)

In one retrospective case-control study of infliximab-treated patients requiring a colectomy, the risks of sepsis, late complications, and the requirement of a 3-stage procedure were greater in patients who had received infliximab, prompting concerns relating to infliximab exposure [15]. However, other studies of infliximab-treated patients, demonstrated no difference in postoperative complications following infliximab exposure [16].

Postoperative use

There is growing evidence to support the use of infliximab in refractory pouchitis with one study demonstrating response in 88% of patients treated with infliximab and concomitant immunomodulators [17] (see Chapter 43).

Conclusions

Infliximab is the only biologic currently with evidence for its use in patients with moderate-to-severe UC. Its present role is in patients who have failed conventional medical therapy; it has demonstrated efficacy and safety when used in the outpatient setting as either monotherapy or concomitant therapy for patients already on 5-aminosalicylates, immunomodulators, or corticosteroids. Use of infliximab in the inpatient setting is evolving, but its benefit may be greatest when used early in the hospitalized patient with severe colitis.

References

1. Baron JH, Connell AM, Kanaghinis TG, et al. Outpatient treatment of ulcerative colitis. Comparison between three doses of oral prednisone. *Br Med J* 1962; **18**: 441–443.
2. Baudet A, Rahmi G, Bretagne AL, et al. Severe ulcerative colitis: present medical treatment strategies. *Expert Opin Pharmacother* 2008; **9**: 447–457.
3. Turner D, Walsh CA, Steinhart AH, et al. Response to corticosteroids in severe ulcerative colitis: a systematic review of the literature and a meta-regression. *Clin Gastroenterol Hepatol* 2007; **5**: 103–110.
4. Rutgeerts P, Sandborn WJ, Feagan BG, et al. Infliximab for induction and maintenance therapy for ulcerative colitis. *N Engl J Med* 2005; **353**: 2462–2476.
5. Sandborn WJ, Rutgeerts P, Feagan BG, et al. Colectomy rate comparison after treatment of ulcerative colitis with placebo or infliximab. *Gastroenterology* 2009; **137**: 1250–1260.
6. Ferrante M, Vermeire S, Fidder H, et al. Long-term outcome after infliximab for refractory ulcerative colitis. *J Crohn's Colitis* 2008; **2**: 219–225.
7. Jarnerot G, Hertervig E, Friis-Liby I, et al. Infliximab as rescue therapy in severe to moderately-severe ulcerative colitis: a randomized, placebo-controlled study. *Gastroenterol* 2005; **128**: 1805–1811.
8. Travis SPL, Farrant Jm, Ricketts C, et al. Predicting outcome in severe ulcerative colitis. *Gut* 1996; **38**: 905–910.
9. Seow CH, Newman A, Irwin SP, et al. Trough serum infliximab: a predictive factor of clinical outcome for infliximab treatment in acute ulcerative colitis. *Gut* 2010; **59**: 49–54.
10. Selvasekar CR, Clima RR, Larson DW, et al. Effect of infliximab on short-term complications in patients undergoing operation for chronic ulcerative colitis. *J Am Coll Surg* 2007; **205**: e3–e4.
11. Maser EA, Deconda D Lichtiger S, et al. Cyclosporine and infliximab as rescue therapy for each other in patients with

steroid-refractory ulcerative colitis. *Clin Gastroenterol Hepatol* 2008; **6**: 1112–1116.

12. Lawson MM, Thomas AG, Akobeng AK. Tumor necrosis factor alpha blocking agents for induction of remission in ulcerative colitis. *Cochrane Database Syst Rev* 2006; **3**: CD005112.

13. Reinisch W, Sandborn W, Hommes D, et al. *Adalimumab for Induction of Clinical Remission in Moderately to Severely Active Ulcerative Colitis.* European Crohn's & Colitis Organization meeting abstracts; 2010.

14. Feagan BG, Greenberg GR, Wild G, et al. Treatment of ulcerative colitis with a humanized antibody to alpha4beta6 integrin. *N Engl J Med* 2005; **353**: 1180–1181.

15. Mor IJ, Vogel JD, da Luz Moreira A, et al. Infliximab in ulcerative colitis is associated with an increased risk of postoperative complications after restorative proctocolectomy. *Dis Colon Rectum* 2008; **51**: 1202–1207.

16. Bordeianou L, Kunitake H, Shellito P. Preoperative infliximab treatment in patients with ulcerative and indeterminate colitis does not increase rate of conversion to emergent and multistep abdominal surgery. *Int J Colorectal Dis* 2009; epub.

17. Ferrante M, D'Haens G, Dewit O, et al. Efficacy of infliximab in refractory pouchitis and Crohn's disease-related complications of the pouch: a Belgian case series. *Inflamm Bowel Dis* 2009; epub.

18. Panaccione R, Ghosh S, Middelton S, et al. Infliximab, azathioprine, or infliximab + azathioprine for treatment of moderate to severe ulcerative colitis : The UC SUCCESS trial. In ECCO Congress Abstracts; 2011 Feb 24–26; Dublin, Ireland. *Journal of Crohn's & Colitis* 2011; **5**(1); Abstract OP13.

19. Sandborn WJ, Van Assche G, Reinsch W, et al. Induction and Maintenance of Clinical REmission by Adalimumab in Patients with Moderate-to-Severe Ulcerative Colitis. In DDW Abstracts; 2011 May 7–10; Chicago, IL. *Gastroenterology* 2011; **140**(5). Abstract #744.

20. Laharie D, Bourreille A, Branche J, et al. Cyclosporin versus Infliximab in Severe Acute Ulcerative Colitis Refractory to Intravenous Steroids: A randomized trial. In DDW Abstracts; 2011 May 7–10; Chicago IL. *Gastroenterology* 2011; **140**(5). Abstract #619.

What can we do with Crohn's patients who fail or lose response to anti-TNF therapy?

David T. Rubin

Inflammatory Bowel Disease Center, University of Chicago Medical Center, Chicago, IL, USA

LEARNING POINTS

- Patients who are considered for anti-TNF therapy should have careful assessment to exclude irritable bowel, infection, and fibrostenotic obstruction prior to the initiation of therapy or when loss of response is suspected.

- Response to anti-TNF therapy is greater in patients with shorter disease duration.

- In patients naïve to immune suppressants and prior biologic therapies, combination therapy with azathioprine and infliximab is superior to either therapy alone.

- Assessment of loss of response to infliximab using serum infliximab levels and antibodies to infliximab can guide decisions regarding dose adjustments and switching to alternative anti-TNF therapies.

- There is little evidence to favor switching to a second anti-TNF therapy after primary nonresponse to loading doses of the first anti-TNF therapy. In such cases, alternative methods of disease control or surgery should be considered.

The development of anti-TNF therapies for Crohn's disease (CD) represented a major revolution in available treatment options for patients with moderately to severely active luminal CD, or with perianal fistulizing disease. Patients who respond to biologic therapies enjoy an improvement in symptoms, a better quality of life, less disability, fatigue and depression, and fewer surgeries and hospitalizations.

There are currently three anti-TNF therapies available in the US (infliximab, adalimumab and certolizumab pegol), and two that are available in Canada and most of Europe (infliximab and adalimumab). Despite the benefits demonstrated with these therapies, there remain a number of clinical challenges, including positioning them at the right time in the treatment algorithm, maximizing their effectiveness, and assessing the patient who either fails to respond or loses response to these therapies. This chapter outlines an approach to patients who fail to respond, or lose response to anti-TNF therapy.

When considering how to deal with the patient who has failed to respond or loses response to anti-TNF therapy, it is important to ensure that appropriate patients are treated and that their chance of responding is maximized.

Treat the patient earlier in their disease course

By virtue of the design of the clinical trials that led to FDA and EMA approvals, Crohn's patients were moderately to severely ill and had failed other medical therapies before receiving the anti-TNF therapy. Therefore, the labeled indication of these agents was for moderately to severely active CD *after failure of conventional treatments*. These labels not only resulted in the constricted use of these therapies, as physicians often waited until patients failed most other therapies before considering anti-TNF therapy, but also contributed to the perception that anti-TNF therapies are *unconventional*. The natural result of "saving" anti-TNF

Clinical Dilemmas in Inflammatory Bowel Disease: New Challenges, Second Edition. Edited by P. Irving, C. Siegel, D. Rampton and F. Shanahan.
© 2011 Blackwell Publishing Ltd. Published 2011 by Blackwell Publishing Ltd.

therapy for the sicker patients who fail other therapies is their use in patients with longer duration of disease. More recent analyses, however, have suggested that patients with shorter disease duration are more likely to respond to anti-TNF therapies.

A study of pediatric patients (under age 17 years) who received infliximab demonstrated substantially higher response and remission rates (REACH: 88% response, 59% remission [1]) than a study of similar design for adult patients with longer disease duration (ACCENT 1: 67% response, 39% remission [2]). Post hoc analysis of the adult trials also demonstrated a trend toward higher response rates in patients with shorter disease duration [3,4]. Therefore, one of the key strategies for maximizing the likelihood of response to an anti-TNF appears to be treating earlier in the disease course, and not "saving" anti-TNF therapies for the patients who fail everything and have suffered from years of untreated or ineffectively treated disease.

Nonetheless, the balance between potential benefit, fear of risks and desire by a physician to preserve the TNF-inhibitor therapy for a time when other therapies have already failed are all significant challenges to making such decisions. More recent emphasis on prognostic markers in Crohn's patients and selection of patients with the potential for poor outcomes (hospitalization, disability, surgery) have led to selection of specific Crohn's patients for earlier use of anti-TNF therapies [5,6].

Use concomitant immune modulation and commit to maintenance therapy

As proteins, all of the biologic therapies have the potential to generate an immune response, and this immunogenicity may be associated with reactions to the drug and attenuation of response. Although this has best been described with infliximab, it likely occurs with all biologic therapies, regardless of how "humanized" they are. A number of strategies for minimization of immunogenicity have been described and recommended, including using loading doses to "tolerize" the immune system, commitment to maintenance therapy, and use of concomitant immunomodulator therapy [7] (see Chapter 24). Although concerns about increased risks of infection and lymphoma with combination therapy are still justified, the long-term benefit of stable medical therapy remains important and must be weighed against such rare side effects.

Confirm active inflammation

Patients with CD may have symptoms and appear to be failing therapies due to multiple mechanisms. It is imperative that the patient with suspected active CD be assessed in an objective and reliable manner before abandoning a treatment strategy. This evaluation should confirm the presence of active inflammation and exclude such common confounders as fibrostenotic disease with bowel obstruction, infection (especially CMV and *Clostridium difficile*), and overlapping irritable bowel syndrome.

Defining primary nonresponse to anti-TNF therapy

In the assessment of non-response to anti-TNF therapy, distinction between primary nonresponse and secondary loss of response is essential. The general approach to initiating therapy with a TNF inhibitor in CD includes loading doses of therapy. **Primary nonresponse** may be defined as nonresponse to infliximab at week 6 after induction dosing of 5 mg/kg at weeks 0 and 2. In the clinical trials, there was little added benefit demonstrated from a third infusion at week 6. Whether an additional dose of 10 mg/kg at week 6 in such patients will capture some patients is untested. For adalimumab and certolizumab pegol, a similar approach of assessing their response after two loading doses should be taken.

Management of the Patient with Primary Nonresponse to TNF inhibitors

At least one-third of patients do not respond initially to an anti-TNF therapy, and many of these have already failed steroids, 6-mercaptopurine/azathioprine, and methotrexate. If primary nonresponse occurs, it seems likely that TNF inhibition may not be effective and alternative strategies should be considered although it may be reasonable to consider a trial of infliximab in primary non-responders to adalimumab or certolizumab pegol on the basis that the intravenous delivery or weight-based dosing may matter for some patients. However, there is no evidence to support this practice, and exposing patients to the risk of a therapy whose mechanism is not effective has not been recommended.

Unfortunately, there is no published controlled trial that looks at anti-TNF primary non-responders. In reviewing medical options for these patients, review of previous therapies and confirmation that their previous treatments were optimized and given for an appropriate amount of time is important. If the patient has exhausted the "conventional" therapies already, natalizumab (where available) may be considered. In clinical trials of natalizumab, post-hoc analysis of the patients who were TNF-naïve compared with those who were previously treated with anti-TNF therapy revealed that there was equal likelihood of response to natalizumab (TNF-naïve remission rate: 55%, TNF-exposed remission rate: 50%) [8]. However, concerns about the risk of progressive multifocal leukoencephalopathy and the availability of this therapy in many parts of the world limit this as an option. Therefore, offering patients ethically appropriate clinical trials is another option. Unfortunately, other off-label medical options (like antibiotics or other immune suppressive therapies) are insufficiently tested in this setting.

A surgical approach must always be considered. A simple resection with primary anastomosis or proctocolectomy with permanent end ileostomy may be a durable, medication-free solution, and the benefits of this approach must be weighed carefully compared to the risks of ongoing medical therapies.

Management of the patient with secondary loss of response or simple relapse

In contrast, the patient who clearly responds to loading and/or maintenance dosing of their first TNF inhibitor and suffers a relapse (*secondary loss of response*) should be reassessed carefully. Patients having ongoing response to maintenance dosing with breakthrough symptoms prior to the next dose, suggesting attenuation of response, are likely to respond to a decrease in the dosing interval or an increase of the dose of anti-TNF agent). On the other hand, patients who have been stable for some time on maintenance therapy who develop active symptoms and recurrent disease that does not respond at all to a dose of anti-TNF may be suffering from a relapse, an infection, fibrostenosis and obstruction, or a problem that is not Crohn's-related. These patients especially require careful review and may ultimately benefit from returning to stable dosing of their original TNF inhibitor. (See Figures 27.1a and b.)

If the patient is on infliximab, drug and antibody levels may be obtained at least 3 weeks after an infusion, although measurement at the nadir, prior to the next infusion is preferred. If infliximab levels are undetectable, it suggests that the drug is being cleared too rapidly. Although seen in patients on stable maintenance dosing, this occurs more often in the patients who received episodic treatment with infliximab or were induced without concomitant immune modulation. Reducing the interval and possibly increasing the dose may improve this pharmacokinetic challenge. Recently, the Mayo Clinic retrospectively reviewed their approach to this problem in 155 patients. They found that in patients with anti-infliximab antibodies, switching to another TNF inhibitor was an effective strategy, with 11/12 patients having a complete or partial response. In patients with subtherapeutic infliximab levels (<12 mcg/mL), 25/29 patients responded to increasing the dose of infliximab, while 2/6 patients responded to switching to another TNF inhibitor [9]. Application of this strategy with the other anti-TNF inhibitors would in theory be similar, provided that such levels could be commercially obtained.

A placebo controlled double blind trial of switching to adalimumab after loss of response or intolerance to infliximab among patients who were previous responders, demonstrated a recapture remission rate at 4 weeks of 21% [10]. Open label follow-up of such patients demonstrated a 40% remission rate at 1 year [11]. Similar results have been found when patients who are previous infliximab responders are switched to certolizumab pegol. An open label trial demonstrated 39% remission at 6 weeks after switching therapy to certolizumab [12]. For those patients who do not respond to such a within-class switching strategy, a different biologic target, methotrexate, or surgery may be necessary. (See Table 27.1.)

Conclusions

In summary, patients with active CD need a careful evaluation to confirm active inflammation and rule out other confounders or conditions before initiation of anti-TNF therapy. In the patient who fails to respond to loading doses of their first anti-TNF drug, alternative methods of disease control (if available) or surgery should be considered. In the patient who responds to anti-TNF therapy and then loses response, the clinician should first distinguish between attenuation of response due to changing pharmacokinetic behavior and a simple disease relapse. In the first situation, drug levels and antibodies to drug (when they are available), may be used to guide the decision between dose adjustment and changing medications within class. In the

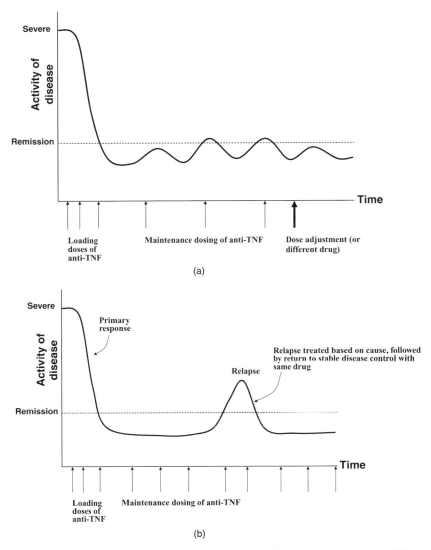

FIGURE 27.1 (a) Secondary loss of response due to attenuation/immunogenicity requires dose change or different drug. (b) Secondary loss of response due to relapse recaptured with treatment of cause.

TABLE 27.1 Interpretation and assessment of infliximab and antibody levels in Crohn's patients losing response (measurement of trough level at nadir or when patient is symptomatic at least 3 weeks post infusion)

Infliximab level	Antibodies to infliximab	Treatment recommendation
Therapeutic	Absent	Switch treatment mechanism
Therapeutic	Present	Unclear. Consider switching to another TNF-inhibitor
Sub-therapeutic	Absent	Adjust dose and/or interval of infliximab
Sub-therapeutic	Present	Switch to another TNF-inhibitor

Source: Adapted from [8].
Note: "Therapeutic" levels are assumed to be >12 mcg/mL.

second situation, it remains possible that a short duration change in management may result in recapture and return to stable disease control. There is a clear need for additional studies of drug optimization and efficient utilization of resources as newer therapies become available.

References

1. Hyams J, Crandall W, Kugathasan S, et al. Induction and maintenance infliximab therapy for the treatment of moderate-to-severe Crohn's disease in children. *Gastroenterology* 2007; **132**(3): 863–873; quiz 1165–6. Epub 2006 Dec 3.

2. Hanauer SB, Feagan BG, Lichtenstein GR, et al. Maintenance infliximab for Crohn's disease: the ACCENT I randomised trial. Lancet 2002; **359**: 1541–1549.

3. Schreiber S, Reinisch W, Colombel JF, et al. Early Crohn's disease shows high levels of remission to therapy with adalimumab: sub-analysis of CHARM. DDW 2007: #985. *Gastroenterology* 2007; **132**(4 Suppl 2): A-147.

4. Schreiber S, Khaliq-Kareemi M, Lawrance IC, et al. Maintenance therapy with certolizumab pegol for Crohn's disease. *N Engl J Med* 2007; **357**(3): 239–250.

5. Beaugerie L, Seksik P, Nion-Larmurier I, et al. Predictors of Crohn's disease. *Gastroenterology* 2006; **130**(3): 650–656.

6. Dubinsky MC, Kugathasan S, Mei L, et al. Increased immune reactivity predicts aggressive complicating Crohn's disease in children. *Clin Gastroenterol Hepatol* 2008; **6**(10): 1105–1111. Epub 2008 Jul 10.

7. Hanauer SB, Wagner CL, Bala M, et al. Incidence and importance of antibody responses to infliximab after maintenance or episodic treatment in Crohn's disease. *Clin Gastroenterol Hepatol* 2004; **2**(7): 542–553.

8. Sandborn WJ, Colombel JF, Enns R, et al. Natalizumab induction and maintenance therapy for Crohn's disease. *N Engl J Med* 2005; **353**(18): 1912–1925. (post-hoc data on file, Elan Pharmaceuticals, San Francisco, Ca.)

9. Afif W, Loftus EV Jr, Faubion WA, et al. Clinical utility of measuring infliximab and human anti-chimeric antibody concentrations in patients with inflammatory bowel disease. *Am J Gastroenterol* 2010; **105**(5): 1133–1139. Epub 2010 Feb 9.

10. Sandborn WJ, Rutgeerts P, Enns R, et al. Adalimumab induction therapy for Crohn's disease previously treated with infliximab: a randomized trial. *Ann Intern Med* 2007; **146**: 829–838.

11. Panaccione R, Sandborn WJ, D'Haens G, et al. Adalimumab maintains long-term remission in moderately to severely active Crohn's disease after infliximab failure: 1-year follow-up of Gain trial. DDW 2008: #920. *Gastroenterology* 2008; **134**(4 Suppl 1): A-133.

12. Sandborn WJ, Abreu MT, D'Haens G, et al. Certolizumab pegol in patients with moderate to severe Crohn's disease and secondary failure to infliximab. *Clin Gastroenterol Hepatol* 2010; **8**(8): 688–695.e2. Epub 2010 May 6.

28 Which extraintestinal manifestations of IBD respond to biologics?

Tina A. Mehta and Chris S.J. Probert

Department of Gastroenterology, Bristol Royal Infirmary, Bristol, Avon, UK

> **LEARNING POINTS**
>
> - Where the activity of extraintestinal manifestations (EIMs) parallels that of IBD (erythema nodosum, peripheral arthritis, and episcleritis) the response to anti-TNF is generally good.
> - Pyoderma gangrenosum is the only EIM for which there is controlled evidence of efficacy for an anti-TNF agent.

About a third of patients with IBD develop extraintestinal manifestations (EIMs) affecting the joints, skin, mouth, eyes, liver, and biliary tree [1,2]. The use of biologics in many of these conditions is in its infancy, with few randomized trials having been reported. We review the evidence for the efficacy of biologics in treating EIMs.

The pathogenesis of EIMs is multifactorial, including genetic, environmental, and immunological factors; a shared epitope between the gastrointestinal tract and the other sites is thought to lead to an immune mediated attack at extraintestinal sites. Thus, drugs that are broadly immunosuppressive, or which suppress the immune response in the intestine, as well as sites of EIM, are likely to be effective for IBD as well as EIMs. Some biologic agents have shown efficacy against EIMs; at present these are mainly anti-TNF agents designed to suppress TNF-mediated diseases, including arthritis.

Musculoskeletal EIMs

Musculoskeletal EIMs occur in 30% of IBD patients and can be divided into peripheral arthropathies, sacroiliitis, and ankylosing spondylitis.

There are two types of peripheral arthropathy. Type 1 affects <5 large joints; it is an acute, self-limiting arthropathy, which is strongly associated with other EIMs, and occurs alongside intestinal inflammation. Type 2 affects >5 peripheral joints; it runs a prolonged course independent of gut inflammation, and is associated with uveitis only. Axial arthropathies, including ankylosing spondylitis and sacroiliitis, present as lower back pain and stiffness in the morning; they improve with exercise, are more common in smokers and are often independent of intestinal inflammation. Treatment is traditionally with NSAIDS and COX-2 inhibitors, but these may exacerbate IBD; sulfasalazine, steroids and methotrexate are often used.

Infliximab, adalimumab and etanercept have each demonstrated efficacy in ankylosing spondylitis in rheumatological studies of non-IBD associated disease; the National Institute for Clinical Excellence recommends adalimumab or etanercept. Infliximab has been reported to show efficacy in IBD-associated joint disease in several small case series [3–6]. An open nonrandomized study of 24 Crohn's disease patients with spondyloarthropathy, of whom 16 had active intestinal disease, assessed induction with infliximab and, if remission was achieved, maintenance; there was a statistically significant benefit in spinal pain and arthritis [7]. A small retrospective study found clinical benefit in spondyloarthropathy when patients were switched to adalimumab after being intolerant of or losing response to infliximab [8]. Etanercept is effective in ankylosing spondylitis, but not effective in IBD. There is no randomized controlled data for infliximab or adalimumab in other IBD-related joint diseases.

Clinical Dilemmas in Inflammatory Bowel Disease: New Challenges, Second Edition. Edited by P. Irving, C. Siegel, D. Rampton and F. Shanahan.
© 2011 Blackwell Publishing Ltd. Published 2011 by Blackwell Publishing Ltd.

TABLE 28.1 EIMs of IBD in which biological therapy (shown in bold) may be efficacious

	Extraintestinal manifestation	Course parallel to IBD	Recommended treatments	Citations	Level of evidence for biologic
Joints	Sacroileitis Ankylosing spondylitis	No	Physiotherapy Sulfasalazine Methotrexate **Infliximab** **Adalimumab**	Kaufman, 2005 Antivalli, 2008	Case series
	Type 1 large joint peripheral arthropathy	Yes	Steroids oral or intraarticular Sulfasalazine	Generini, 2004 Herfarth, 2002	Case series
	Type 2 small joint peripheral arthropathy	No	Immunomodulators **Infliximab**		
Skin	Pyoderma gangrenosum	No	Oral steroids Ciclosporin **Infliximab**	Brooklyn, 2006	RCT
	Erythema nodosum	Yes	Treatment of IBD flare **Infliximab**		Case reports
	Sweets syndrome		Steroids **Infliximab**	Vanbiervliet, 2002	Case report
	Aphthous ulcers		Topical steroids Oral steroids **Infliximab**	Kaufman, 2005	Case series
Liver	PSC	No	Transplant		
Eyes	Uveitis	No	Steroids ciclosporin **Infliximab**	Fries, 2002	Case report
	Episcleritis	Yes	Topical steroids		

Skin manifestations

Skin manifestations occur in up to 20% of IBD patients.

Pyoderma gangrenosum

Pyoderma gangrenosum classically presents in the ulcerative form as pain, a pustule and then a rapidly developing painful ulcer with a serpiginous bluish edge, often on extensor surfaces, especially the legs. It can be peristomal or perianal and 50% of patients have pathergy [1]. It occurs in up to 2% of IBD patients with equal sex distribution. Treatment includes moist wound management, topical steroids, topical tacrolimus, and intralesional steroids. High-dose, prolonged courses of oral steroids and ciclosporin are the best documented treatments; azathioprine, sulfasalazine, tacrolimus, and minocycline have also been used.

In 2006, the first multicentre, randomized controlled trial of any treatment in pyoderma gangrenosum showed that infliximab, in 30 patients of whom 19 had IBD, pro-

duced a statistically significant advantage over placebo [9]: 69% had a beneficial clinical response. Case reports of the use of other biologics include adalimumab and etanercept [10,11].

Erythema nodosum

Erythema nodosum presents as multiple, bilateral, warm, tender violaceous nodules on the shins, but can occur on the calves, trunk, and face. It has a female sex preponderance. Systemic symptoms may occur. A 3- to 6-week course is usually associated with an IBD flare [1]. Treatment includes leg elevation, NSAIDs, and potassium iodide. The most important management of erythema nodosum is the treatment of the IBD flare; corticosteroids are very effective in patients needing them for their active gut disease. The literature reports that erythema nodosum may arise as a complication of infliximab, but other reports describe the use of infliximab to treat erythema nodosum [12].

Sweet's syndrome

Sweet's syndrome is an acute febrile neutrophilic dermatitis with associated pathergy. Treatment is most commonly with topical or oral steroids; potassium iodide, colchicine, and metronidazole may all have a role but infliximab, as second-line treatment, is reportedly effective [13].

Oral manifestations

Oral manifestations occur in up to 10% of patients; these include aphthous ulcers, angular stomatitis, mucosal nodularity (cobblestoning), and pyostomatitis vegetans. Aphthous ulcers are treated by management of the underlying disease in conjunction with topical steroids or NSAIDS; in severe cases oral steroids may be used. There is limited literature on biologics in aphthous ulceration; an open prospective study included three cases with completion resolution after a single infliximab dose [3].

Ocular complications of IBD

Ocular complications of IBD occur in up to 6% of cases; episcleritis and uveitis are more common than scleritis. Episcleritis is a painless hyperemia of the sclera occurring with flares of intestinal disease; it responds to topical steroid treatment and causes no visual disturbance. Scleritis is inflammation of deep scleral vessels causing erythema, pain, and visual disturbance. Uveitis runs a course independent of intestinal disease and presents as an acute painful eye, with visual disturbance that can progress to blindness if not managed early with steroids, and if refractory, ciclosporin.

There are retrospective case series showing benefits with infliximab in isolated ocular disease, but none in IBD-associated ocular disease. Ninety patients receiving infliximab in published trials for ankylosing spondylitis were reviewed by Braun et al; there was a significant reduction in anterior uveitis flares [14]. Infliximab therapy has been reported to resolve uveitis fully in a young CD patient [15]; we found no case reports evaluating other biologics in IBD-related ocular complications.

Hepatobiliary complications of IBD

Hepatobiliary complications of IBD include primary sclerosing cholangitis, autoimmune hepatitis, autoimmune pancreatitis, and gallstones. There are no large case series or randomized controlled trials of the use of biologics for any of these indications.

Conclusion

There is an evolving body of evidence for the use of biologics in the management of EIMs of IBD; Table 28.1 summarizes this evidence. The current evidence supports the use of anti-TNF agents in those EIMs whose activity is concurrent with intestinal inflammation. When planning further clinical trials of biologics in IBD, it will be useful to capture data on the impact of these drugs on EIM. However, investigators must be aware of the mechanism of action of biologic agents—newer agents that target gut-specific pathways are unlikely to impact on EIMs.

References

1. Trost LB, McDonnell JK. Important cutaneous manifestations of inflammatory bowel disease. *Postgrad Med J* 2005; **81**: 580–585.
2. Barrie A, Reguiero M. Biologic therapy in the management of extra-intestinal manifestations of inflammatory bowel disease. *Inflamm Bowel Dis* 2007; **13**(11): 1424–1429.
3. Kaufman I, Caspi D, Yeshurun D, Dotan I, Elkayam O. The effect of infliximab on extra-intestinal manifestations of Crohn's disease. *Rheumatol Int* 2005; **25**: 406–410.
4. Herfarth H, Obermeier F, Andus T, et al. Improvement of arthritis and arthralgia after treatment with infliximab (Remicade) in a German prospective, open-label, multi-centre trial in refractory Crohn's disease. *Am J Gastroenterol* 2002; **97**(10): 2688–2690.
5. Ellman MH, Hanauer S, Citrin M, Cohen R. Crohn's disease arthritis treated with infliximab. *J Clin Rheum* 2201; **7**(2): 67–71.
6. Rispo A, Scarpa R, Di Girolamo E, et al. Infliximab in the treatment of extra-intestinal manifestations of crohn's disease. *Scand J Rheumatol* 2005; **34**(5): 387–391.
7. Generini S, Giacomelli R, Fedi R, et al. Infliximab in spondyloarthropathy associated with crohn's disease: an open study on the efficacy of inducing and maintaining remission of musculoskeletal and gut manifestations. *Ann Rheumatol Dis* 2004; **63**(3): 1664–1669.
8. Antivalli M, Bertani L, Atzeni F, et al. Disease activity and quality of life in Crohns-associated spondyloarthropathy after switching from infliximab to adalimumab. *Clin Exp Rheum* 2008; **26**: 746.
9. Brooklyn TN, Dunnill MG, Shetty A, et al. Infliximab for the treatment of pyoderma gangrenosum: a randomised, double blind, placebo controlled trial. *Gut* 2006; **55**(4): 505–509.

10. Fonder MA, Cummins DL, Ehst BD, Anhalt GJ, Meyerle GH. Adalimumab therapy for recalcitrant pyoderma gangrenosum. *J Burns Wounds* 2006; **5**: 66–67.

11. McGowan JW, Johnson CA, Lynn A. Treatment of pyoderma gangrenosum with etanercept. *J Drugs Dermol* 2004; **3**(4): 441–444.

12. Rosen T, Martinelli P. Erythema nodosum associated with infliximab therapy. *Dermatol Online J* 2008; **14**(4): 3.

13. Vanbiervliet G, Anty R, Schneider S, Arab K, Rampal P, Hebuterne X. Sweet's syndrome and erythema nodosum associated with crohn's disease treated with infliximab. *Gastro Clin Biol* 2002; **26**: 295–297.

14. Braun J, Baraliakos X, Listing J, Sieper J. Decreased incidence of anterior uveitis in patients with ankylosing spondylitis treated with the anti tumor necrosis factor agents infliximab and etanercept. *Arthritis Rheum* 2005; **52**: 2447–2451.

15. Fries W, Giofre MR, Catanoso M, Lo Gullo R. Treatment of acute uveitis associated with Crohn's disease and sacro-ileitis with infliximab. *Am J Gastroenterol* 2002; **97**: 499–500.

29 Use and abuse of biologics in pregnancy

Marla C. Dubinsky

Pediatric IBD Center, Cedars Sinai Medical Center, Los Angeles, CA, USA

LEARNING POINTS

- Disease remission is critical for conception.
- Anti-TNF-α therapies are considered FDA Category B. (Animal studies have revealed no evidence of harm to the fetus; however, there are no adequate and well-controlled studies in pregnant women. OR Animal studies have shown an adverse effect, but adequate and well-controlled studies in pregnant women have failed to demonstrate a risk to the fetus in any trimester.)
- Anti-TNF-α therapies appear to be safe in pregnancy.
- Dosing frequency of Anti-TNFs may need to be adjusted during pregnancy.
- Placental transfer must be considered when using anti-TNFs.
- Anti-TNFs can be used when breastfeeding.

Use of biologics during pregnancy

The key to a successful pregnancy for women with IBD is to conceive in a state of disease remission so as to go into pregnancy with the highest likelihood of staying in remission throughout the gestational period. It should be noted that the majority of medications used for the treatment of IBD are not associated with significant adverse outcomes on the pregnancy or with congenital anomalies.

Biologics have certainly improved outcome and disease activity in IBD and this has translated to more women being healthy enough to consider starting a family. The most commonly used biologics are the anti-TNF therapies, which are classified as pregnancy category B (Animal stud- ies have revealed no evidence of harm to the fetus; however, there are no adequate and well-controlled studies in pregnant women. OR Animal studies have shown an adverse effect, but adequate and well-controlled studies in pregnant women have failed to demonstrate a risk to the fetus in any trimester). Infliximab, adalimumab, and certolizumab are currently approved for use in Crohn's disease (CD). Both infliximab and adalimumab are IgG1 antibodies that do not cross the placenta in the first trimester, but do so efficiently in the third trimester [1]. The lack of transfer in the first trimester protects the fetus from drug exposure during the period of organogenesis. Reports confirm that these medications cross the placenta easily in the third trimester and, based on data from infliximab, are present in the infant for several months from birth [2,3]. However, it does not appear that fetal exposure impacts the outcome of the pregnancy for either the mother or the fetus.

Infliximab

Initial knowledge was based on case reports of infliximab exposure in patients with CD [4], all but one of which had a successful outcome. The two largest series are from the TREAT Registry [5] and the Infliximab Safety Database [6] maintained by Centocor (Malvern, PA). Of the close to 6000 patients enrolled in the prospective TREAT registry, 36 pregnancies with prior infliximab exposure were reported. Congenital malformations did not occur in any of the pregnancies. Additionally, miscarriage (11.1% versus 7.1%; $P = 0.53$) and neonatal complications rates (8.3% versus 7.1%; $P = 0.78$) were not significantly different between infliximab-treated and infliximab-naïve patients,

Clinical Dilemmas in Inflammatory Bowel Disease: New Challenges, Second Edition. Edited by P. Irving, C. Siegel, D. Rampton and F. Shanahan.
© 2011 Blackwell Publishing Ltd. Published 2011 by Blackwell Publishing Ltd.

respectively. The infliximab safety database reported that the expected versus observed outcomes among women exposed to infliximab were not different from those of the general population. This retrospective database described the pregnancy outcomes for 96 women with exposure to infliximab, primarily during conception and the first trimester.

Mahadevan et al. were the first to report on the intentional use of maintenance infliximab in a series of ten women [7]. All ten pregnancies ended in live births, with no reported congenital malformations. However, there was a recent review of the FDA database from 1999 through December of 2005, which reviewed over 120,000 adverse events and reported on a number of congenital anomalies that were part of the VACTERL spectrum in fetuses exposed to anti-TNF (either infliximab or etanercept). They concluded that these congenital anomalies were occurring at a rate higher than historical controls [8]. By the nature of the FDA database, there is no clear denominator of exposed patients, so comparisons to expected rates are suspect, and further data are needed to examine this potential association.

Adalimumab

Initial case reports also document the successful use of adalimumab to treat CD during pregnancy [9]. OTIS (Organization for Teratology Information Specialists) reported that the rate of spontaneous abortion and stillbirth, as well as congenital abnormalities, in adalimumab-exposed patients was similar to disease controls not on adalimumab and the general population [10].

Certolizumab

Certolizumab pegol is a PEGylated Fab' fragment of a humanized anti-TNF monoclonal antibody. A study of pregnant rats receiving a murinized IgG1 antibody of TNF and a PEGylated FAB' fragment of this antibody, demonstrated much lower levels of drug in the infant and in breast milk with the Fab' fragment compared to the full antibody [11]. Human studies have confirmed low to negligible levels of drug are seen in either the cord blood or serum of newborn [12]. However, one concern is that the Fab' fragment may cross the placenta in low levels in the first trimester as well, which IgG1 antibodies (infliximab/adalimumab) should not do. Early reports suggest that, like adalimumab and infliximab, newborns outcomes are favorable.

How should anti-TNF therapy be modified in the third trimester?

More data are needed to better understand the impact of the lack of placental transfer in the third trimester before choosing certolizumab for all patients considering pregnancy. Until such data are available, clinicians can consider discontinuing infliximab early in the third trimester to decrease the degree of placental transfer and thereby decrease levels in the newborn. Infliximab can then be resumed immediately after delivery, as the postpartum period may be associated with increased disease activity. The dosing schedule of adalimumab (every other week) may preclude clinicians from stopping the agent very early in the third trimester. Physicians may want to consider stopping adalimumab 6–8 weeks before expected delivery date, although no consensus has been reached on this.

Natalizumab

Natalizumab is a category C drug (Animal studies have shown an adverse effect and there are no adequate and well-controlled studies in pregnant women. **OR** No animal studies have been conducted and there are no adequate and well-controlled studies in pregnant women) and to date there are no reports of exposure during pregnancy in IBD patients. There is currently a pregnancy registry in patients with multiple sclerosis, which will likely also be initiated for CD.

Use of biologics and breastfeeding (see Chapter 20)

To date there are limited data available on the safety of anti-TNF therapies during breastfeeding. Two studies have been published reporting the absence of measurable infliximab levels in breast milk [2,13] and one study showed absence of certolizumab levels in breast milk [12]. A recent report describes detection of adalimumab in breast milk, albeit at very low levels [14]. In general, anti-TNF treatment should be continued during breastfeeding.

Use of biologics and newborn management

The implications of measurable drug levels of anti-TNFs in newborns and how, if at all, these medications impact upon the ontogeny of the fetal and infant immune systems remains unknown. Infliximab levels are measurable in cord blood and up to 6 months after birth in infants born to mothers receiving infliximab throughout pregnancy [2,3].

The half-life of the IgG subclass1 molecules in the infant is approximately 4 weeks.

Animal model studies have suggested that TNF-α is necessary in utero and in the postnatal period for the effective development of the humoral immune system [15]. However, babies exposed to infliximab in utero and via breastfeeding demonstrate an age-appropriate protective immune response to routine vaccinations [2,16]. It is recommended that all exposed newborns receive the killed or attenuated vaccines such as hemophilus influenza type B, tetanus, diphtheria, pertussis, and hepatitis B. It may also be worth assessing vaccination response by measuring antibody titers to tetanus toxoid and hemophilus influenza type B in biologic-exposed newborns. If they are undetectable, the infant should receive a booster shot and can be retested to assess protection. The infant can also be checked to ensure there are no measurable infliximab drug levels at the same time.

However, as is the case in all patients with IBD receiving immunosuppressive therapies, live vaccines could present a problem for infants exposed to biologics in utero and during lactation. For example, in the United States, the live rotavirus vaccine is recommended for infants at 8 weeks of age. Despite the paucity of data to support abnormal immune responses, it is recommended that biologic-exposed infants should not receive this vaccine. This recommendation must of course be balanced with the risk of rotavirus to high-risk infants. Other live vaccinations (varicella and measles, mumps and rubella (MMR) are not administered until 12 months of age and these should, therefore, be given despite in utero or lactation exposure.

Conclusions

Advances in therapies for IBD patients have afforded more women the opportunity to conceive and successfully carry out a full-term pregnancy. The biologic therapies are considered to be safe during pregnancy for both the mother and the fetus. Ongoing clinical experience and research including national registries will help elucidate the benefits and safety of biologics during pregnancy.

References

1. Simister NE. Placental transport of immunoglobulin G. *Vaccine* 2003; **21**: 3365–3369.
2. Vasiliauskas EA, Church JA, Silverman N, et al. Case report: evidence for transplacental transfer of maternally administered infliximab to the newborn. *Clin Gastroenterol Hepatol* 2006; **4**: 1255–1258.
3. Mahadevan U, Terdiman JP, Church J, et al. Infliximab levels in infants born to women with inflammatory bowel disease. *Gastroenterology* 2007; **132**: A144.
4. Srinivasan R. Infliximab treatment and pregnancy outcome in active Crohn's disease. *Am J Gastroenterol* 2001; **96**: 2274–2275.
5. Lichtenstein GR, Feagan BG, Cohen RD, et al. Serious infections and mortality in association with therapies for Crohn's disease: TREAT registry. *Clin Gastroenterol Hepatol* 2006; **4**: 621–630.
6. Katz JA, Antoni C, Keenan GF, et al. Outcome of pregnancy in women receiving infliximab for the treatment of Crohn's disease and rheumatoid arthritis. *Am J Gastroenterol* 2004; **99**: 2385–2392.
7. Mahadevan U, Kane S, Sandborn WJ, et al. Intentional infliximab use during pregnancy for induction or maintenance of remission in Crohn's disease. *Aliment Pharmacol Ther* 2005; **21**: 733–738.
8. Carter JD. Ladhani A, Ricca LR, et al. A safety assessment of tumor necrosis factor antagonists during pregnancy: a review of the Food and Drug Administration database. *J Rheumatol* 2009; **36**: 635–641.
9. Mishkin DS, Van Deinse W, Becker JM, et al. Successful use of adalimumab (Humira) for Crohn's disease in pregnancy. *Inflamm Bowel Dis* 2006; **12**: 827–828.
10. Chambers CD, Johnson DL, Jones KL. Pregnancy Outcomes in Women Exposed to Adalimumab: The OTIS Autoimmune Diseases in Pregnancy Project. Personal communication July 13, 2007.
11. Nesbitt A, Brown D, Stephens S, Foulkes R. Placental transfer and accumulation in milk of the anti-TNF antibody TN3 in rats: immunoglobulin G1 versus PEGylated Fab'. *Am J Gastroenterol* 2006; Abstract 119.
12. Mahadevan U, Siegel C, Abreu M. Certolizumab use in pregnancy: low levels detected in cord blood. *Gastroenterology* 2009; Abstract 960.
13. Kane S, Ford J, Cohen R, et al. Absence of infliximab in infants and breast milk from nursing mothers receiving therapy for Crohn's disease before and after delivery. *J Clin Gastroenterol* 2009; **43**: 613–616.
14. Ben-Horin S, Yavzori M, Katz L, et al. Adalimumab level in breast milk of a nursing mother. *Clin Gastroenterol Hepatol* 2010; **8**: 475–476.
15. Hunt JS, Chen Hua-Lin, Miller Lance. Tumour necrosis factor: pivotal components of pregnancy? *Biol Reprod* 1996; **54**: 554–562.
16. Mahadevan U, Kane S, Church JA, et al. The effect of maternal peripartum infliximab use on neonatal immune response. *Gastroenterology* 2008; Abstract 302.

30 Is anti-TNF therapy safe to use in people with a history of malignancy?

Mark Lust[1] and Simon Travis[2]

[1]Translational Gastroenterology Unit, John Radcliffe Hospital, Oxford, UK
[2]Translational Gastroenterology Unit, John Radcliffe Hospital, Oxford, UK

LEARNING POINTS

- Drugs that inhibit the action of tumor necrosis factor theoretically increase the risk of development or progression of malignant disease.

- Cancers developing after treatment with anti-TNF agents have been reported but the risk appears to be small.

- In patients with a history of malignant or premalignant disease, the risk of cancer progression or recurrence after treatment with anti-TNF therapy is unknown.

- In all patients, the potential benefits of anti-TNF therapy need to be balanced against the risks of malignancy

- Decisions regarding the use of anti-TNF agents in patients with a history of malignant or premalignant disease need to be individualized after careful discussion with the patient and appropriate specialists.

Introduction

Initially recognized for its ability to lyse tumor cells, tumor necrosis factor (TNF) is required for natural killer cell and CD8 lymphocyte-mediated tumor cell death [1]. Drugs that inhibit the action of TNF may, therefore, increase the risk of development or progression of malignancy. While these agents have revolutionized the treatment of inflammatory bowel disease (IBD), their use in patients with a previous history of malignancy raises alarm bells and their safety in this context remains uncertain. Some studies have highlighted the potential for an increased risk of malignant disease in patients receiving anti-TNF therapy, but no study has specifically asked whether TNF blockade increases the risk of recurren cancer in patients with previous malignancy.

What is the risk of malignancy in patients treated with anti-TNF antibodies?

There are several reports of cancer developing after anti-TNF therapy [2–6], but proving a link between drug exposure and tumor development is difficult. Patients treated with anti-TNF therapy may already be predisposed to cancer as a consequence of their underlying disease. For example, patients with rheumatoid arthritis (RA) have an increased risk of lymphoma [7], while patients with long-standing ulcerative colitis have an increased risk of colon cancer [8]. Furthermore, patients with immune-mediated disorders have often been exposed to other immunomodulators that could independently increase the risk of cancer.

Malignancy in RCTs of anti-TNF therapy for IBD

Malignancy has been reported in randomized controlled clinical trials (RCTs) of anti-TNF therapy in IBD, but rates are no higher than in controls. A meta-analysis of all six anti-TNF agents (infliximab (IFX), adalimumab, certolizumab, etanercept, onercept, and CDP571) evaluated in RCTs in 3955 patients with Crohn's disease (CD) showed no difference in the frequency of malignancy between anti-TNF and control groups [5]. According to safety data from clinical trial experience with adalimumab, which included 2228 patients with CD treated for a total of 2373 patient-years, the absolute risk of any malignancy was 1.3 per 100 patient-years of treatment [9]. While reassuring, these results should be interpreted with caution as RCTs have

Clinical Dilemmas in Inflammatory Bowel Disease: New Challenges, Second Edition. Edited by P. Irving, C. Siegel, D. Rampton and F. Shanahan.
© 2011 Blackwell Publishing Ltd. Published 2011 by Blackwell Publishing Ltd.

stringent inclusion and exclusion criteria, which may not represent clinical practice. Furthermore, many of the "control patients" in these trials received an induction course of therapy prior to randomization, these studies were not powered to detect differences in adverse events, and the duration of follow-up may be too short to detect rare serious events, such as malignancy.

Malignancy in IBD practice

Postmarketing surveillance provides data from larger numbers of patients, more representative of the population treated and potentially followed over longer periods of time. However, such data are limited by incomplete or selective reporting and documentation. Similarly to the RCTs, several large cohort studies have reported the development of malignant disease in patients receiving anti-TNF therapy, however, at no greater rate than in patients not exposed to anti-TNF agents [10–14].

Lymphoma in IBD

A recent meta-analysis assessing the risk of non-Hodgkin lymphoma (NHL) included RCTs and observational studies with nearly 9000 patients and 22,000 patient-years of exposure to anti-TNF therapy [15]. An absolute rate of non-Hodgkin lymphoma (NHL) of 6.1 per 10,000 patient-years was calculated, resulting in an SIR of 3.23 (95% confidence interval (CI) 1.5–6.9) compared to the expected rate in the general population. However, most of the patents with NHL also had exposure to immunomodulators, so it is difficult to sort out the risk attributable to anti-TNF therapy, immunomodulators, or combination therapy.

Of great concern is the potential for the development of a rare but aggressive and often fatal subtype of NHL, hepatosplenic T-cell lymphoma (HSTCL). HSTCL occurs predominantly in young male patients with CD treated with anti-TNF therapy and a thiopurine [3]. Nineteen cases have been reported to date (Q2 2010), but no case has occurred without combination immunosuppression.

Malignancy in RCTs of anti-TNF therapy for other disease

In RA, a meta-analysis of nine clinical trials reported a dose-dependent increased risk of malignancy in 3493 patients treated with IFX or adalimumab compared to 1512 patients receiving placebo [2]. None of the trials in this meta-analysis included patients with preexisting malignancy. In contrast, two large cohort studies failed to demonstrate an increased risk of malignancy associated with the use of anti-TNF

therapy in patients with RA [16,17]. A longitudinal study of 19,591 patients with RA with 89,710 patient-years of follow-up demonstrated no increased risk of lymphoma in patients that were treated with IFX [6].

Results from a placebo-controlled trial of IFX in patients with chronic obstructive pulmonary disease caused some concern. After 6 months of follow-up, ten cancers had been diagnosed in 157 patients given IFX compared to only one cancer in the placebo group of 77 patients [18]. Most cancers involved the respiratory tract and it is possible that anti-TNF therapy accelerated the growth of preexisting cancers in a smoking population already at high risk. However, the small sample size makes it difficult to draw any firm conclusions.

What is the risk of cancer recurrence or progression after anti-TNF therapy?

There are very few data on the risk of anti-TNF therapy in patients with previous malignancy. One abstract reports data from the British Society of Rheumatology Biologics' Register to assess the potential risk of malignancy associated with starting anti-TNF therapy in patients with RA who had preexisting cancer [19]. Patients who had a malignancy prior to starting anti-TNF therapy had an increased risk of a further malignancy after commencing treatment, compared to those with no previous malignancy. 6/154 patients (4%) with RA and a previous malignancy developed a new cancer, compared to 158/9844 patients (1.6%) with RA but no previous malignancy (incidence risk ratio 2.5; 95% CI 1.2–5.8). Of the six cancers that developed in patients with a history of previous malignancy, three occurred in patients who had a malignancy >10 years before starting anti-TNF therapy. Only one was a local recurrence or metastatic spread.

Other data are anecdotal. Two cases of metastatic colorectal carcinoma are reported after treatment with IFX in patients with CD and previous colonic neoplasia [4]. Of most concern is that both patients had colonoscopies prior to treatment with IFX and developed metastatic colon cancer within 2 years.

Should patients with previous malignancy be treated with anti-TNF therapy?

Apart from anecdotes and case reports, this is an evidence-free zone. While there is a theoretical risk that anti-TNF therapy will increase the risk of tumor progression or recurrence in patients with malignant or premalignant disease, controlled data are lacking. The British Society of Rheumatology (BSR) recommends caution before using anti-TNF therapy in patients with previous malignancy or premalignant conditions such as Barrett's esophagus, cervical dysplasia, or colonic polyps [20]. The BSR says that there is no established contraindication to anti-TNF therapy for patients who have been free of recurrence of their malignancy for 10 years, although this "cancer-free window" of 10 years is arbitrary.

The potential benefits of anti-TNF therapy need to be balanced against the potential risks of malignancy and decisions have to be tailored to the individual.

- In *normal circumstances*, the risk of a new malignancy appears so low that it is almost always outweighed by the benefits of treatment in patients with active IBD refractory to other therapy.
- For patients with *premalignant conditions* (including Barrett's esophagus without dysplasia or colonic polyps), the same would generally apply.
- For *established dysplasia*, the balance tilts against anti-TNF therapy. However, a situation in which a patient with cervical dysplasia and debilitating symptoms from IBD can readily be conceived. In this example, anti-TNF therapy in conjunction with treatment of the cervical dysplasia may be reasonable after discussion with other specialists (e.g., gynecology and oncology).
- For patients with a *past history of malignancy* (other than a basal cell carcinoma or curative resection of a squamous cell carcinoma), anti-TNF therapy should generally be avoided, unless there are compelling reasons that it presents the only practical therapeutic option. Specialist advice is again advisable, including consideration of whether surgery or other medical therapy is more appropriate for treating the IBD.
- Anti-TNF therapy should almost always be avoided in patients with *active malignant disease*, because of the risk of accelerating tumor progression and spread.

The principle of *primum non nocere* (first, do no harm), espoused by William Osler, is sound. However, the risk of anti-TNF therapy in patients with a previous malignancy or premalignant condition is simply not known. Discussion with the patient about all therapeutic options and appropriate specialist advice is necessary before an informed mutual decision can be reached.

References

1. Carswell EA, Old LJ, Kassel RL, Green S, Fiore N, Williamson B. An endotoxin-induced serum factor that causes necrosis of tumors. *Proc Natl Acad Sci USA* 1975; **72**: 3666–3670.
2. Bongartz T, Sutton AJ, Sweeting MJ, Buchan I, Matteson EL, Montori V. Anti-TNF antibody therapy in rheumatoid arthritis and the risk of serious infections and malignancies: systematic review and meta-analysis of rare harmful effects in randomized controlled trials. *Jama* 2006; **295**: 2275–2285.
3. Mackey AC, Green L, Liang LC, Dinndorf P, Avigan M. Hepatosplenic T cell lymphoma associated with infliximab use in young patients treated for inflammatory bowel disease. *J Pediatr Gastroenterol Nutr* 2007; **44**: 265–267.
4. Nicholson T, Orangio GR, Brandenburg D, Wolf DC, Pennington EE. Crohn's colitis presenting with node-negative colon cancer and liver metastasis after therapy with infliximab: report of two cases. *Dis Colon Rectum* 2005; **48**: 1651–1655.
5. Peyrin-Biroulet L, Deltenre P, de Suray N, Branche J, Sandborn WJ, Colombel JF. Efficacy and safety of tumor necrosis factor antagonists in Crohn's disease: meta-analysis of placebo-controlled trials. *Clin Gastroenterol Hepatol* 2008; **6**: 644–653.
6. Wolfe F, Michaud K. The effect of methotrexate and anti-tumor necrosis factor therapy on the risk of lymphoma in rheumatoid arthritis in 19,562 patients during 89,710 person-years of observation. *Arthritis Rheum* 2007; **56**: 1433–1439.
7. Gridley G, McLaughlin JK, Ekbom A, et al. Incidence of cancer among patients with rheumatoid arthritis. *J Natl Cancer Inst* 1993; **85**: 307–311.
8. Ekbom A, Helmick C, Zack M, Adami HO. Ulcerative colitis and colorectal cancer. A population-based study. *N Engl J Med* 1990; **323**: 1228–1233.
9. Burmester GR, Mease PJ, Dijkmans BA, et al. Adalimumab safety and mortality rates from global clinical trials of six immune-mediated inflammatory diseases. *Ann Rheum Dis* 2009; **68**(12): 1863–1869.
10. Biancone L, Orlando A, Kohn A, et al. Infliximab and newly diagnosed neoplasia in Crohn's disease: a multicentre matched pair study. *Gut* 2006; **55**: 228–233.
11. Caspersen S, Elkjaer M, Riis L, et al. Infliximab for inflammatory bowel disease in Denmark 1999–2005: clinical outcome and follow-up evaluation of malignancy and mortality. *Clin Gastroenterol Hepatol* 2008; **6**: 1212–1217; quiz 1176.
12. Colombel JF, Loftus EV, Jr., Tremaine WJ, et al. The safety profile of infliximab in patients with Crohn's disease: the Mayo clinic experience in 500 patients. *Gastroenterology* 2004; **126**: 19–31.

13. Fidder H, Schnitzler F, Ferrante M, et al. Long-term safety of infliximab for the treatment of inflammatory bowel disease: a single-centre cohort study. *Gut* 2009; **58**: 501–508.

14. Lichtenstein G, Cohen R, Feagan B, et al. Safety of infliximab and other Crohn's disease therapies: Treat™ registry data with 24,575 patient-years of follow-up. *Am J Gastroenterol* 2008; **103**: S436.

15. Siegel CA, Marden SM, Persing SM, Larson RJ, Sands BE. Risk of lymphoma associated with combination anti-tumor necrosis factor and immunomodulator therapy for the treatment of Crohn's disease: a meta-analysis. *Clin Gastroenterol Hepatol* 2009;7:874–881.

16. Askling J, Fored CM, Brandt L, et al. Risks of solid cancers in patients with rheumatoid arthritis and after treatment with tumour necrosis factor antagonists. *Ann Rheum Dis* 2005; **64**: 1421–1426.

17. Setoguchi S, Solomon DH, Weinblatt ME, et al. Tumor necrosis factor alpha antagonist use and cancer in patients with rheumatoid arthritis. *Arthritis Rheum* 2006; **54**: 2757–2764.

18. Rennard SI, Fogarty C, Kelsen S, et al. The safety and efficacy of infliximab in moderate to severe chronic obstructive pulmonary disease. *Am J Respir Crit Care Med* 2007; **175**: 926–934.

19. Dixon WG, Watson KD, Lunt M, et al. Influence of anti-tumor necrosis factor therapy on cancer incidence in patients with rheumatoid arthritis who have had a prior malignancy: results from the British Society for Rheumatology Biologics Register. *Arthritis Care Res* 2010;**62**:755–763.

20. Ledingham J, Deighton C. Update on the British Society for Rheumatology guidelines for prescribing TNFalpha blockers in adults with rheumatoid arthritis (update of previous guidelines of April 2001). *Rheumatology (Oxford)* 2005; **44**: 157–163.

31 The risks of immunomodulators and biologics: what should we tell patients?

Corey A. Siegel

Inflammatory Bowel Disease Center, Dartmouth–Hitchcock Medical Center, Section of Gastroenterology and Hepatology, Lebanon, NH, USA

LEARNING POINTS

- Immunomodulators and anti-TNF agents offer substantial benefit to patients with IBD, but decisions about their use need to be balanced against the risks of therapy.

- Both thiopurines and anti-TNF agents are associated with very small, but probably real increased risks of serious infections and non-Hodgkin's lymphoma.

- The risks of anti-TNF monotherapy (without any prior thiopurine use) are not well understood.

- Natalizumab is associated with an approximately 1 per 1000 risk of progressive multifocal leukoencephalopathy.

- When discussing risks of therapy with patients, it is important also to review the risks of poorly treated disease.

- When communicating probability of adverse events to patients, present absolute numbers in a format that is easy to comprehend rather than relative risk or odds ratios (e.g., 6 out of 10,000 rather than 0.06% or a standardized incidence ratio of 3.23).

Introduction

Many patients with inflammatory bowel disease (IBD) are prescribed immune suppressant medications to treat their symptoms and keep them off of corticosteroids. The most commonly prescribed of these are the immunomodulators including 6-mercaptopurine (6MP), azathioprine (AZA), and methotrexate, and the biologics including the anti-tumor necrosis factor (TNF) agents (adalimumab, cer-

tolizumab pegol, and infliximab) and the anti-integrin molecule natalizumab. While there is little question that these medications are effective, there are still many questions about their safety. With every prescription written, clinicians are faced with the challenge of what to tell patients about the safety of these medications, and how best to communicate this information. This chapter aims to give an updated review of the risks of immunomodulators and biologics for the treatment of IBD, and to offer some advice on how to discuss this with your patients.

What to tell patients about possible side effects

Descriptions and rates of adverse events associated with immunomodulators have been fairly consistent over time (Table 31.1).

Thiopurines

The more common side effects directly related to exposure to thiopurines include allergic reactions, nausea, pancreatitis, hepatitis, and bone marrow suppression [1]. Between 6% and 22% of patients need to stop thiopurine therapy because of side effects [2]. Serious adverse events that can occur indirectly due to immune suppression include serious infections and malignancy. The most common malignancies seen with the thiopurines are skin cancers, specifically squamous cell carcinomas. The rate of non-Hodgkin's lymphoma also appears to be increased. A meta-analysis studying the risk of lymphoma in IBD patients treated with thiopurines reported a 4-fold increased risk of lymphoma compared to the expected rate [3]. More recently, a large

Clinical Dilemmas in Inflammatory Bowel Disease: New Challenges, Second Edition. Edited by P. Irving, C. Siegel, D. Rampton and F. Shanahan.
© 2011 Blackwell Publishing Ltd. Published 2011 by Blackwell Publishing Ltd.

Event	Estimated frequency (annual)
Thiopurines [2,3]	
Stopping therapy due to lack of tolerance	6%–22%
Havingan an allergic reaction	3%
Getting pancreatitis	3%
Getting a serious infection	5%
Getting Non-Hodgkin's Lymphoma	0.04% (4 per 10,000)
Antitumor necrosis factor agents [7,8]	
Stopping therapy due to lack of tolerance	10%
Infusion or injection site reactions	3%–20%
Getting a serious infection	3%
Tuberculosis	0.05% (5 per 10,000)
Getting Non-Hodgkin's Lymphoma	0.06%(6 per 10,000)

TABLE 31.1 Estimated risks of thiopurines and anti-TNF agents

population-based study from France reported a rate of lymphoproliferative disorders of 9 per 10,000 patient-years for those taking thiopurines versus 2.6 per 10,000 patient-years for IBD patients never exposed to thiopurines (Hazard ratio 5.28, 96% CI 2.01–13.9, $p = 0.0007$) [4]. Interestingly, in this study many of the lymphomas that developed in patients receiving thiopurines were pathologically similar to those seen in posttransplant lymphoproliferative disorder (PTLD). PTLD is typically driven by Epstein–Barr Virus (EBV), and this phenomenon has also been described in lymphomas seen in other patients with IBD [5].

Methotrexate

In many parts of the world methotrexate has a reputation for being "unsafe" or difficult to tolerate, but in fact may have fewer side effects than the thiopurines (see Chapter 21). Nausea and fatigue are not uncommon, but typically can be managed easily. Suppression of the white blood cell count is unusual, and although serious infections have been reported, fortunately they appear rare. Non-Hodgkin's lymphomas are also reported in the literature, but there is a suspicion that this is at a lower rate than that associated with thiopurines. Although hypersensitivity pneumonitis is well-reported in patients with rheumatoid arthritis, there are only a few reports of this occurring in IBD patients [2]. Liver toxicity is often a fear of using methotrexate, but fortunately, IBD patients are not at the same risk as other patients groups (e.g., psoriasis) treated with this drug [6]. Methotrexate is teratogenic and should be avoided in women of childbearing potential who are not using birth control. There is uncertainty about the effect of methotrex-

ate on sperm, and some experts recommend stopping this medication for three months prior to trying to conceive.

Anti-TNF therapy

Anti-TNF agents are typically well tolerated, with approximately 10% of patients having to stop therapy due to adverse events [7]. Common but minor side effects include hypersensitivity reactions (injection or infusion site reactions, or delayed hypersensitivity reactions), headache, rash, and minor infections. More severe, but fortunately rare adverse events include: serious infections and sepsis related to both typical and opportunistic infections; demyelinating disorders; heart failure (in predisposed individuals); drug-induced lupus; hepatotoxicity; and malignancy (Table 31.1). Death associated with anti-TNF use has been reported; most cases due to sepsis. A systematic review found the rate of death from sepsis thought attributable to anti-TNF use to be 4 patients per 1000 patient-years [7]. Although this rate seems high, the subgroup affected was typically older (average age 63), was taking concomitant corticosteroids and had multiple comorbidities. Non-Hodgkin's lymphoma has also been associated with anti-TNF therapy and a recent meta-analysis estimated the rate to be 6 per 10,000 patient-years [8]. When compared to the expected rate in the general population the standardized incidence ratio (SIR) is 3.23 (95% CI 1.5–6.9). Most of the patients in this study who developed non-Hodgkin's lymphoma also had previous exposure to immunomodulators, thus making it difficult to determine whether anti-TNF monotherapy is associated with lymphoma. Perhaps anti-TNF agents are not associated with lymphoma at all and it is the immunomodulators driving the increased risk. Since so few patients have been treated with anti-TNF therapy without prior exposure to immunomodulators, this question has been very difficult to answer.

Hepatosplenic T-cell lymphoma (HSTCL) is a subtype of non-Hodgkin's lymphoma

As opposed to Hodgkin's and non-Hodgkin's lymphoma, which are reasonably curable, HSTCL is universally fatal. It has been reported in IBD patients receiving immunomodulator monotherapy and with combination immunomodulator and anti-TNF therapy. The patients affected have been young (average age in the 20s) and almost all patients have been male. Although cases continue to be reported, the denominator of patients exposed to these likely offending medications is very large (over 1 million patients have received anti-TNF therapy worldwide, and many more exposed to immunomodulators). It is difficult to calculate estimates of the rate of HSTCL, but most likely it occurs less often than standard non-Hodgkin's lymphoma.

Anti-integrin therapy

Natalizumab is the newest biologic available for the treatment of patients with Crohn's disease (CD). Excitement about the therapeutic potential of this drug has been tempered by reports of cases of progressive multifocal leukoencephalopathy (PML). The rate of developing PML if exposed to natalizumab is approximately 1 per 1000 patient-years. Although the majority of these reports have been in patients with multiple sclerosis, it is not safe to assume that Crohn's patients are not also at risk [9].

How to tell patients about the risk of side effects

Even when armed with the appropriate data, it is still difficult to clearly communicate all of this information to patients. There are a number of complex problems to overcome when explaining risk to patients, but the most basic is the general difficulty in comprehending small numbers. For example, in one study patients, had great difficulty converting percentages into fractions (e.g., 0.06% to 6 per 10,000) and comparing numbers with differing denominators (e.g., which is a higher risk, 1 in 27 or 1 in 37?) [10]. Concerningly, medical students also had a hard time with similar tasks [11].

Some general rules in communicating numbers to patients include the following [12]:

- Avoid descriptive words such as "rare" or "common"—these are interpreted in different ways by different people.
- Do not use relative terms such as relative risk, odds ratios, or numbers needed to treat, instead present absolute numbers.
- Change small number percentages (0.06%) to "X out of 1000" or 10,000 (e.g., 6 per 10,000).
- Keep denominators consistent, instead of 6 per 10,000 versus 0.9 per 1000 use 6 versus 9 per 10,000.

The risk of medication side effects needs to be presented in perspective with risks of their disease and other life risks. The risk of poorly treated CD and/or steroid use is associated with higher rates of mortality when compared to patients receiving immunomodulators [13]. In addition, the risks of dying from any cancer over the course of a lifetime is approximately 1 in 8, and the chance in the United States of dying in a car accident about 1 in 300 [14]. Surely, the very low rate of lymphoma and other serious adverse events associated with medical therapy needs to be compared with other risks our patients are taking daily.

Patients can be overwhelmed with the amount of information available about side effects of medical therapy. Package inserts are required to list all possible associated adverse events recorded in clinical trials and postmarketing experience, and the internet allows easy access to case reports and patient anecdotes. A clinician's role should be to focus on the most common and most feared risks, and it is appropriate to admit uncertainty that we do not know everything about these medications.

Documentation of a discussion regarding risks and benefits is prudent; however, signed informed consent is not necessary and may send the wrong message to patients.

Conclusion

Although we have come a long way in understanding the risks of immunomodulators and biologics, there is still a lot to learn. The point estimates above typically report annual rates, and it is difficult to extrapolate beyond this time period on the basis of the available data. A critical unanswered question is whether most of the risk is up-front soon after exposure or cumulative over time. In addition, since the vast majority of patients in the world who receive anti-TNF agents have previously been exposed to immunomodulators, we really do not know much about the risks of anti-TNF monotherapy. We will need to stay tuned as time goes on, be willing to admit uncertainty to ourselves and our patients, and be flexible in our opinions as data evolve. For now, we should present the available information as clearly as possible to our patients, remember also to present the risks of poorly treated disease and corticosteroids, and help our patients make reasoned decisions that fit with their personal preferences for treatment.

References

1. Present DH, Meltzer SJ, Krumholz MP, Wolke A, Korelitz BI. 6-Mercaptopurine in the management of inflammatory bowel disease: short- and long-term toxicity. *Ann Intern Med* 1989; **111**(8): 641–649.

2. Siegel CA, Sands BE. Review article: practical management of inflammatory bowel disease patients taking immunomodulators. *Aliment Pharmacol Ther* 2005; **22**(1): 1–16.

3. Kandiel A, Fraser AG, Korelitz BI, Brensinger C, Lewis JD. Increased risk of lymphoma among inflammatory bowel disease patients treated with azathioprine and 6-mercaptopurine. *Gut* 2005; **54**(8): 1121–1125.

4. Beaugerie L, Brousse N, Bouvier AM, et al. Lymphoproliferative disorders in patients receiving thiopurines for inflammatory bowel disease: a prospective observational cohort study. *Lancet* 2009; **374**(9701): 1617–1625.

5. Dayharsh GA, Loftus EV, Jr., Sandborn WJ, et al. Epstein-Barr virus-positive lymphoma in patients with inflammatory bowel disease treated with azathioprine or 6-mercaptopurine. *Gastroenterology* 2002; **122**(1): 72–77.

6. Te HS, Schiano TD, Kuan SF, Hanauer SB, Conjeevaram HS, Baker AL. Hepatic effects of long-term methotrexate use in the treatment of inflammatory bowel disease. *Am J Gastroenterol* 2000; **95**(11): 3150–3156.

7. Siegel CA, Hur C, Korzenik JR, Gazelle GS, Sands BE. Risks and benefits of infliximab for the treatment of Crohn's disease. *Clin Gastroenterol Hepatol* 2006; **4**(8): 1017–1024.

8. Siegel CA, Marden SM, Persing SM, Larson RJ, Sands BE. Risk of lymphoma associated with combination anti-tumor necrosis factor and immunomodulator therapy for the treatment of Crohn's disease: a meta-analysis. *Clin Gastroenterol Hepatol* 2009; **7**(8): 874–881.

9. Van Assche G, Van Ranst M, Sciot R, et al. Progressive multifocal leukoencephalopathy after natalizumab therapy for Crohn's disease. *N Engl J Med* 2005; **353**(4): 362–368.

10. Schwartz LM, Woloshin S, Black WC, Welch HG. The role of numeracy in understanding the benefit of screening mammography. *Ann Intern Med* 1997; **127**(11): 966–972.

11. Sheridan SL, Pignone M. Numeracy and the medical student's ability to interpret data. *Eff Clin Pract* 2002; **5**(1): 35–40.

12. Lipkus IM. Numeric, verbal, and visual formats of conveying health risks: suggested best practices and future recommendations. *Med Decis Making* 2007; **27**(5): 696–713.

13. Lewis JD, Gelfand JM, Troxel AB, et al. Immunosuppressant medications and mortality in inflammatory bowel disease. *Am J Gastroenterol* 2008; **103**(6): 1428–1435; quiz 36.

14. Odds of Dying, National Safety Council. Available at: http://www.nsc.org/lrs/statinfo/odds.htm (accessed July 22, 2006).

32 When, how, and in whom should we stop biologics?

Edouard Louis, Jacques Belaiche, and Catherine Reenaers

Department of gastroenterology, CHU Liège and GIGA Research University of Liège, Liège, Belgium

LEARNING POINTS

- Patients with Crohn's disease may obtain prolonged benefit from anti-TNF treatment.

- Safety of anti-TNF up to 5 years has been adequately assessed and is good.

- Because of remaining concerns about long-term safety and in order to save costs, anti-TNF discontinuation may be considered in patients in prolonged steroid-free remission.

- Risk factors for relapse after discontinuation of anti-TNF include the following:

  ○ Lack of mucosal healing

  ○ Persistent elevation of C-reactive protein

  ○ Persistent elevation of fecal calprotectin.

Introduction

To the question "when, how, and in whom should we stop biologics," an easy answer would be that one should never stop a drug that is effective and well tolerated in inflammatory bowel disease (IBD). Indeed, recent data from routine practice in experienced centers and from registries have shown both a sustained benefit in up to two-third of patients and a good safety record without significant increase of severe infections, cancers or mortality after up to 5 years of anti-TNF treatment [1,2]. Nevertheless, treatment discontinuation may be considered for several reasons, including cost, remaining uncertainties about long-term safety, and in specific situations, such as pregnancy. The decision to discontinue anti-TNF therapy should be assessed on a case-by-case basis and should take into account both cost and risk/benefit ratio. In Crohn's disease (CD), recent data contribute to such assessments and assist in making appropriate decisions. In ulcerative colitis (UC), due to its different natural history and the potential benefit of surgery, the situation may be very different and specific studies are required to delineate the best options.

Reasons for stopping anti-TNF

The main reasons for contemplating anti-TNF discontinuation include uncertainties about long-term safety, cost issues, and specific situations, including pregnancy. While short- and medium-term safety and tolerance of anti-TNF is usually very good, the fear of long-term complications is generally the reason why both patients and physicians would like to stop the drug once long-term remission has been achieved. The best documented side effects are the increased risk of tuberculosis [3] and of other infections, mainly due to intracellular pathogens (such as mycobacteria, listeria, histoplasmosis), as well as a probable slight increase in the risk of lymphoma [4].

Cost studies in CD have essentially included direct medical costs. These studies have suggested that a therapeutic strategy that decreases the number of hospitalizations and/or surgeries in CD might have an impact on direct medical costs [5]. Prospective studies with both infliximab and adalimumab given for induction and maintenance of remission have shown a significant decrease in both hospitalizations and surgeries and potential cost-efficacy after 1 year of treatment [6]. However, beyond 1 year of treatment, the cost-effectiveness of continuous

---

Clinical Dilemmas in Inflammatory Bowel Disease: New Challenges, Second Edition. Edited by P. Irving, C. Siegel, D. Rampton and F. Shanahan.
© 2011 Blackwell Publishing Ltd. Published 2011 by Blackwell Publishing Ltd.

scheduled anti-TNF treatment would require marked superiority of this strategy compared to maintenance with immunosuppressive treatment and/or on demand anti-TNF.

IBD often affects adults in their reproductive years. Therefore, the impact of such treatment on the outcome of pregnancy must be addressed. Available data on pregnancies in women exposed to anti-TNF therapies are limited (reviewed in [7] and see Chapter 29). No strong signal for an increased risk of malformation or poor outcome has been detected.

Available studies on anti-TNF treatment cessation in IBD

The earliest data regarding the use of infliximab in CD relate to its use to induce remission. Initially, single infusions were used and it is striking to note that some patients had a very prolonged clinical response or even remission with this strategy [8]. Even in these initial studies, these data suggested that prolonged treatment was probably not necessary in all patients. However, since then it has become clear that such one off treatment was not a good option for the majority of patients; the median time to relapse was 10 weeks and, furthermore, reuse of infliximab more than 4 months after a single infusion was associated with a high risk of allergic reaction.

More recently, the GETAID "bridge" study explored the idea of a three-dose regimen of infliximab as induction therapy given in parallel with an immunosuppressant that would then maintain the remission [9]. The results of this study were rather disappointing. While the short-term effect of infliximab was good, the maintenance effect with immunosuppressant was less impressive. After 1 year, the overall sustained remission rate in these patients was low and not significantly greater than those who received placebo induction. Only in patients who were immunosuppressant-naïve at the time of infliximab induction was the benefit more consistent, with a 40% remission rate after 1 year of treatment. This study demonstrates that in patients who have failed to respond to an immunosuppressant, a longer period of anti-TNF treatment is necessary to obtain a durable remission before considering treatment cessation.

Long-term results of the large Leuven cohort of patients treated with infliximab indicate that a significant propor-tion of patients (around 20%) remain in sustained remission after infliximab cessation [1]. This possibility has been explored in a recent GETAID study, STORI [10]. In this prospective cohort study, 115 patients with a stable remission on combined immunosuppressant-infliximab therapy for more than 1 year discontinued treatment with infliximab, while continuing immunosuppressive treatment. After 1 year, more than half of the patients were still in sustained remission. Factors at baseline associated with a low risk of relapse included low CDAI, low highly sensitive CRP, low fecal calprotectin, high hemoglobin levels, and nonsmoking. These features indicate that the patients with a low risk of relapse are the ones who are in a deep clinical, endoscopic, and biological remission. In these patients (representing 20–25% of the cohort), when continuing immunosuppressive treatment, the relapse rate was around 10% over 1 year. Another important finding of the STORI trial was that the relapsing patients could be safely and effectively retreated with infliximab. No acute infusion reaction was observed, and only a few patients were not in remission after the second retreatment infusion.

It is possible that this scenario is more likely if the anti-TNF is started earlier in the disease as has been suggested both in CD and in rheumatoid arthritis (RA). In the pioneering Belgian–Dutch study comparing step-up to top-down treatment in CD, prolonged remission using immunosuppressants was reached in a substantial proportion of patients who were treated early in the disease with three infliximab infusions [11]. In another pioneering study in RA, a significant proportion of patients with poor prognostic factors at diagnosis and treated from the start with combined therapy with infliximab and methotrexate, remained in remission despite infliximab discontinuation after 1 year of treatment [12]. While promising, the case for using biologics early in the disease in an attempt to alter outcome remains to be proved.

Practical considerations when stopping anti-TNF treatment in CD

The minimal duration of anti-TNF treatment that will induce sustained remission is not known and probably varies from person to person. However, when considering discontinuation of anti-TNF therapy, the duration of stable, steroid-free remission is probably a more valid criterion. Empirically, one could consider that at least a 6–12 months' quiescent period without steroid may reflect a deep and stable remission. However, as highlighted by the recent GETAID study [10], this alone is not sufficient to identify those at low risk of relapse upon anti-TNF cessation. These patients must also be assessed by the measurement of stool and blood biomarkers, as well as by endoscopy and/or medical imaging, depending on the disease location. Of the blood markers, the association between a low C-reactive protein (CRP) concentration and a low risk of relapse has been confirmed in different clinical situations. With anti-TNF cessation, the threshold discriminating patients with a lower risk of relapse was very low (<5 mg/dL) and might be better assessed using highly sensitive CRP (hsCRP). A low fecal calprotectin level has also been associated with a lower risk of relapse in IBD and, according to the recent GETAID study, a level of <250 μg/g, when used in conjunction with hsCRP may identify low-risk patients [10]. In patients with ileocolonic disease, complete mucosal healing assessed by endoscopy, or at least disappearance of any deep ulcer, with a CDEIS <2 also identifies low-risk patients. Patients with more proximal small bowel lesions inaccessible to ileocolonoscopy have not been adequately evaluated in previous studies. Small bowel MRI is a possible candidate to assess such patients [13] and while the absence of mucosal lesions is not always easy to detect using this technique, contrast enhancement of the bowel wall or the mesentery could be interpreted as tissue healing. Small bowel capsule endoscopy may represent another option to assess mucosal healing, although the risk of retention, the difficulty of precise assessment of extent and location of the lesions, as well as the lack of a validated scoring system represent current limitations [14].

Conclusions

The decision to discontinue or prolong anti-TNF treatment in CD must be based on a case-by-case assessment of the risk/benefit ratio in conjunction with cost of the drug. In patients with unstable chronic active disease, stopping an effective treatment will put the patients at risk of worsening disease and the development of complications and should not be attempted. However, in patients in prolonged stable remission, a careful assessment of the clinical, biological, and endoscopic situation will enable the patient and their physician to consider the risks and benefits of discontinuing treatment.

References

1. Schnitzler F, Fidder H, Ferrante M, et al. Long-term outcome of treatment with infliximab in 614 patients with Crohn's disease: results from a single-centre cohort. *Gut* 2009; **58**: 492–500.
2. Lichtenstein GR, Feagan BG, Cohen RD, et al. Serious infections and mortality in association with therapies for Crohn's disease: TREAT registry. *Clin Gastroenterol Hepatol* 2006; **4**: 621–630.
3. Keane J, Gershon S, Wise R, et al. Tuberculosis associated with infliximab, a tumor necrosis factor alpha-neutralizing agent. *N Engl J Med* 2001; **345**: 1098–1104.
4. Siegel CA, Marden SM, Persing SM, Larson RJ, Sands BE. Risk of lymphoma associated with combination anti-tumor necrosis factor and immunomodulator therapy for the treatment of Crohn's disease: a meta-analysis. *Clin Gastroenterol Hepatol* 2009; **7**: 874–881.
5. Silverstein MD, Loftus EV, Sandborn WJ, et al. Clinical course and costs of care for Crohn's disease: Markov model analysis of a population-based cohort. *Gastroenterology* 1999; **117**: 49–57.
6. Feagan BG, Panaccione R, Sandborn WJ, et al. Effects of adalimumab therapy on incidence of hospitalization and surgery in Crohn's disease: results from the CHARM study. *Gastroenterology* 2008; **135**: 1493–1499.
7. Gisbert JP. Saftey of immunomodulators and biologics for the treatment of inflammatory bowel disease during pregnancy and breast-feeding. *Inflam Bowel Dis* 2009; Nov 2. Epub ahead of print.
8. Rutgeerts P, D'Haens G, Targan S, et al. Efficacy and safety of retreatment with anti-tumor necrosis factor antibody (infliximab) to maintain remission in Crohn's disease. *Gastroenterology* 1999; **117**: 761–769.
9. Lémann M, Mary JY, Duclos B, et al. Infliximab plus azathioprine for steroid-dependent Crohn's disease patients: a randomized placebo-controlled trial. *Gastroenterology* 2006; **130**: 1054–1061.
10. Louis E, Vernier-Massouille G, Grimaud J, et al. Infliximab discontinuation in Crohn's disease patients in stable remission of combined therapy with immunosuppressors: interim analysis of a prospective cohort study. *Gut* 2008; **57**(sII): A66.
11. D'Haens G, Baert F, van Assche G, et al. Early combined immunosuppression or conventional management in patients with newly diagnosed Crohn's disease: an open randomised trial. *Lancet* 2008; **371**: 660–667.

12. Quinn MA, Conaghan PG, O'Connor PJ, et al. Very early treatment with infliximab in addition to methotrexate in early, poor-prognosis rheumatoid arthritis reduces magnetic resonance imaging evidence of synovitis and damage, with sustained benefit after infliximab withdrawal: results from a twelve-month randomized, double-blind, placebo-controlled trial. *Arthritis Rheum* 2005; **52**: 27–35.

13. Rimola J, Rodriguez S, García-Bosch O, et al. Magnetic resonance for assessment of disease activity and severity in ileocolonic Crohn's disease. *Gut* 2009; **58**: 1113–1120.

14. Bourreille A, Ignjatovic A, Aabakken L, et al. Role of small-bowel endoscopy in the management of patients with inflammatory bowel disease: an international OMED-ECCO consensus. *Endoscopy* 2009; **41**: 618–637.

PART V:
Other Treatments

33 Avoiding drug interactions

Tim Elliott and Peter M. Irving

Department of Gastroenterology, Guys and St. Thomas' Hospital, London, UK

LEARNING POINTS

- Patients with IBD often take a combination of drugs. Therefore, clinicians need to be aware of adverse drug interactions.
- Some drug interactions can be of therapeutic benefit in IBD.
- Evidence about the clinical importance and frequency of drug interactions is often sparse.
- Ongoing collection of drug interaction data for reporting systems is important.

Introduction

Patients with inflammatory bowel disease (IBD) often require a combination of drugs to control their disease, making the possibility of clinically important drug interactions of real concern. In this chapter, we address the most common and serious adverse interactions as well as some that may, conversely, be of therapeutic benefit. Particular attention is paid to interactions that occur where both drugs are commonly used in patients with IBD, others are summarized in Table 33.1. We have provided possible mechanisms for most of the drug interactions, although many of these are speculative given that the evidence is sparse.

Drug interactions

Sulfasalazine/5-aminosalicylates (5-ASAs) (see also cyclosporine)

Azathioprine/Mercaptopurine

Sulfasalazine and 5-ASAs may potentiate the effects of thiopurines; their use in people taking thiopurines results in higher 6-thioguanine nucleotide (6-TGN) levels and potentially leukopenia [1]. The mechanism for this may be inhibition of thiopurine methyltransferase (TPMT) [2,3]; however, it appears that, with the possible exception of sulfasalazine, the concentration of these drugs necessary to inhibit TPMT in vivo are above those reached with standard doses [4]. Therefore, if 5-ASA dose changes are made, the interval between monitoring blood tests should be reduced, and should include measurement of 6-TGN if possible.

An increased risk of leukopenia may not be the only side effect of this combination. A recent audit of 95 IBD patients on azathioprine monotherapy compared with 104 patients on azathioprine/mesalamine dual therapy also described an increase in other adverse events in those on dual therapy (abdominal symptoms, pancreatitis) as well as higher relapse rates [5]. The risks of these interactions must be weighed against the potential chemopreventive effects of 5-ASA in patients with colonic IBD.

Antibiotics

Ciprofloxacin inhibits CYP1A2, a member of the CYP450 family and, therefore, can increase the bioavailability of other drugs metabolized by CYP1A2, such as amitriptyline, clozapine, olanzapine, paracetamol, propranolol, verapamil, and warfarin [6].

Probiotics

Probiotics used in IBD therapeutic trials such as *Lactobacilli* and *Bifidobacteria* have variable sensitivities to antibiotics used commonly in IBD such as ciprofloxacin and metronidazole, and therefore the concurrent use of these antibiotics with probiotics could limit their efficacy [1].

Clinical Dilemmas in Inflammatory Bowel Disease: New Challenges, Second Edition. Edited by P. Irving, C. Siegel, D. Rampton and F. Shanahan.
© 2011 Blackwell Publishing Ltd. Published 2011 by Blackwell Publishing Ltd.

TABLE 33.1 Some further potentially important interactions of drugs used in IBD

IBD Drug	Drug	Potential effects	Explanation	Comments
Sulfasalazine	Folate, digoxin, talinolol	Low folate Decreased digoxin levels Decreased effect of talinolol	Decreased absorption of drugs (Folate; also inhibition of dihydrofolate reductase)	Monitor folate and digoxin levels Consider folate supplementation
	Cholestyramine, iron	Decreased effect of sulfasalazine	Drugs bind sulfasalazine	Separate doses by 2 h
Azo-bonded 5-ASA	Antibiotics (rifampin, and ampicillin)	Alter release of 5-ASA	Alter colonic bacterial flora	
Ciprofloxacin	Nutritional supplements and antacids	Decreased bioavailability of ciprofloxacin	Ciprofloxacin forms insoluble compounds with divalent cations such as calcium, iron, zinc, magnesium	Do not take nutritional supplements/antacids containing these substances within 2 h of ciprofloxacin
	Ursodeoxycholic acid	Possible decreased bioavailability of ciprofloxacin	Decreased absorption	Single case report only
Metronidazole	Liver enzyme inducers/inhibitors	Altered levels of metronidazole	Liver enzyme induction/inhibition	Probably not clinically important
Corticosteroids	Oral contraceptives	Increased plasma levels of prednisolone		Does not occur with budesonide
	Loop/thiazide diuretics	Hypokalemia	Mineralocorticoid effects of corticosteroids	Lesser effect with prednisolone than hydrocortisone Monitor/supplement potassium, or use potassium-sparing diuretic if necessary
	Grapefruit juice	Increased bioavailability of budesonide	CYP450 inhibition	Inform patients of interaction
	Food, acid suppressing medication	Altered bioavailability of budesonide	Altered absorption of budesonide	Interactions probably not clinically relevant
	Antacids	Decreased bioavailability of prednisolone	Decreased absorption of prednisolone	Not clinically significant with standard doses of antacids
Thiopurines	ACE inhibitors	Leukopenia and anemia	Additive effect of thiopurines on leukopenia Anaemia due to decreased levels of erythropoietin or insulin-like growth factor-1.	Only reported in renal transplant patients, but could be relevant in IBD

TABLE 33.1 *(Continued)*

IBD Drug	Drug	Potential effects	Explanation	Comments
Methotrexate	Antibiotics (penicillins and tetracycline)	Methotrexate toxicity	Unknown: Possibly impaired renal excretion of methotrexate	Only rarely reported
	Cholestyramine	Decreased levels of methotrexate	Methotrexate undergoes enterohepatic circulation. Therefore, cholestyramine can increase excretion of methotrexate.	Interaction independent of route of administration of methotrexate
	Proton pump inhibitors	Myalgia	Unknown: Possibly decreased renal excretion of 7-hydroxymethotrexate	
Cyclosporine	Renally excreted drugs	Increased levels of, for example, digoxin	Cyclosporine-induced renal impairment	Predictable decrease in GFR induced by cyclosporine—monitor levels of digoxin if starting cyclosporine
	Grapefruit juice	Increased levels of oral, but not intravenous cyclosporine	Probably via inhibition of (enteral, rather than hepatic) CYP450	

Source: Adapted from [1].

Corticosteroids (see also cyclosporine)

Nonsteroidal anti-inflammatory drugs (NSAIDs), cyclooxygenase-2 (COX-2) inhibitors

The risk of upper gastrointestinal (GI) bleeding associated with NSAIDs is increased by concomitant usage of corticosteroids [7]. COX-2 inhibitors are probably no safer than nonselective NSAIDs regarding serious upper GI side effects [8]. Prophylactic proton pump inhibitor use is advised when these drugs are used in combination.

Thiopurines (see also 5-ASA, infliximab, and adalimumab)

Allopurinol

Allopurinol is a xanthine oxidase (XO) inhibitor used to treat gout. As thiopurines are partly metabolized by XO, allopurinol increases mercaptopurine levels potentially leading to life-threatening leukopenia [1]. Therefore, coprescription of these drugs is generally contraindicated. However, recently allopurinol has been used deliberately

and cautiously, with reduced dose thiopurine, in patients not responding to standard thiopurine monotherapy, to increase 6-TGN levels via this interaction (see Chapter 18).

Methotrexate

Methotrexate inhibits XO and when used with azathioprine in patients with acute lymphoblastic leukemia, results in increased levels of 6-TGNs [1]. This may increase the risk of profound myelosuppression. Furthermore, given that in 19 patients with IBD, this combination was no more effective clinically than methotrexate alone, and was associated with an increase in adverse events [9], it should be avoided.

Methotrexate (see also thiopurines and infliximab)

Aspirin and NSAIDs

There are reports of pancytopenia, some fatal, induced by coadministration of aspirin or NSAIDs with methotrexate. However, at the low dose used in IBD, such interactions appear to be of limited clinical relevance [10]. Isolated thrombocytopenia induced by a combination of low-dose methotrexate and NSAIDs can normally be corrected by omitting the NSAIDs on the day methotrexate is taken [1]. Nevertheless, the British National Formulary (March 2009) advises that patients taking methotrexate should avoid self-medication with aspirin or ibuprofen.

Trimethoprim

The combination of trimethoprim (or co-trimoxazole) and low-dose methotrexate can cause fatal pancytopenia [1] and, therefore, coadministration of these drugs should be avoided. As both drugs inhibit dihydrofolate reductase, the interaction may result in functional folate deficiency and bone marrow suppression.

Ciprofloxacin

Renal tubular transport of methotrexate may be inhibited by concomitant administration of ciprofloxacin potentially leading to increased plasma levels of methotrexate and consequent clinical toxicity such as pancytopenia or liver dysfunction [11]. Therefore, patients taking methotrexate should be carefully monitored when concomitant ciprofloxacin therapy is indicated.

Cyclosporine

Cyclosporine has a narrow therapeutic range and interacts with many drugs [1]. It is metabolized by the CYP450 family of proteins (predominantly by CYP3A4). This enzyme is induced by a variety of drugs and foods and competitively inhibited by others.

Corticosteroids, thiopurines, and methotrexate

There is conflicting or limited data regarding the presence of interactions between cyclosporine and these IBD medications; however, close monitoring is prudent when any of them is used with cyclosporine [1].

Statins (HMG coA reductase inhibitors)

Plasma levels of statins can be markedly increased by cyclosporine and resultant rhabdomyolysis, which can be fatal, as has been reported [1]; statins should be reduced to a minimum dose if given with cyclosporine.

Colchicine

Colchicine, if coprescribed with cyclosporine is reported to cause myopathy, multiorgan failure, and death [1]. The interaction might be mediated by P-glycoprotein, resulting in toxic levels of colchicine [12]. This combination of drugs should be avoided.

Antitumor necrosis factor (Anti-TNF) therapy (infliximab and adalimumab)

Thiopurines

Fatal hepatosplenic T-cell lymphomas (HSTCLs) have been reported in more than 20, predominantly male, IBD patients receiving infliximab or adalimumab with thiopurines [13]. However, HSTCL remains rare and has also been reported in IBD patients on thiopurine monotherapy [14]. The risk of non-Hodgkins lymphoma (NHL) in IBD patients on concomitant thiopurine/anti-TNF therapy was examined recently in a meta-analysis of over 8000 patients treated with anti-TNF therapy (most of whom also had prior or concurrent immunomodulatory therapy). Thirteen cases of NHL were identified, giving a case rate of 6.1 per 10,000 patient years [15], higher than the expected rate in Crohn's disease (CD) patients, but still a low absolute risk. The reduced formation of antibodies to biologics in patients taking both biologics and immunomodulators is an example of a beneficial drug interaction [1]. Therefore, the risk/benefit ratio of combination therapy must be considered in each patient individually, particularly in view of recent evidence of its superior efficacy compared with either drug alone (see Chapter 24) [16].

Warfarin

Thromboembolism is increased in IBD and, therefore, drug interactions between warfarin and IBD drugs are important. Metronidazole, thiopurines, prednisolone, 5-ASA-containing drugs, and ciprofloxacin have been reported to interact with warfarin [1], therefore, changes in therapy of these drugs in warfarinized patients should prompt more frequent monitoring of the international normalized ratio (INR).

Smoking cessation

Smoking cessation provides clear benefits for patients with CD [17]. However, polycyclic aromatic hydrocarbons within cigarette smoke potently inhibit CYP1A2; therefore, in patients who are giving up smoking, doses of drugs metabolized by this enzyme (see Section "Ciprofloxacin") may need to be decreased to avoid toxicity [18].

Conclusion

There is a wide range of potentially serious drug interactions that can occur when managing patients with IBD. In contrast, a minority of interactions can be to patients' benefit. Reference works such as Drug Interaction Facts, the British National Formulary, and Stockley's Drug Interactions provide invaluable information about drug interactions. For these to remain up to date, healthcare professionals must be diligent in their use of reporting systems (e.g., Yellow Card System, United Kingdom and MedWatch, United States), when they encounter possible drug interactions.

References

1. Irving PM, Shanahan F, Rampton DS. Drug interactions in inflammatory bowel disease. *Am J Gastroenterol* 2008; **103**: 207–219.

2. Szumlanski CL, Weinshilboum RM. Sulphasalazine inhibition of thiopurine methyltransferase: possible mechanism for interaction with 6-mercaptopurine and azathioprine. *Br J Clin Pharmacol* 1995; **39**: 456–459.

3. Lowry PW, Szumlanski CL, Weinshilbourn RM, et al. Balsalazide and azathioprine or 6-mercaptopurine: evidence for a potentially serious drug interaction. *Gastroenterology* 1999; **116**: 1505–1506.

4. Green JR. Balsalazide and azathioprine or 6-mercaptopurine. *Gastroenterology* 1999; **117**: 1513–1514.

5. Shah JA, Edwards CM, Probert CS. Should azathioprine and 5-aminosalicylates be coprescribed in inflammatory bowel disease?: an audit of adverse events and outcome. *Euro J Gastroenterol Hepatol* 2008; **20**: 169–173.

6. Website; http://medicine.iupui.edu/clinpharm/ddis/

7. Piper JM, Ray WA, Daugherty JR, et al. Corticosteroid use and peptic ulcer disease: Role of nonsteroidal anti-inflammatory drugs. *Ann Intern Med* 1991; **114**: 735–740.

8. Laine L, Curtis SP, Cryer B, et al. Assessment of upper gastrointestinal safety of etoricoxib and diclofenac in patients with osteoarthritis and rheumatoid arthritis in the Multinational Etoricoxib and Diclofenac Arthritis Long-term (MEDAL) programme: a randomized comparison. *Lancet* 2007; **369**: 465–473.

9. Soon SY, Ansari A, Yaneza M, et al. Experience with the use of low-dose methotrexate for inflammatory bowel disease. *Eur J Gastroenterol Hepatol* 2004; **16**: 921–926.

10. Zachariae H. Methotrexate and non-steroidal anti-inflammatory drugs. *Br J Dermatol* 1992; **126**: 95.

11. Dalle JH, Auvrignon A, Vassal G, et al. Interaction between methotrexate and ciprofloxacin. *J Pediatr Hematol Oncol* 2002; **24**(5): 321–322.

12. Gruberg L, Har-Zahav Y, Agranat O, et al. Acute myopathy induced by colchicine in a cyclosporine treated heart transplant recipient: possible role of the multidrug resistance transporter. *Transplant Proc* 1999; **31**: 2157–2158.

13. Kotlyar D, Blonski W, Mendizabal M, et al. Case Report of Trisomy 13 in Bone Marrow in a case of hepatosplenic T-cell lymphoma (HSTCL) and inflammatory bowel disease (IBD). *Gastroenterology* 2009; **136**(Suppl. I): A146.

14. Shale M, Kanfer E, Panaccione R, et al. Hepatosplenic T cell lymphoma in inflammatory bowel disease. *Gut* 2008; **57**; 1639–1641.

15. Siegel CA, Marden F, Persing F, et al. Risk of lymphoma associated with combination anti-tumour necrosis factor and immunomodulator therapy for the treatment of Crohn's disease: a meta-analysis. *Clin Gastroenterol Hepatol* 2009; **7**(8): 874–881.

16. Colombel JF, Sandborn WJ, Weinisch W, et al. Infliximab, azathioprine, or combination therapy for Crohn's disease. *N Engl J Med.* 2010; **362**(15):1383–1395.

17. Johnson GJ, Cosnes J, Mansfield JC. Review article: smoking cessation as primary therapy to modify the course of Crohn's disease. *Aliment Pharm Ther* 2005; **21**: 921–931.

18. Kroon LA. Drug interactions with smoking. *Am J Health Syst Pharm* 2007; **64**(18): 1917–1921.

34 Is there still a role for ursodeoxycholic acid treatment in patients with inflammatory bowel disease associated with primary sclerosing cholangitis?

Emmanouil Sinakos and Keith D. Lindor

Division of Gastroenterology and Hepatology, Mayo Clinic Rochester, MN, USA

LEARNING POINTS

- Ursodeoxycholic acid (UDCA) improves liver biochemistry, but not the course of primary sclerosing cholangitis (PSC).

- A recent randomized, controlled trial of high-dose UDCA in PSC failed to demonstrate improvement in survival, and was associated with increased rates of serious adverse events.

- UDCA may act as a chemopreventive agent against colorectal cancer in patients with PSC and inflammatory bowel disease (IBD).

- On the basis of existing data, UDCA cannot be generally recommended to treat PSC in patients with IBD. However, such patients may benefit from its chemopreventive action.

Introduction

Primary sclerosing cholangitis (PSC) is a chronic cholestatic liver disease characterized by inflammation and destruction of the extrahepatic and/or intrahepatic bile ducts. It may result in biliary cirrhosis and need for liver transplantation, and often leads to a reduced life expectancy. Up until now there are no reports of a medical therapy that is able to halt disease progression. Ursodeoxycholic acid (UDCA) represents a hydrophilic dihydroxy (3α, 7β-dihydroxy-5β-cholan-24-oic acid) bile acid, which is shown to have some beneficial effects as measured by liver biochemistry [1].

PSC has an intriguing association with inflammatory bowel disease (IBD). The prevalence of IBD, mainly ulcerative colitis (UC), in patients with PSC ranges from 21% to 80%, depending on the methods of disease screening and the study population [2]. Conversely, PSC is present in 2–7% of patients with IBD. There is evidence that certain disease characteristics predominate when the two entities coexist compared to a separate presentation of each disease.

The PSC–IBD relationship

IBD in patients with PSC is often mild or asymptomatic and is associated with rectal sparing and backwash ileitis [3]. Moreover, patients with UC and concomitant PSC have an increased risk for developing colorectal cancer (CRC) compared to UC alone [4]. Proctocolectomy as a treatment for chronic UC appears to have no effect on liver biochemistry, histology or survival of patients with PSC; however, pouchitis is far more common after colectomy and ileoanal pouch formation in patents with UC and PSC compared to UC alone [5].

In contrast, on the basis of existing data, PSC in patients with IBD does not seem to constitute a disease separate from that seen in patients without IBD. Nevertheless, one study showed that patients with PSC and concomitant IBD are more likely to be male, to present with abnormal liver function as the first manifestation of their liver disease and to have combined intrahepatic and extrahepatic bile duct

Clinical Dilemmas in Inflammatory Bowel Disease: New Challenges, Second Edition. Edited by P. Irving, C. Siegel, D. Rampton and F. Shanahan.
© 2011 Blackwell Publishing Ltd. Published 2011 by Blackwell Publishing Ltd.

strictures [6]. Finally, transplanted patients with PSC and IBD have a variable UC course, and continue to carry the same increased risk of developing CRC after transplantation [5].

Effectiveness of UDCA in PSC

UDCA exerts multiple potentially beneficial effects for chronic cholestasis, including an expansion of the hydrophilic bile acid pool, hypercholeresis, immunomodulation, and cytoprotection [7]. Several studies with varying drug doses have shown that administration of UDCA in patients with PSC is well tolerated and has a favorable outcome, generally limited to biochemical parameters of the disease (Table 34.1). Data emerging from these studies have implied that higher drug doses could possibly increase survival rates as well. However, a recently published randomized, double-blind controlled trial of high-dose UDCA (28–30 mg/kg/day) versus placebo failed to demonstrate improvement in survival and was associated with increased rates of serious adverse events [8]. In this study, which was terminated early because of futility, more patients developed varices, died, or became eligible for liver transplantation in the group receiving UDCA than in that given placebo. It is unclear why a drug thought to be extremely safe resulted in such outcomes: it has been speculated that an alteration in the composition of the bile acid pool or a direct toxic effect could be implicated.

IBD has been present in a considerable percentage of the PSC patients in all published studies of the therapeutic potential of UDCA, and the results obtained were similar to those in PSC patients without IBD. Furthermore, no IBD-related adverse events were reported, even in the most recent high-dose UDCA trial. Therefore, medical treatment of PSC itself in patients with concomitant IBD is currently considered to be identical to treatment of PSC in general, at least in terms of efficacy.

Chemopreventive effect of UDCA

Patients with IBD and PSC carry an important risk of developing colorectal or hepatobiliary malignancy. UDCA in vitro inhibits growth, stimulated by deoxycholic acid, in several tumor cell lines [9]. Based on this observation, UDCA has subsequently been studied as a chemopreventive strategy against CRC. Two retrospective studies showed a lower risk of developing colorectal dysplasia in patients with PSC who were taking UDCA compared to in those not doing so [10,11]. By following a cohort of patients drawn from an earlier randomized, placebo-controlled trial, Pardi et al. documented that UDCA-treated patients with PSC have a significantly lower risk of developing colorectal dysplasia or cancer [12].

However, the evidence for a beneficial effect of UDCA on the risk of developing cholangiocarcinoma in patients with PSC is limited. Thus, it seems reasonable that UDCA chemoprevention treatment in the setting of PSC should be offered only to patients at high risk for CRC development, such as those with a family history of CRC, previous colorectal neoplasia, or long-standing extensive colitis, as the recent guidelines published by the European Association for the Study of the Liver advised [13].

TABLE 34.1 Clinical trials of ursodeoxycholic acid (UDCA) treatment in primary sclerosing cholangitis (PSC)

First author	Journal, year	RCT	n	Duration (years)	UDCA dose	IBD (%)	LFTs improved	Histology improved
Beuers	*Hepatology*, 1992	Y	14	1	13–15 mg/kg	83	Y	Y
Stiehl	*J Hepatol*, 1994	Y	20	0.25	750 mg	90	Y	Y
Lindor	*N Engl J Med*, 1997	Y	102	2.2	13–15 mg/kg	77	Y	N
Harnois	*Am J Gastroenterol*, 2001	N	30	1	25–30 mg/kg	77	Y	NA
Mitchell	*Gastroenterology*, 2001	Y	26	2	20–25 mg/kg	84	Y	Y
Olsson	*Gastroenterology*, 2005	Y	219	5	17–23 mg/kg	84	Y	NA
Cullen	*J Hepatol*, 2008	Y	31	2	10–30 mg/kg	84	Y	N
Lindor	*Hepatology*, 2009	Y	150	5	25–30 mg/kg	72	Y	N

RCT, randomized controlled trial; LFTs, liver function tests; Y, yes; N, no; NA, not available.

Conclusions

PSC in association with IBD is an extremely interesting disease combination with unique characteristics. The liver component cannot currently be effectively treated. UDCA seems to improve the biochemical characteristics of the disease, but is not associated with an improvement in survival. However, this drug has an excellent safety profile associated with its use in PSC–IBD patients and possibly exerts a chemopreventive effect against colon cancer. Furthermore, 24-*nor*UDCA, a novel bile acid chemically related to UDCA, has recently been shown in an animal model to have beneficial effects in cholestasis [14]: it may be worth further evaluation in patients with PSC.

Taking all the available information into consideration, we think that there is insufficient evidence to support the general use of UDCA in patients with IBD and PSC. However, further studies need to be performed before drawing any final conclusions on the possible roles of bile acid therapy in the prevention of progression of the hepatobiliary disease itself, and as chemoprotection against biliary and colonic malignancy in patients with PSC and IBD.

References

1. Lindor KD. Ursodiol for primary sclerosing cholangitis. Mayo primary sclerosing cholangitis-ursodeoxycholic acid study group. *N Engl J Med* 1997; **336**(10): 691–695.

2. Broome U and Bergquist A. Primary sclerosing cholangitis, inflammatory bowel disease, and colon cancer. *Semin Liver Dis* 2006; **26**(1): 31–41.

3. Loftus EV, Jr, Harewood GC, Loftus CG, et al. PSC-IBD: A unique form of inflammatory bowel disease associated with primary sclerosing cholangitis. *Gut* 2005; **54**(1): 91–96.

4. Soetikno RM, Lin OS, Heidenreich PA, et al. Increased risk of colorectal neoplasia in patients with primary sclerosing cholangitis and ulcerative colitis: A meta-analysis. *Gastrointest Endosc* 2002; **56**(1): 48–54.

5. Saich R, Chapman R. Primary sclerosing cholangitis, autoimmune hepatitis and overlap syndromes in inflammatory bowel disease. *World J Gastroenterol* 2008; **14**(3): 331–337.

6. Rabinovitz M, Gavaler JS, Schade RR, et al. Does primary sclerosing cholangitis occurring in association with inflammatory bowel disease differ from that occurring in the absence of inflammatory bowel disease? A study of sixty-six subjects. *Hepatology* 1990; **11**(1): 7–11.

7. Lazaridis KN, Gores GJ, Lindor KD. Ursodeoxycholic acid 'mechanisms of action and clinical use in hepatobiliary disorders'. *J Hepatol* 2001; **35**(1): 134–146.

8. Lindor KD, Kowdley KV, Luketic VA, et al. High-dose ursodeoxycholic acid for the treatment of primary sclerosing cholangitis. *Hepatology* 2009; **50**(3): 808–814.

9. Martinez JD, Stratagoules ED, LaRue JM, et al. Different bile acids exhibit distinct biological effects: the tumor promoter deoxycholic acid induces apoptosis and the chemopreventive agent ursodeoxycholic acid inhibits cell proliferation. *Nutr Cancer* 1998; **31**(2): 111–118.

10. Tung BY, Emond MJ, Haggitt RC, et al. Ursodiol use is associated with lower prevalence of colonic neoplasia in patients with ulcerative colitis and primary sclerosing cholangitis. *Ann Intern Med* 2001; **134**(2): 89–95.

11. Wolf JM, Rybicki LA, Lashner BA. The impact of ursodeoxycholic acid on cancer, dysplasia and mortality in ulcerative colitis patients with primary sclerosing cholangitis. *Aliment Pharmacol Ther* 2005; **22**(9): 783–788.

12. Pardi DS, Loftus EV, Jr, Kremers WK, et al. Ursodeoxycholic acid as a chemopreventive agent in patients with ulcerative colitis and primary sclerosing cholangitis. *Gastroenterology* 2003; **124**(4): 889–893.

13. EASL Clinical Practice Guidelines: management of cholestatic liver diseases. *J Hepatol* 2009; **51**(2): 237–267.

14. Halilbasic E, Fiorotto R, Fickert P, et al. Side chain structure determines unique physiologic and therapeutic properties of norursodeoxycholic acid in Mdr2-/- Mice. *Hepatology* 2009; **49**(6): 1972–1981.

35 Stem cell transplantation for Crohn's: will it fulfill its promise?

Venkataraman Subramanian[1] and Christopher J. Hawkey[2]

[1] Nottingham Digestive Diseases Centre, Queens Medical Centre, Nottingham University Hospitals NHS Trust, Nottingham, UK
[2] University Hospital, Queen's Medical Centre, Nottingham University Hospitals NHS Trust, Nottingham, UK

LEARNING POINTS

- Sustained remission has occurred in most patients with Crohn's disease (CD) who have undergone hematologous stem cell transplantation (HSCT).

- The high mortality from HSCT for other autoimmune conditions suggests that its use in CD should be limited at present to patients with no other treatment options.

- Local inoculation of adipose tissue-derived mesenchymal stem cells is a promising new treatment of fistulas in patients with CD.

- Systemic infusion of stem cells does not require toxic conditioning regimens and is currently being evaluated in clinical trials.

Introduction

Patients with Crohn's disease (CD) who have failed to respond to available medical therapies are commonly referred to tertiary centers for investigational studies. Autologous stem cell transplantation is being explored as a potential therapy for a variety of autoimmune diseases such as rheumatoid arthritis, multiple sclerosis, and systemic lupus erythematosus. The serendipitous discovery of long-standing remission in patients with CD undergoing bone marrow transplantation for other indications has led to the hope that hematopoietic stem cell transplantation (HSCT) could lead to a "cure" for this often refractory condition [1].

What are stem cells?

Stem cells have the unique capacity for self-renewal and the ability to give rise to one or more types of differentiated progeny. Of late, there is some evidence that stem cells could also have immunomodulatory properties. The bone marrow is the major source of stem cells, but while they are known to exist in several different tissues, their role and identity in these is unclear. Bone marrow-derived CD34-positive stem cells are committed to differentiate into erythroid, lymphoid, and myeloid lineages. A distinct lineage of stem cells called mesenchymal stem (or stromal) cells (MSC) are thought to support hematopoiesis, but their role is unclear. These cells also migrate to areas of tissue injury and give rise to cell lineages, including epithelial cells, adipocytes, astrocytes, osteoblasts, and myocytes. MSCs have also been isolated from other tissues including skin, adipose tissue, cartilage, and placenta.

Rationale for stem cell transplantation in Crohn's disease

CD is characterized by a loss of immune tolerance in the gastrointestinal tract and a T-helper 1 (Th1) cell-mediated inflammatory response. The discovery of several specific mutations predisposing to CD, including NOD2, IL23R, and ATG16L1, has led to the belief that phenotypic expression of CD is mediated by an interaction between genetic and environmental factors (such as smoking, luminal bacteria, early childhood infections) and that this interaction is mediated by the immune system [2].

Clinical Dilemmas in Inflammatory Bowel Disease: New Challenges, Second Edition. Edited by P. Irving, C. Siegel, D. Rampton and F. Shanahan.
© 2011 Blackwell Publishing Ltd. Published 2011 by Blackwell Publishing Ltd.

Allogenic HSCT could benefit patients by replacing the genetic predisposition to CD in circulating leukocytes. Autologous HSCT would not change the genetic predisposition but might "reset" the immune system by eliminating autoreactive cells in the recipient and restoring the patient to the status quo of being predisposed to CD, but not suffering from it. Therefore, although the susceptibility to relapse of CD is not eliminated, the patient may remain in remission so long as he/she is not exposed to the appropriate trigger in the future. The efficacy of bone marrow and HSCT in other immune-mediated diseases [3] also suggests that it may be of value for patients with CD.

Hematopoietic stem cell transplantation

HSCT is principally used for hematologic and lymphoproliferative disorders; autologous HSCT has been performed in more than 700 patients with autoimmune diseases [3]. The first report of bone marrow transplantation in a patient with CD was in 1993 [4], when a patient who underwent autologous transplant for lymphoma stayed in remission from his Crohn's during 6 months' follow-up. Subsequently, there have been over 40 reported autologous and allogenic HSCTs in patients who coincidentally had CD (Table 35.1).

This experience has led to some groups offering HSCT specifically for CD. Apart from case reports, the largest study

TABLE 35.1 Published studies on hematopoietic stem cell transplantation (HSCT) for patients with Crohn's disease [1,5,6,7,8]

Author	Year of publication	Type of HSCT	Number	Primary indication	Outcome	Follow-up
Drakos	1993	Autologous	1	Non-Hodgkin's lymphoma	Remission	6 months
Castro	1996	Autologous	2 (1 CD and 1 UC)	Breast cancer	Off therapy, Mild colitis on follow-up colonoscopy	3 years
Kashyap	1998	Autologous	1	Non-Hodgkin's lymphoma	Remission	7 years
Lopez-Cubero	1998	Allogenic	6	Leukemia	4 in remission 1 died at day 97 (sepsis) 1 relapse at 1.5 years	4.5–15.3 years
Talbot	1998	Allogenic	1	Leukemia	Remission	8 years
Musso	2000	Autologous	1	Hodgkin's lymphoma	Remission	3 years
Soderholm	2002	Allogenic	1	Leukemia	Remission	5 years
Ditschkowski	2003	Autologous	11 (7 CD and 4 UC)	Leukemia (10) MDS (1)	10 in remission 1 died (fungal infection)	Median 34 months
Hawkey	2004	Autologous	1	Small bowel lymphoma	Remission	18 months
Anumakonda	2007	Autologous	1	Non-Hodgkin's lymphoma	Remission	12 years
Burt	2003	Autologous	2	Refractory CD	Remission	1 year
Kreisel	2003	Autologous	1	Refractory CD	Clinical and histological improvement	9 months
Scime	2004	Autologous	1	Refractory CD	Remission	5 months
Oyama	2005	Autologous	12	Refractory CD	Remission in 11/12	7–37 months
Duijvestein	2008	Autologous	3	Refractory CD	Remission (1 had mobilization only)	8 weeks to 2 years
Cassinotti	2008	Autologous	4	Refractory CD	3 patients had complete response, 1 had partial response	11–20 months

reporting HSCT specifically for CD was a Phase 1 study of 12 patients with refractory CD who had failed therapy with infliximab: 11 entered sustained remission (CDAI < 150) over a median follow-up of 18 months [5].

Despite these clinical studies, there is still uncertainty on which component of this complex therapeutic process has the most benefit. Allogenic HSCT usually involves high-dose immunoablative therapy or conditioning (e.g., cyclophosphamide and total body irradiation) followed by HSCT from a human leukocyte antigen (HLA) matched donor, while autologous HSCT involves a mobilization phase (usually with cyclophosphamide and G-CSF) followed by leukapheresis (when the autologous stem cells are collected and stored) and conditioning (e.g., cyclophosphamide, antithymocyte globulin) followed by HSCT (of stem cells collected at leukapheresis). An initial beneficial effect might be expected from the eradication of autoreactive T cells and memory cells produced by the lymphoablative effects of the conditioning regimen. There have been reports that improvement of CD occurs after the mobilization phase of HSCT [5,9], but this is not universally accepted [6]. HSCT may simply enable immunosuppression to be more intense with subsequent long-term benefit arising through reinstated immunoregulation.

The ASTIC trial (Autologous stem cell transplant for Crohn's), is an ongoing multicenter, prospective, randomized Phase III study conducted by the European Crohn's and Colitis Organisation (ECCO), sponsored by the Autoimmune Disease Working Party of the European Group for Blood and Marrow Transplantation (EBMT). This trial aims to compare the benefit of HSCT with mobilization, immunoablation, and HSCT between patients who have immediate and delayed (1 year) autologous HSCT after mobilization. So far 14 patients have been included and 7 have completed HSCT (http://www.nottingham.ac.uk/icr/astic/). Final results are expected in 2011.

Safety of HSCT in Crohn's disease

There has been no transplant-related mortality in HSCT done for refractory CD so far. Data from HSCT done for other autoimmune conditions are not so reassuring. Data collated from multiple centers in 2000 on 390 patients undergoing autologous HSCT for various autoimmune conditions showed a mobilization-associated mortality of 1.5% and an overall procedure-related mortality of 9% [10]. The EBMT/EULAR (European Group for Blood and Marrow Transplantation and the European League Against Rheumatism) registry report in 2005 on 473 patients also undergoing autologous HSCT for autoimmune disease revealed an overall mortality of 11% and a transplant-related mortality of 7%, the latter mainly being due to infection [11].

CD is associated with an increased risk of translocation of bacteria from the inflamed gut and from residual sites of infection in patients with perianal disease, which could increase the risk of transplant-related infections. Polymorphisms in the *NOD2* gene have been shown to predict increased 1-year transplant-related mortality in patients undergoing allogenic HSCT, with a trend towards increased risk of bacteremia with coagulase-negative *Staphylococci* [12]. Given the considerable mortality rate for other autoimmune diseases, HSCT should perhaps be limited to CD patient's refractory to all immunosuppressive drugs including biologics, and in whom there are no current surgical options.

Mesenchymal stem cell transplantation

MSCs were first identified as an adherent fibroblast-like population of cells in the bone marrow by Friedenstein et al. [13]. MSCs can be derived from virtually any connective tissue including bone marrow, adipose tissue, and cartilage. Animal studies have indicated that MSCs have immunomodulatory functions in addition to their pluripotent (stem cell like) properties [14]. MSCs derived from adipose tissue inhibit peripheral blood mononuclear-cell proliferation and interferon-γ production, while increasing interleukin-10 secretion; they also ameliorate trinitrobenzene sulfonic acid-induced colitis in mice and inhibit mucosal and systemic proinflammatory cytokine production [15].

In a Phase 1 study using local inoculation of autologous adipose tissue-derived MSCs for fistulizing CD, 75% of fistulas were healed in 8 weeks [16]. Another observational Phase 1 study also showed that 3 of 4 CD patients with fistulas treated with autologous expanded adipose-derived stem cells (ASCs) had complete healing compared with 1 of 4 such patients treated with a lipoaspirate alone [17]. A Phase 2 study on the use of ASCs in patients with complex perianal fistulas showed healing in 17 of 24 patients who received ASCs in addition to fibrin glue compared with 4 of 25 patients given fibrin glue alone (relative risk for healing, 4.43; confidence interval (CI), 1.74–11.27; $P < 0.001$) [18].

One of the advantages of using MSCs for transplantation is that it does not require conditioning chemotherapy. Osiris Therapeutics reported in 2006 results of a Phase 2 study of patients with moderate-to-severe CD given MSCs derived from healthy bone marrow volunteer donors (Prochymal™): there was a clinical response in only 3 of 9 patients (http://www.osiristx.com/pdf/Crohn's_Ph_II_Handout.pdf). A Phase 3 trial is underway, but recruitment has been stopped due to higher than expected placebo response rates during an interim analysis of the first 210 patients recruited (http://www.reuters.com/article/idUSBNG41270520090327). Phase I trials by Celgene on their placental derived stem cell, in patients with moderate to severe CD, have been released to the press in April 2010 and apparently showed that 4 of 6 patients receiving low dose of the cells had clinical remission (better than the high dose group). (http://www.reuters.com/article/idUSN0822182420100408). Although no mortality has been reported in patients receiving MSCs for autoimmune disease, there are some reports suggesting that MSCs stimulate the growth of cancers in mice and promote metastasis [19]. Reports on the long-term effects of MSC transplantation in humans are still awaited.

Conclusions

There has been rapid progress in stem cell therapy for patients with CD over the past decade. Autologous HSCT has been evaluated for severe refractory CD, but is currently indicated only in carefully selected patients who have run out of conventional treatment options. The use of MSCs derived from adipose tissue has been evaluated in fistulizing CD with some success. Data on the use of systemically infused MSCs for luminal CD are awaited. With improvements in transplantation techniques and reduction in transplant-related morbidity, there could be an expansion in the role of both HSCT and MSC transplants for patients with CD.

References

1. Hawkey CJ. Stem cell transplantation for Crohn's disease. *Best.Pract.Res.Clin.Haematol* 2004; **17**: 317–325.
2. Watts DA, Satsangi J. The genetic jigsaw of inflammatory bowel disease. *Gut* 2002; **50**(Suppl 3): III31–III36.
3. van Laar JM, Tyndall A. Adult stem cells in the treatment of autoimmune diseases. *Rheumatology* (Oxford) 2006; **45**: 1187–1193.
4. Drakos PE, Nagler A, Or R. Case of Crohn's disease in bone marrow transplantation. *Am.J.Hematol* 1993; **43**: 157–158.
5. Oyama Y, Craig RM, Traynor AE, et al. Autologous hematopoietic stem cell transplantation in patients with refractory Crohn's disease. *Gastroenterology* 2005; **128**: 552–563.
6. Cassinotti A, Annaloro C, Ardizzone S, et al. Autologous haematopoietic stem cell transplantation without CD34+ cell selection in refractory Crohn's disease. *Gut* 2008; **57**: 211–117.
7. Duijvestein M, van den Brink GR, Hommes DW. Stem cells as potential novel therapuetic strategy for inflammatory bowel disease. *Journal of Crohn's and Colitis* 2008; **2**: 99–106.
8. Fortun PJ, Hawkey CJ. The role of stem cell transplantation in inflammatory bowel disease. *Autoimmunity* 2008; **41**: 654–659.
9. Scime R, Cavallaro AM, Tringali S, et al. Complete clinical remission after high-dose immune suppression and autologous hematopoietic stem cell transplantation in severe Crohn's disease refractory to immunosuppressive and immunomodulator therapy. *Inflamm Bowel Dis* 2004; **10**: 892–894.
10. Tyndall A, Passweg J, Gratwohl A. Haemopoietic stem cell transplantation in the treatment of severe autoimmune diseases 2000. *Ann Rheum Dis* 2001; **60**: 702–707,
11. Gratwohl A, Passweg J, Bocelli-Tyndall C, et al. Autologous hematopoietic stem cell transplantation for autoimmune diseases. *Bone Marrow Transplant* 2005; **35**: 869–879.
12. van der Velden WJ, Blijlevens NM, Maas FM, et al. NOD2 polymorphisms predict severe acute graft-versus-host and treatment-related mortality in T-cell-depleted haematopoietic stem cell transplantation. *Bone Marrow Transplant* 2009; **44**: 243–248.
13. Friedenstein AJ, Deriglasova UF, Kulagina NN, et al. Precursors for fibroblasts in different populations of hematopoietic cells as detected by the in vitro colony assay method. *Exp Hematol* 1974; **2**: 83–92.
14. Bernardo ME, Locatelli F, Fibbe WE. Mesenchymal stromal cells. *Ann.N.Y.Acad.Sci* 2009; **1176**: 101–117.
15. Gonzalez MA, Gonzalez-Rey E, Rico L, Buscher D, Delgado M. Adipose-derived mesenchymal stem cells alleviate experimental colitis by inhibiting inflammatory and autoimmune responses. *Gastroenterology* 2009; **136**: 978–989.
16. Garcia-Olmo D, Garcia-Arranz M, Herreros D, Pascual I, Peiro C, Rodriguez-Montes JA. A phase I clinical trial of the treatment of Crohn's fistula by adipose mesenchymal stem cell transplantation. *Dis Colon Rectum* 2005; **48**: 1416–1423.
17. Garcia-Olmo D, Herreros D, Pascual M, Pascual I, De La Quintana P, Trebol J et al. Treatment of enterocutaneous

fistula in Crohn's Disease with adipose-derived stem cells: a comparison of protocols with and without cell expansion. *Int.J.Colorectal Dis* 2009; **24**: 27–30.

18. Garcia-Olmo D, Herreros D, Pascual I, et al. Expanded adipose-derived stem cells for the treatment of complex perianal fistula: a phase II clinical trial. *Dis Colon Rectum* 2009; **52**: 79–86.

19. Karnoub AE, Dash AB, Vo AP, et al. Mesenchymal stem cells within tumour stroma promote breast cancer metastasis. *Nature* 2007; **449**: 557–563.

Complementary therapy: is there a needle in the haystack?

Shane M. Devlin

Division of Gastroenterology, Inflammatory Bowel Disease Clinic, The University of Calgary, Calgary, AB, Canada

LEARNING POINTS

- Many patients with IBD use complementary and alternative medicine.

- Complementary and alternative therapy is widely believed by patients to be safer than traditional pharmacologic approaches.

- There is a paucity of randomized controlled data evaluating complementary therapy in IBD despite there being a wide range of therapies available to patients in an unregulated fashion.

- The available evidence supports the use of oral curcumin as a maintenance agent for quiescent ulcerative colitis and may support the use of *Artemisia absinthium* (wormwood) as a steroid-sparing agent for Crohn's disease but further study is needed.

- There is a need for larger randomized trials with rigorous endpoints before the use of most complementary therapies can be advocated.

- While the potential toxicity of herbal or other potions should be addressed, clinicians should avoid dismissive responses to patients' suggestions regarding harmless remedies.

- Complementary therapy may confer a sense of control for the patient over their disease.

How often and why is CAM used in IBD?

Complementary and alternative medicine (CAM) encompasses a broad range of therapies that extend well beyond the standard notion of herbal therapy that many people would associate with CAM (see Table 36.1). These treatments do not generally require a prescription and are widely available to patients in an unregulated fashion. Moreover, patients regard them as safer therapies with only 16% of patients reporting adverse events related to their use [1].

CAM is widely used by patients with inflammatory bowel disease (IBD), a phenomenon common to other chronic diseases [1]. Studies encompassing both patients with Crohn's disease (CD) and ulcerative colitis (UC) from a wide range of geographic distributions report frequencies of CAM use ranging from 21–53% with homeopathy and herbal therapies being the most commonly used [1]. This phenomenon is not limited to adults with IBD as a recent American study demonstrated, revealing that 50% of pediatric patients were using CAM [2].

The rationale behind the use of CAM seems to vary widely among patients. Studies that have examined why patients choose to use CAM have demonstrated a variety of reasons that cross all spectra of disease activity and lifestyle choices [3–6]. Factors associated with CAM use included, among others, severe disease, high corticosteroid usage, a desire to feel in control, and a lack of confidence in their physician.

Finding the needle in the haystack: what is the evidence for CAM in IBD?

Despite the wide range of potential CAM available to patients with IBD, there is a relative paucity of agents for which there is high-level evidence. Importantly, among controlled studies there is considerable heterogeneity in terms of defined end points, study length, and the presence of blinding, so that interpretation is challenging. Although

Clinical Dilemmas in Inflammatory Bowel Disease: New Challenges, Second Edition. Edited by P. Irving, C. Siegel, D. Rampton and F. Shanahan.
© 2011 Blackwell Publishing Ltd. Published 2011 by Blackwell Publishing Ltd.

TABLE 36.1 Types of complementary and alternative medicine

Domain	Alternative medical system
Whole medical systems	Homeopathic medicine Naturopathic medicine Ayurvedic medicine[a] Traditional Chinese medicine (including acupuncture/ moxibustion)
Mind–body medicine	Meditation Prayer Art, music, dance
Biologically based therapy	Herbal therapy Dietary supplements Vitamins
Manipulative and body-based practices	Chiropractic Osteopathic manipulation Massage
Energy medicine	Bioelectromagnetic field therapy Therapeutic touch, Reiki

Source: http://www.nccam.nih.gov/health/whatiscam.
[a] A form of traditional medicine native to the Indian subcontinent.

beyond the limited scope of this chapter, excellent reviews exist that summarize a greater breadth of animal and human studies of CAM in IBD and explore the possible biologic mechanisms of the agents discussed in this chapter as well as other potential therapies [1,7]. This chapter will focus only on blinded, randomized controlled trials: note that all of the published studies are small, ranging in size from 23–89 patients [8–14]. The largest randomized controlled trial, recently published in abstract form only, studied the effectiveness of an extract of *Andrographis paniculata* in 223 patients with mild to moderately active UC [15].

Boswellia serrata

In Europe, *Boswellia serrata* is a frequently used remedy that is a common component of incense. In a randomized, double-blind placebo-controlled trial, *B. serrata* H15 extract was shown to be comparable to mesalamine for active CD [8]. However, as mesalamine is now often considered ineffective in CD, the value of this therapy for this indication is questionable.

Wheat grass juice

The use of wheat grass juice was evaluated in a double-blind randomized placebo-controlled trial in 24 patients with mild-to-moderate distal UC [9]. After 1 month of 100 mL daily of wheat grass juice, there was a statistically significant improvement in rectal bleeding, the disease activity index (DAI), and the physicians' global assessment versus those treated with placebo. There was an improvement in the sigmoidoscopic subscore of the DAI in 78% of those treated with wheat grass juice versus 30% in the placebo arm, but this was not statistically significant.

Aloe vera gel

Aloe vera gel is a commonly used complementary therapy and is purported to have anti-inflammatory and antioxidant properties. The use of oral aloe vera gel was evaluated in a 4-week, double-blind, placebo-controlled trial of mild-to-moderately active UC [10]. Forty-four patients were randomized 2:1 to 100 mL of aloe vera gel orally twice daily or placebo for 4 weeks. The primary end point was remission based on the simple clinical colitis activity index (CAI) at week 4 with secondary end points being changes in inflammatory bowel disease questionnaire (IBDQ) and improvements in sigmoidoscopic and histologic scores. There was a numerical but not statistically significant difference in the proportion of patients in remission, and there was no difference in sigmoidoscopic or histologic scores at 4 weeks.

Traditional acupuncture and moxibustion (TAM)

Traditional acupuncture and moxibustion (the application of heat to acupuncture points) is commonly used by patients with a number of ailments, though its mechanism of action is not known. An intriguing study in an animal model of UC demonstrated reduced levels of interleukin-1β (IL-1β), IL-6, and TNF-α associated with acupuncture, but the relevance of this to human disease is unknown [16]. In a single-blind randomized controlled trial, 51 patients with active CD were treated with either 10 TAM sessions ($N = 27$) or 10 sham acupuncture sessions ($N = 24$) (acupuncture in nonacupuncture points) over 4 weeks [11]. Patients included in the study had relatively mild disease with a CD activity index (CDAI) of between 150 and 350, they could be on no more than 15 mg of prednisone and were not on immunosuppressant agents. TAM was associated with a statistically greater mean reduction in CDAI than sham acupuncture (78 versus 26), which was no longer significant 12 weeks posttreatment. There was a similar improvement in the IBDQ in both groups, perhaps implying a strong placebo effect.

The same authors evaluated TAM in 29 active UC patients in a nearly identical study design [12]. The primary end point was reduction in the CAI at 5 weeks. There was a statistically significant reduction in the CAI in both groups with the decrease being significantly larger in the TAM arm. There were significant improvements in the IBDQ and a patient-generated visual analog scale of self-assessed disease severity in both arms, again perhaps implying a significant placebo effect.

Curcumin

The largest and most rigorously conducted study of CAM therapy in IBD is a multicenter, double-blind randomized placebo-controlled trial of curcumin for maintenance of remission of quiescent UC [13]. Curcumin is the yellow pigment in turmeric and is known to exert anti-inflammatory properties and, more specifically, suppresses activation of transcription factor NF-κB [1, 7]. In this study, 89 patients were randomized to 1 g orally twice daily of curcumin or placebo in combination with 1.0–3.0 g/day of sulfasalazine or 1.5–3.0 g/day of mesalamine. Patients continued the therapy for 6 months, at which point the curcumin and placebo were withdrawn and patients were studied for an additional 6 months on aminosalicylates alone. Patients requiring immunosuppressant agents were excluded from the study.

By intention to treat analysis, there was a significantly lower rate of relapse at 6 months in those treated with curcumin *versus* placebo. The endoscopic score improved in the curcumin group compared to baseline while there was a nonsignificant deterioration in the endoscopic score in the placebo group.

Wormwood

The most recent study of CAM in IBD is a double-blind placebo-controlled study of wormwood (*Artemisia absinthium*) as a steroid-sparing agent in CD [14]. In this multicenter trial, 40 patients with a CDAI of 170 or greater, on 40 mg or less of prednisone and stable concomitant medications which could include mesalamine or immunosuppressants (excluding biologic therapy) were randomized to a standardized preparation of wormwood (SedaCrohn®, Noorherbals, Hockessin, Delaware) 500 mg orally three times daily or placebo for 10 weeks. The primary end points were steroid dose, CDAI, and IBDQ after 10 weeks of treatment and 10 weeks posttreatment. Though there was no rigorous statistical comparison, there was a sustained decrease in CDAI, a numerical reduction in steroid dose, and an improvement in IBDQ at 20 weeks in patients treated with wormwood implying some sustained beneficial effect.

Andrographis paniculata

Though only published thus far in abstract form, a rigorously performed randomized controlled trial evaluating an extract of the *A. paniculata* plant was done in patients with mild to moderately active UC. A dose of 1800 mg/day was associated with statistically significant differences in clinical response, remission, and mucosal healing at 8 weeks over placebo-treated patients [15]. The full manuscript of this study is eagerly anticipated.

What should we tell our patients?

It is important to recognize that many of our patients are using CAM and they will seek our expertise in guiding them. Though most physicians will lack any specific training in CAM, an awareness of those treatments that have been studied can only serve to enhance the therapeutic relationship between physicians and those patients who have an interest in CAM. However, it is important to convey to patients that any therapy that exerts a biologic effect is, by definition, a drug that can have toxicity and potential drug interactions. Furthermore, in those instances when patients are using CAM under the care of an allied health care provider (such as a naturopath) communication between the physician and allied health care provider, for example to examine for potential drug interactions, is vital.

Conclusions

So, is there a needle in the haystack? In considering the varied study designs and heterogeneous end points and small sample sizes of the above studies, the use of curcumin as a maintenance therapy for quiescent UC is attractive and warrants further study. The use of a standardized extract of *A. paniculata* as a therapy for mild-to-moderate UC seems similarly attractive and, when published, will represent the largest randomized controlled trial ever done with a complementary therapy. However, its use cannot yet be advocated given the limited data available. The use of wormwood for CD and wheat grass juice for distal UC is intriguing but certainly needs more rigorous study. At this point, on the basis of the available evidence, the use of TAM, *B. serrata,* and aloe vera gel cannot be advocated. However, these studies have taken the first steps toward enhancing our understanding of therapies that have been part of medical folklore for hundreds of years and indeed with further study we may find therapies that are not only safe but also effective. Ultimately, better standardization of products and more robust safety data will be needed before these therapies will gain widespread acceptance by practitioners.

References

1. Rahimi R, Mozaffari S, Abdollahi M. On the use of herbal medicines in management of inflammatory bowel diseases: a systematic review of animal and human studies. *Dig Dis Sci* 2009; **54**(3): 471–480.

2. Wong AP, Clark AL, Garnett EA, et al. Use of complementary medicine in pediatric patients with inflammatory bowel disease: results from a multicenter survey. *J Pediatr Gastroenterol Nutr* 2009; **48**(1): 55–60.

3. Li FX, Verhoef MJ, Best A, Otley A, Hilsden RJ. Why patients with inflammatory bowel disease use or do not use complementary and alternative medicine: a Canadian national survey. *Can J Gastroenterol* 2005; **19**(9): 567–573.

4. Moser G, Tillinger W, Sachs G, et al. Relationship between the use of unconventional therapies and disease-related concerns: a study of patients with inflammatory bowel disease. *J Psychosom Res* 1996; **40**(5): 503–509.

5. Langhorst J, Anthonisen IB, Steder-Neukamm U, et al. Amount of systemic steroid medication is a strong predictor for the use of complementary and alternative medicine in patients with inflammatory bowel disease: results from a German national survey. *Inflamm Bowel Dis* 2005; **11**(3): 287–295.

6. Langhorst J, Anthonisen IB, Steder-Neukamm U, et al. Patterns of complementary and alternative medicine (CAM) use in patients with inflammatory bowel disease: perceived stress is a potential indicator for CAM use. *Complement Ther Med* 2007; **15**(1): 30–37.

7. Langmead L, Rampton DS. Review article: complementary and alternative therapies for inflammatory bowel disease. *Aliment Pharmacol Ther* 2006; **23**(3): 341–349.

8. Gerhardt H, Seifert F, Buvari P, Vogelsang H, Repges R. [Therapy of active Crohn disease with Boswellia serrata extract H 15]. *Z Gastroenterol* 2001; **39**(1): 11–17.

9. Ben-Arye E, Goldin E, Wengrower D, Stamper A, Kohn R, Berry E. Wheat grass juice in the treatment of active distal ulcerative colitis: a randomized double-blind placebo-controlled trial. *Scand J Gastroenterol* 2002; **37**(4): 444–449.

10. Langmead L, Feakins RM, Goldthorpe S, et al. Randomized, double-blind, placebo-controlled trial of oral aloe vera gel for active ulcerative colitis. *Aliment Pharmacol Ther* 2004; **19**(7): 739–747.

11. Joos S, Brinkhaus B, Maluche C, et al. Acupuncture and moxibustion in the treatment of active Crohn's disease: a randomized controlled study. *Digestion* 2004; **69**(3): 131–139.

12. Joos S, Wildau N, Kohnen R, et al. Acupuncture and moxibustion in the treatment of ulcerative colitis: a randomized controlled study. *Scand J Gastroenterol* 2006; **41**(9): 1056–1063.

13. Hanai H, Iida T, Takeuchi K, et al. Curcumin maintenance therapy for ulcerative colitis: randomized, multicenter, double-blind, placebo-controlled trial. *Clin Gastroenterol Hepatol* 2006; **4**(12): 1502–1506.

14. Omer B, Krebs S, Omer H, Noor TO. Steroid-sparing effect of wormwood (Artemisia absinthium) in Crohn's disease: a double-blind placebo-controlled study. *Phytomedicine* 2007; **14**(2–3): 87–95.

15. Sandborn WJ, Targan SR, Byers VS, Yan X, Tang T. 847x Double Blind Placebo Controlled Phase IIB Trial of HMPL-004 (Andrographis Paniculata Extract) in Active Mild to Moderate Ulcerative Colitis (UC). *Gastroenterology* 2010; **138**(5): S115–116.

16. Wu HG, Liu HR, Tan LY, et al. Electroacupuncture and moxibustion promote neutrophil apoptosis and improve ulcerative colitis in rats. *Dig Dis Sci* 2007; **52**(2): 379–384.

PART VI:
Surgical Dilemmas in IBD

37 Optimizing IBD patients for surgery and recovery

Jonathan M. Wilson and Alastair Windsor

Department of Colorectal Surgery, University College London Hospitals, London, UK

LEARNING POINTS

- Postoperative outcomes can be improved using a multidisciplinary team approach.
- High-quality imaging allows accurate preoperative mapping of the extent of disease, identification of complications, and drainage of sepsis.
- "Down staging" of disease with optimized medical management allows more conservative surgery and reduces the need for stoma formation.
- Preoperative risk stratification can identify patients needing specific perioperative management strategies.
- Undernourished patients may benefit from perioperative nutritional supplementation.
- Thromboembolic prophylaxis is essential.
- Laparoscopic techniques have better short-term postoperative outcomes than open surgery.
- The combined principles of "enhanced recovery after surgery (ERAS)/fast track" surgery reduce postoperative complication and hospital stays.

Introduction

In this chapter, we focus on the perioperative optimization of inflammatory bowel disease (IBD) patients undergoing elective surgery whose disease has proved refractory to medical treatment. The surgical management of acute IBD complications, such as obstruction, perforation, hemorrhage, fulminant colitis, and toxic megacolon, is beyond the remit of this chapter.

Preoperative care

Excellent perioperative care is essential for good results in IBD surgery, and an effective multidisciplinary team approach is likely to improve recovery and postoperative outcomes. Thorough preoperative counseling is obligatory, and in doing so, adjusting expectations will improve patients' compliance and overall experience. Key areas in this discussion should include the likely time course of recovery, potentially serious complications, the possibility of a stoma being necessary (by preoperative discussion with a specialist stoma nurse and including skin marking where appropriate), functional outcomes, and the possibility of a need for ongoing medical treatment after surgery. Deep vein thrombosis prophylaxis is mandatory as these patients are at increased risk of thromboembolic complication. Perioperative low molecular weight heparin, graduated compression stockings, intraoperative intermittent pneumatic calf compression devices, and early mobilization will suffice in most cases. In patients with a history of recent systemic steroid usage, the possibility of adrenal suppression should be considered and perioperative intravenous steroid cover ("stress dose") administered.

"Down-staging" of Crohn's disease (CD) with optimized medical management allows more conservative resection with a reduced risk of stoma formation [1]. This should be given due consideration routinely to minimize the incidence of postoperative intestinal failure through "short gut," especially given the statistics that a significant proportion of these patients will go onto require further surgical resections. In steroid-dependant patients, every attempt should be made to reduce the dose, as higher doses of

---

Clinical Dilemmas in Inflammatory Bowel Disease: New Challenges, Second Edition. Edited by P. Irving, C. Siegel, D. Rampton and F. Shanahan.
© 2011 Blackwell Publishing Ltd. Published 2011 by Blackwell Publishing Ltd.

preoperative steroids (≥20 mg prednisolone daily or equivalent for >6 weeks) are associated with increased postoperative septic complications. This is especially true when considering complex surgery, such as restorative proctocolectomy (ileal pouch-anal anastomosis) [2].

Azathioprine can safely be continued in the perioperative period and beyond. However, whether or not there is a higher rate of postoperative complications during or after anti-TNF therapy remains controversial. There is no consensus between experts as to the optimum timing between treatment and surgery, with some authors suggesting 1 month, some longer, and some maintaining that it is not important (see Chapter 41) [2].

The role of preoperative imaging, using CT scanning, MR enterography, barium studies, ileocolonoscopy, and/or wireless capsule endoscopy as appropriate, is several fold: (1) disease mapping within the gastrointestinal tract; (2) identifying areas of active inflammation that may benefit from "down-staging" with alternative/additional medical therapy; (3) identification of complications (phlegmon, fistulation, perforation/abscess), which may alter the modality and magnitude of surgery offered; (4) preoperative guided drainage of sepsis to allow more timely elective resection with reduced overall complication rates [3].

Correction of significant malnutrition in elective IBD surgery reduces postoperative complications and should be employed routinely [4]. In addition, the risk of adverse outcome in patients undergoing major surgery is affected by both cardiorespiratory fitness and the presence and severity of comorbidities. Accurate preoperative risk stratification may help in the identification of patients who may benefit from specific perioperative management strategies or from an augmented level of perioperative care. An example of this is the use of cardiopulmonary exercise testing (calculated anaerobic thresholds) to triage high-risk patients to the "postanesthesia care unit" (PACU) in order to reduce postoperative morbidity and mortality [5].

"Enhanced recovery after surgery" (ERAS) represents an evidence-based multimodality shift away from traditional perioperative management after intestinal resection with a resulting reduced postoperative morbidity and mortality [6]. A fortuitous by-product of the quicker postoperative recovery is a reduced length of hospital stay, which has resulted in the pseudonym "fast track" surgery, with its obvious financial attractions. Much of the evidence for ERAS in gastrointestinal surgery comes from studies in elective resectional colorectal surgery, with relatively little described specifically for IBD; therefore, many parallels are assumed and randomized controlled trials are necessary to confirm them. We will discuss some of the key elements of ERAS in turn. It has always been assumed that any patient undergoing elective left-sided colonic and rectal resectional surgery would require formal preoperative mechanical bowel preparation to minimize the possibility of anastomotic disruption and the clinical sequelae of anastomotic leak. However, this often results in patients becoming dehydrated and being found to have electrolyte derangement on the morning of surgery. Several well-conducted meta-analyses have now demonstrated that these patients do not benefit from mechanical bowel preparation, and may actually experience slightly higher leak rates than those undergoing surgery with unprepared colon [7]. The normal physiological response to surgical operative stress includes postoperative insulin resistance, hyperglycemia, and a catabolic state. This in turn is associated with impaired immune function, an exaggerated inflammatory response, and increased postoperative infective complications and mortality rates [8]. There is now good evidence that preoperative oral carbohydrate loading with commercially available supplement drinks up to 2 hours before induction of anesthesia (on the morning of surgery) is associated with a reduction in postoperative insulin resistance and an earlier return of normal gut function [9]. There is also good evidence that reducing the magnitude of surgical insult (minimally invasive surgery) and postoperative pain (thoracic epidural anesthesia) may also reduce the degree of postoperative insulin resistance with improved outcomes.

Operative care

While the therapeutic options for the medical treatment of IBD have bourgeoned in the last decade, the development of new surgical procedures has perhaps lagged behind [1]. That is to say, aside from a few notable exceptions such as the extended isoperistaltic strictureplasty and anal fistula plug, we are still performing the same operations as 10 years ago. However, there has been a huge change in surgical approach (minimally invasive techniques) and surgical process (risk stratification, perioperative optimization, ERAS). There is now an abundance of data demonstrating that laparoscopic surgery (LS) in intestinal resection is safe and has significant advantages in several postoperative outcomes compared with open surgery. In patients undergoing elective resection for colorectal cancer, LS reduces intraoperative blood loss and postoperative pain, and results in a faster return of bowel function with an associated reduced length of hospital stay [10]. Although the body of evidence is much smaller for LS in IBD patients, similarly improved short-term outcomes have been demonstrated over the open technique without increased complication rates; however, case selection is critical [11]. With regard to the anastomotic configuration following resection, a recent meta-analysis demonstrated that side-to-side anastomosis might lead to fewer anastomotic leaks and overall postoperative complications, a shorter hospital stay, and a perianastomotic recurrence rate comparable to end-to-end anastomosis [12].

"Natural orifice transluminal endoscopic surgery" (NOTES) and "single incision laparoscopic surgery" (SILS) are two innovative surgical approaches that aim to reduce surgical trauma even further than existing LS. However, these techniques are still in their infancy and their role in IBD surgery has yet to be investigated.

Postoperative care

There is increasing evidence that restrictive perioperative fluid management and goal-directed intraoperative fluid therapy guided by oesophageal Doppler cardiac output monitoring rather than conventional hemodynamic variables, reduces morbidity after elective colorectal resection [13]. Randomized controlled trials have also shown that a midthoracic epidural commenced preoperatively containing local anesthesia in combination with a low-dose opioid is superior to purely opioid-based parenteral regimes in terms of postoperative nausea and vomiting, pain control, duration of ileus, and improved pulmonary function after elective colorectal surgery [14]. Early postoperative feeding has been shown to be safe and associated with an earlier return of normal intestinal motility without compromising anastomoses. Other contemporary moves away from traditional postoperative care, which have been shown to be safe and effective, include the cessation of routine use of nasogastric tubes and abdominal drains, and early mobilization.

Several randomized studies have shown that postoperative treatment with anti-TNF agents, and to a lesser extent immunomodulators such as azathioprine and 6-mercaptopurine, reduce postoperative recurrence of CD. The majority of these studies have commenced therapy

immediately after surgery without any significant increase in postoperative complications [15].

Therefore, there appears to be a growing body of evidence that utilizing an enhanced recovery protocol in colorectal surgery improves outcome and shortens hospital stay. These protocols have been successfully applied to IBD surgery and this approach is increasingly accepted as "gold standard of care." Remaining challenges include identifying what constitutes the best enhanced recovery protocol, standardizing this approach, and making it a mandatory part of perioperative surgical care in IBD.

References

1. Roses RE, Rombeau JL. Recent trends in the surgical management of inflammatory bowel disease. *World J Gastroenterol* 2008; **14**(3): 408–412.

2. Dignass A, Van Assche G, Lindsay JO, et al. The second European evidence-based consensus on the diagnosis and management of Crohn's disease: Current management. *J Crohns Colitis* 2010; **4**: 28–62.

3. Da Luz Moreira A, Stocchi L, Tan E, Tekkis PP, Fazio VW. Outcomes of Crohn's disease presenting with abdominopelvic abscess. *Dis Colon Rectum* 2009; **52**(5): 906–912.

4. Smedh K, Andersson M, Johansson H, Hagberg T. Preoperative management is more important than choice of sutured or stapled anastomosis in Crohn's disease. *Eur J Surg* 2002; **168**(3): 154–157.

5. Moonesinghe SR, Mythen MG, Grocott MP. Patient-related risk factors for postoperative adverse events. *Curr Opin Crit Care* 2009; **15**(4): 320–327.

6. Gouvas N, Tan E, Windsor A, Xynos E, Tekkis PP. Fast-track vs standard care in colorectal surgery: a meta-analysis update. *Int J Colorectal Dis* 2009; **24**(10): 1119–1131.

7. Guenaga KK, Matos D, Wille-Jorgensen P. Mechanical bowel preparation for elective colorectal surgery. *Cochrane Database Syst Rev* 2009; (1): CD001544.

8. Doenst T, Wijeysundera D, Karkouti K, et al. Hyperglycemia during cardiopulmonary bypass is an independent risk factor for mortality in patients undergoing cardiac surgery. *J Thorac Cardiovasc Surg* 2005; **130**(4): 1144.

9. Noblett SE, Watson DS, Huong H, Davison B, Hainsworth PJ, Horgan AF. Pre-operative oral carbohydrate loading in colorectal surgery: a randomized controlled trial. *Colorectal Dis* 2006; **8**(7): 563–569.

10. Reza MM, Blasco JA, Andradas E, Cantero R, Mayol J. Systematic review of laparoscopic versus open surgery for colorectal cancer. *Br J Surg* 2006; **93**(8): 921–928.

11. Ananthakrishnan AN, McGinley EL, Saeian K, Binion DG. Laparoscopic resection for inflammatory bowel disease: outcomes from a nationwide sample. *J Gastrointest Surg* 2009; **14**(1): 58–65.

12. Simillis C, Purkayastha S, Yamamoto T, Strong SA, Darzi AW, Tekkis PP. A meta-analysis comparing conventional end-to-end anastomosis vs. other anastomotic configurations after resection in Crohn's disease. *Dis Colon Rectum* 2007; **50**(10): 1674–1687.

13. Rahbari NN, Zimmermann JB, Schmidt T, Koch M, Weigand MA, Weitz J. Meta-analysis of standard, restrictive and supplemental fluid administration in colorectal surgery. *Br J Surg* 2009; **96**(4): 331–341.

14. Gendall KA, Kennedy RR, Watson AJ, Frizelle FA. The effect of epidural analgesia on postoperative outcome after colorectal surgery. *Colorectal Dis* 2007; **9**(7): 584–598.

15. Regueiro M, Schraut W, Baidoo L, et al. Infliximab prevents Crohn's disease recurrence after ileal resection. *Gastroenterology* 2009; **136**(2): 441–450.

38 Is surgery the best initial treatment for limited ileocecal Crohn's disease?

Tom Øresland

Department of GI Surgery, Akershus University Hospital, University of Oslo, Lørenskog, Norway

LEARNING POINTS

- Failure of medical therapy remains the standard indication for surgery in Crohn's disease, but an early surgical approach merits consideration when disease is localized, particularly at the ileocecal junction.

- Recurrent disease requiring another surgery may occur in up to 50% over time, but the recurrence tends to mimic the initial disease in type and extent.

- Therefore, the threshold for surgery could be lower in patients with a short segment affected.

- The primacy of medical therapy over surgery should be challenged in localized ileocecal disease, but the evidence base to support a clinical decision in this situation remains to be established.

- The risk of short bowel syndrome after a limited elective resection is minimal.

- Prospective long-term studies of bowel function and quality of life comparing initial surgery with medical therapy are needed in well-characterized patients stratified for smoking status and other risk factors for relapse.

Introduction

Surgery was once the primary treatment for ileocecal Crohn's disease (CD). However, as the number of pharmacological modalities has grown, surgery has become a secondary or tertiary option. Despite this, the lifetime risk of a patient with CD requiring surgery [1] is still more than 70%. CD can lead to symptomatic lesions anywhere in the gastrointestinal tract. Recurrence after surgery tends to occur just upstream of the anastomosis. The timing of surgery is a common question with efforts made to offer the best quality of life with lowest long-term risks.

Medical treatment

There are no good data stating that the long-term quality of life of patients with limited ileocecal CD has improved as a result of new therapies. Such evidence is very hard to obtain considering the unpredictable course of the disease in individual patients. Long-term follow-up over years and decades is scarce with respect to patients who have never been operated upon. What we know for sure is that some of these therapies are very expensive and most pharmacological therapies demand careful follow-up of patients since they have associated side effects that can be severe, or life-threatening. Also, the effectiveness of medical therapies can be debated. The disease has a tendency to get more complicated with time. The natural course is such that a majority of patients can eventually expect obstruction, abdominal sepsis, or fistulas to adjacent bowel loops, to genitourinary organs, or to the skin.

Medical therapy may delay these complications, but when they occur the risks of poor quality of life, irrespective of the treatment options used, are high. Even with biological therapies, fistulas continue to be a major problem. In the much quoted ACCENT study, at 1 year, the number needed to treat with infliximab was six, so that one patient should have diminished the number of draining fistula openings by 50% [2]. From a surgeon's point of view, this is not an impressive effect, particularly for a costly therapy. Fibrostenotic disease is another complication of CD, where medical therapy has been suboptimal.

Clinical Dilemmas in Inflammatory Bowel Disease: New Challenges, Second Edition. Edited by P. Irving, C. Siegel, D. Rampton and F. Shanahan.
© 2011 Blackwell Publishing Ltd. Published 2011 by Blackwell Publishing Ltd.

Surgical treatment

Modern surgery focuses on dealing with the part of the diseased bowel giving rise to symptoms; the use of wide resection margins has long since been abandoned [3,4]. Today, the risks of patients eventually having a short bowel syndrome due to surgical resections are minimal. Those who end up in this situation are patients operated upon with bad timing, late in the course of disease with septic complications. The outcome is often characterized by further complications and reoperations with further resections. Complications are five times more likely in a patient having surgery with ongoing complications than in one without septic complications [5,6].

An elective ileocecal resection in a patient without septic complications is thus a relatively minor procedure with low surgical risk and leaving little or no functional disability. Indeed, to retain diseased bowel is often more of a disadvantage to the patient than having it resected. Although, resection is a definitive and irreversible procedure which in older studies carries a risk of needing later further surgery of about 50%, the loss of up to 1 meter of terminal ileum, which implies one or two reresections for recurrent disease, will in a majority of patients still be compatible with a reasonably good quality of life. Although, resection is a definitive and irreversible procedure which in older studies carried a risk of needing further surgery in about 50%, the loss of up to 1 meter of terminal ileum, which implies one or two reresections for recurrent disease, will still be compatible with a reasonably good quality of life in the majority of patients. However, dietary and medical modulation of bowel function will be needed in most patients. With the increasing confidence in strictureplasties, even in the setting of primary ileocecal CD, and with the increasing evidence that bowel handled in this way will regain its normal appearance and, maybe, also functional capabilities, it might be that in the future we will no longer resect, but instead will just widen the diseased segment using both traditional and nonconventional strictureplasties [7,8]. There is also the issue of defining recurrence. From a practical point of view, it seems that symptoms in need of further treatment are a good definition. This is not to deny that subclinical recurrences, which are almost universally seen when patients are colonoscoped in the months after surgery, might have an impact on the risk of developing later clinical disease and also on the decision about further medical therapies [9,10]. A possible way forward would be to have effective medication for subclinical disease preventing symptomatic recurrences after surgery.

So is primary resection of ileocecal disease an option for all patients? The main issue would then be to distinguish patients with a high risk of recurrent disease after surgery, a group that might, therefore, benefit more from medical treatment. Studies on this subject have, to a large extent, given inconclusive results. However, it is well established that smokers and those with perianal disease are at a greater risk, as are those with more extensive disease [11]. On the other hand, it seems that recurrent disease after surgery has a strong tendency to mimic the initial disease both in type and extent [12]. So from this point of view, the threshold for surgery could be lower in limited short segment ileocecal disease. Prepubertal patients with significant growth retardation despite appropriate medical therapy should also be considered for early surgery. Since medical therapies offer no guarantee that the natural history of the disease will be changed, it has been suggested that surgical intervention should be early rather than late to avoid the complications of the disease [7]. This reasoning might be particularly relevant in limited ileocecal CD.

Conclusion

There are no firm data supporting surgery as the best initial treatment for limited ileocecal CD. However, if a patient is uncomfortable with medical treatment, a resection as primary treatment is fully justifiable. The question of whether this should be a primary offer to all patients with limited ileocecal CD deserves further studies. One such study is currently underway.

References

1. Cosnes J, Nion-Larmurier I, Beaugerie L, Afchain P, Tiret E, Gendre JP. Impact of the increasing use of immunosuppressants in Crohn's disease on the need for intestinal surgery. *Gut* 2005; **54**: 237–241.
2. Sands BE, Anderson FH, Bernstein CN, et al. Infliximab maintenance therapy for fistulizing Crohn's disease. *N Engl J Med* 2004; **350**: 876–885.
3. Strong SA, Koltun WA, Hyman NH, Buie WD. Practice parameters for the surgical management of Crohn's disease. *Dis Colon Rectum* 2007; **50**: 1735–1746.
4. Fazio VW, Marchetti F, Church M, et al. Effect of resection margins on the recurrence of Crohn's disease in the small

bowel. A randomized controlled trial. *Ann Surg* 1996; **224**: 563–571.

5. Yamamoto T, Allan RN, Keighley MR. Risk factors for intra-abdominal sepsis after surgery in Crohn's disease. *Dis Colon Rectum* 2000; **43**: 1141–1145.

6. Hulten L. Surgical treatment of Crohn's disease of the small bowel or ileocecum. *World J Surg* 1988; **12**: 180–185.

7. Sampietro GM, Cristaldi M, Maconi G et al. A prospective, longitudinal study of nonconventional strictureplasty in Crohn's disease. *J Am Coll Surg* 2004; **199**: 8–20.

8. Michelassi F, Upadhyay GA. Side-to-side isoperistaltic strictureplasty in the treatment of extensive Crohn's disease. *J Surg Res* 2004; **117**: 71–78.

9. Rutgeerts P, Goboes K, Peeters M, et al. Effect of faecal stream diversion on recurrence of Crohn's disease in the neoterminal ileum. *Lancet* 1991; **338**: 771–774.

10. Olaison G, Smedh K, Sjodahl R. Natural course of Crohn's disease after ileocolic resection: endoscopically visualised ileal ulcers preceding symptoms. *Gut* 1992; **33**: 331–335.

11. Bernell O, Lapidus A, Hellers G. Risk factors for surgery and recurrence in 907 patients with primary ileocaecal Crohn's disease. *Br J Surg* 2000; **87**: 1697–1701.

12. D'Haens GR, Gasparaitis AE, Hanauer SB. Duration of recurrent ileitis after ileocolonic resection correlates with presurgical extent of Crohn's disease. *Gut* 1995; **36**: 715–717.

Laparoscopic or open surgery for IBD?

Donna Appleton and Michael Hershman

Department of General and Colorectal Surgery, Stafford General Hospital, Stafford, UK

LEARNING POINTS

- Almost all colorectal procedures are feasible and safe when performed laparoscopically.

- The main advantage of laparoscopic surgery is superior cosmesis.

- Traditionally, short-term improvements, particularly reduced hospital stay and costs, are used as endpoints when comparing laparoscopic surgery with open surgery. This may need to be reassessed with the introduction of enhanced recovery programs.

- The true benefit of laparoscopic surgery compared to open surgery must be sought in long-term results e.g., reductions in recurrence rate in Crohn's disease, incisional hernia, postoperative adhesions, and postoperative infertility.

Introduction

Laparoscopic surgery for IBD is technically difficult in patients who have fragile tissue, thickened mesentery, dense adhesions, and skip lesions and in those who are malnourished or immunosuppressed. Despite these concerns, multiple early reports document advantages of laparoscopic surgery over open surgery for IBD. Laparoscopic surgery is performed more frequently for Crohn's disease (CD) than for ulcerative colitis (UC).

In recent years, advances in technology and surgical laparoscopic skills have lead to increased use of laparoscopic surgery in IBD including in more complex procedures.

Laparoscopy for Crohn's disease

Ileocolectomy

Although there have been few randomized controlled trials, multiple reports have shown advantages of laparoscopic ileocecal resection over open surgery for primary CD [1,2]. Milsom et al. [3] randomized 60 patients with ileocecal Crohn's to have laparoscopic surgery or open surgery: the laparoscopic surgery group had better postoperative pulmonary function, morbidity, and reduced length of stay. In addition, the laparoscopic surgery group had earlier return of bowel function, a finding replicated elsewhere [2,4]. Postoperative pain and analgesia requirements are also significantly reduced by laparoscopic surgery [4]. This enables earlier hospital discharge and reduced direct and indirect costs [1]. Performing ileocolectomy totally laparoscopically as compared to laparoscopy assisted, in which the bowel is mobilized laparoscopically and then delivered and resected extracorporeally, has no advantage and increases operating time and cost [5].

Other studies report that laparoscopic surgery reduces blood loss [6], wound infection, intra-abdominal abscess formation [1], and postoperative bowel obstruction [7]. However, most studies report only short-term outcomes and many of these may need to be reassessed with the increasing introduction of enhanced recovery programs, which enable quicker recovery of both laparoscopic surgery and open surgery patients.

In the future, studies will need to focus on the long-term benefits of laparoscopic surgery. The most obvious benefit is cosmesis [8], which is particularly important for young

---

Clinical Dilemmas in Inflammatory Bowel Disease: New Challenges, Second Edition. Edited by P. Irving, C. Siegel, D. Rampton and F. Shanahan.
© 2011 Blackwell Publishing Ltd. Published 2011 by Blackwell Publishing Ltd.

patients with CD. Data regarding both short- and long-term quality of life (QOL) following laparoscopic ileocolic resection for CD is surprisingly scarce. Although some studies found body image to correlate strongly with cosmesis, others report no difference in quality of life between laparoscopic surgery and open surgery patients [1,8].

With regard to recurrence of CD after primary resection, a meta-analysis reported reduced recurrence after laparoscopic surgery as compared to open surgery [7]. The meantime of recurrence was similar: 60 and 62 months, respectively. However, a more recent meta-analysis reported similar recurrence rates [9].

Conversion rates to an open procedure vary from 0 to 16.7% [10]. Risk factors for conversion are the indicators of more complex and hence more technically challenging disease. They include internal fistulae, a palpable mass, recurrent disease, smoking, steroids, extracecal colonic disease, and preoperative malnutrition. As surgical experience increases, it is likely that conversion rates will decrease. However, timely conversion to an open procedure should not be seen as a failure.

Small bowel resection and strictureplasty

This is a straightforward laparoscopic surgery procedure, but all of the small bowel must be assessed for coexisting strictures. This is usually done by "walking down the bowel" between two laparoscopic instruments.

Fecal diversion (stoma formation)

Fecal diversion by ileostomy or colostomy using laparoscopic surgery has the advantages reported above over open surgery, as no incision except for the stoma is made.

Colonic resection

Segmental colectomy for isolated disease, proctocolectomy for pancolitis or ileo-rectal anastomosis (synchronous or delayed) have all been performed by laparoscopic surgery. Although there are few reports in the literature, laparoscopic surgery appears to permit shorter hospital stay and quicker return to baseline partial and full activity and employment than open surgery [11]. In addition, in the short-term, recurrent disease requiring further surgery may be reduced after laparoscopic surgery compared to open surgery [11].

There are conflicting reports in the literature relating to operating time although it is generally agreed that laparoscopic surgery takes longer than open surgery.

Laparoscopic surgery for complex Crohn's disease

Complex CD, including recurrent disease, fistulae, abscesses, or phlegmon represents a challenge even for very experienced surgeons. Laparoscopic resections can be performed safely without unacceptable conversion rates. Factors that increase the conversion risk include: intraoperative intestinal injury and fistulating disease [12], particularly with duodenal or vaginal involvement. Importantly, conversion does not increase morbidity [12]. Conversion rates are greater in patients with an increased body mass index.

A successful initial laparoscopic resection for CD increases the likelihood that surgery for recurrent disease will also be possible laparoscopically and allows the benefits of laparoscopic surgery to be maintained [13].

Laparoscopy for ulcerative colitis

Experience with laparoscopic surgery for ulcerative colitis is less than that for Crohn's due to the complex nature of these procedures and the steep learning curve.

Subtotal colectomy and panproctocolectomy

Laparoscopic subtotal colectomy confers short term benefits over open surgery including reduced hospital stay, blood loss, and faster return of GI function, even in medically refractory acute severe colitis [2,14] but it has significantly longer operating times, which decrease with greater experience. Hand-assisted laparoscopic surgery, where one hand is inserted in the abdomen within a gas tight glove, enables reduced operative time with similar postoperative recovery and morbidity rates when compared to laparoscopically assisted surgery.

When laparoscopic total colectomy is performed as the initial stage of a three-stage restorative proctocolectomy, patients can proceed to subsequent restorative proctocolectomy and have their ileostomy closure done sooner than patients undergoing open surgery [15].

The arguments for laparoscopic panproctocolectomy are similar to those for ileal pouch-anal anastomosis.

Ileal pouch-anal anastomosis (IPAA)

Restorative proctocolectomy with ileal pouch-anal anastomosis (IPAA) has evolved into the standard of care in selected patients with intractable ulcerative colitis. Laparoscopic surgery can be performed either in a totally laparoscopic fashion or hand assisted. Total laparoscopic IPAA has not been shown to have any significant short-term benefits over hand-assisted techniques [16]. Some surgeons perform the proctectomy through a small incision, whilst other prefer to perform it totally laparoscopically, which has been made possible by the recent development of laparoscopic angulated staplers to cross-staple the distal rectum. No data exists on the safety of this laparoscopic cross-stapling [17]. The pouch is usually formed extracorporeally.

Early series comparing IPAA by laparoscopic surgery compared to open surgery were very discouraging with a doubling of operating time, transfusion requirement and morbidity without reduction in hospital stay [17]. These results may reflect the learning curve for advanced laparoscopic surgery. A recent meta-analysis [18] concluded that laparoscopic IPAA resulted in reduced blood loss and hospital stay as compared with open surgery. However, a Cochrane review of 2009 [19] found no difference in mortality or morbidity between laparoscopic surgery and open surgery and significantly longer operating time for laparoscopic surgery than open surgery. It also reported no difference in pouch function with laparoscopic surgery or open surgery. Other recent studies have shown limited short-term advantages of laparoscopic surgery, despite increased operating time. It is possible that these differences would not have occurred if enhanced recovery protocols were used [17].

The main benefit of laparoscopic surgery is better cosmesis. When laparoscopic surgery was compared to open surgery, cosmesis was better in both sexes and body image was preserved, particularly in women. In the future, the true benefit of laparoscopic surgery for IPPA must focus on long-term outcomes. Recent evidence suggests that incisional herniae occur less frequently after laparoscopic surgery and that adhesion-related obstruction may be reduced [20]. In addition, the reduction in fertility seen after open surgery may be lesser when laparoscopic surgery is used. Future studies will need to assess sexual function after laparoscopic IPAA.

If these studies confirm the anticipated long-term benefits of laparoscopic surgery for IPAA, it will become the "gold standard," particularly for young patients.

Conclusion

Numerous short-term advantages have been discussed for laparoscopic surgery as compared to open surgery for both CD and UC. However, the literature is lacking in quality randomized controlled trials. It will be interesting to see what effect, if any, enhanced recovery programs have on standard outcome measures such as return of gastrointestinal function and hospital stay; reported to be shorter with laparoscopic techniques. Nevertheless, laparoscopic surgery for these procedures is likely to be increasingly adopted with advantages outweighing any arguments about cost and operative time as experience increases and cohorts of surgeons trained in laparoscopic surgery at the onset of training become consultants.

References

1. Maartense S, Dunker MS, Slors JF, et al. Laparoscopic-assisted versus open ileocolic resection for Crohn's disease: a randomized trial. *Ann Surg* 2006; **243**: 143–149.
2. Tilney HS, Constantinides VA, Heriot AG, et al. Comparison of laparoscopic and open ileocecal resection for Crohn's disease: a metaanalysis. *Surg Endosc* 2006; **20**: 1036–1044.
3. Milsom JW, Hammerhofer KA, Bohm B, et al. Prospective, randomized trial comparing laparoscopic versus conventional surgery for refractory ileocolic Crohn's disease. *Dis Colon Rectum* 2001; **44**: 1–8.
4. Sica GS, Iaculli E, Benavoli D, et al. Laparoscopic versus open ileo-colonic resection in Crohn's disease: short- and long-term results from a prospective longitudinal study. *J Gastrointest Surg* 2008; **12**: 1094–1102.
5. Wexner SD, ed. *Laparoscopic colorectal surgery.* New York: Wiley-Liss; 1999.
6. Tanaka S, Matsuo K, Sasaki T, Nakano M, Shimura H, Yamashita Y. Clinical outcomes and advantages of laparoscopic surgery for primary Crohn's disease: are they significant? *Hepatogastroenterology* 2009; **56**: 416–420.
7. Rosman AS, Melis M, Fichera A. Metaanalysis of trials comparing laparoscopic and open surgery for Crohn's disease. *Surg Endosc* 2005; **19**: 1549–1555.
8. Eshuis EJ, Polle SW, Slors JF, et al. Long-term surgical recurrence, morbidity, quality of life, and body image of laparoscopic-assisted vs open ileocolic resection for Crohn's disease: a comparative study. *Dis Colon Rectum* 2008; **51**: 858–867.
9. Tan JJ, Tjandra JJ. Laparoscopic surgery for Crohn's disease: a meta-analysis. *Dis Colon Rectum* 2007; **50**: 576–585.
10. Polle SW, Wind J, Ubbink DT, Hommes DW, Gouma DJ, Bemelman WA. Short-term outcomes after laparoscopic ileocolic resection for Crohn's disease. A systematic review. *Dig Surg* 2006; **23**: 346–357.
11. da Luz Moreira A, Stocchi L, Remzi FH, Geisler D, Hammel J, Fazio VW. Laparoscopic surgery for patients with Crohn's colitis: a case-matched study. *J Gastrointest Surg* 2007; **11**: 1529–1533.

12. Brouquet A, Bretagnol F, Soprani A, Valleur P, Bouhnik Y, Panis Y. A laparoscopic approach to iterative ileocolonic resection for the recurrence of Crohn's disease. *Surg Endosc* 2009; 24(4): 879–887.

13. Lawes DA, Motson RW. Avoidance of laparotomy for recurrent disease is a long-term benefit of laparoscopic resection for Crohn's disease. *Br J Surg* 2006; **93**: 607–608.

14. Watanabe K, Funayama Y, Fukushima K, Shibata C, Takahashi K, Sasaki I. Hand-assisted laparoscopic vs open subtotal colectomy for severe ulcerative colitis. *Dis Colon Rectum* 2009; **52**: 640–645.

15. Chung TP, Fleshman JW, Birnbaum EH, et al. Laparoscopic vs open total abdominal colectomy for severe colitis: impact on recovery and subsequent completion restorative proctectomy. *Dis Colon Rectum* 2009; **52**: 4–10.

16. Polle SW, van Berge Henegouwen MI, Slors JF, Cuesta MA, Gouma DJ, Bemelman WA. Total laparoscopic restorative proctocolectomy: are there advantages compared with the open and hand-assisted approaches? *Dis Colon Rectum* 2008; **51**: 541–548.

17. Bemelman WA. Laparoscopic ileoanal pouch surgery. *Br J Surg* 2010; **97**: 2–3.

18. Tilney HS, Lovegrove RE, Heriot AG, et al. Comparison of short-term outcomes of laparoscopic vs open approaches to ileal pouch surgery. *Int J Colorectal Dis* 2007; **22**: 531–542.

19. Ahmed Ali U, Keus F, Heikens JT, et al. Open versus laparoscopic (assisted) ileo pouch anal anastomosis for ulcerative colitis and familial adenomatous polyposis. *Cochrane Database Syst Rev* 2009; (1):CD006267.

20. Eshuis EJ, Slors JF, Stokkers PC, et al. Long-term outcomes following laparoscopically assisted versus open ileocolic resection for Crohn's disease. *Br J Surg* 2010; **97**: 563–568.

40 Optimizing management of perianal Crohn's disease

David A. Schwartz and Norman R. Clark III

Division of Gastroenterology, Vanderbilt University Medical Center, Nashville, TN, USA

LEARNING POINTS

- Perianal manifestations occur in 40% of patients with Crohn's disease (CD) and may precede intestinal disease.

- Management is determined by the pathology, location, and severity of both the perianal manifestations and the luminal disease.

- Newer imaging modalities such as endoscopic ultrasound and pelvic magnetic resonance imaging are invaluable in diagnosing and evaluating perianal disease.

- For fistulizing disease, a combination of medical and surgical therapies has proven most effective

- With the advent of anti-TNF antibodies, the goal of treatment for fistulizing Crohn's has shifted from reduction of fistula drainage to resolution and even fibrosis of the fistula tracks.

Introduction

Patients with Crohn's have a predisposition for the development of perianal complications, namely, skin tags, strictures, ulcers, fissures, abscesses, and fistulas. Approximately 40% of patients with Crohn's disease (CD) suffer from these manifestations over the course of their illness, which may precede intestinal disease and seriously impair quality of life [1]. However, advances in the understanding of the disease have led to an expanded arsenal of both medical and surgical treatment modalities, with most patients responding well to therapy. This chapter outlines common pathology of the perianum associated with CD and discusses the current available treatment options.

Skin tags and hemorrhoids

Patients with Crohn's often develop perianal skin tags and/or hemorrhoids. Though relatively benign, these lesions frequently result in postoperative complications (e.g., poor healing), and are, therefore, managed conservatively. Routine excision or biopsy is not advised [2]. Clinicians should consider investigating occult luminal disease in patients who have a history of nonhealing lesions without a confirmed diagnosis of Crohn's.

Strictures

Anorectal stricturing or stenosis can arise from chronic inflammation. When symptomatic, patients often complain of tenesmus, urgency, incontinence, or even difficulty in passing stool. Treatment options include gentle dilation during digital rectal exam (DRE) or mechanical dilation with a dilator or balloon. Patients often require repeat dilations and can be trained to do so at home. Refractory symptomatic strictures may require proctectomy [3].

Fissures

Anal fissures are tears in the lining of the anal canal, commonly seen in patients with perianal CD. After a fissure develops, the exposed sphincter can go into spasm; along with inflammation, bacterial overgrowth, and mechanical trauma from stool passage, a cycle of injury ensues. Although fissures are typically asymptomatic and heal spontaneously, bleeding and pain on evacuation may occur [4]. Prolonged pain should raise suspicion of an underlying abscess or developing fistula.

Clinical Dilemmas in Inflammatory Bowel Disease: New Challenges, Second Edition. Edited by P. Irving, C. Siegel, D. Rampton and F. Shanahan.
© 2011 Blackwell Publishing Ltd. Published 2011 by Blackwell Publishing Ltd.

Symptomatic treatments, aimed at reducing pain and discomfort, work by decreasing sphincter tension and thus aid in healing. Antidiarrheals, warm sitz baths, and gentle cleansing are generally recommended in order to keep the affected area as free from soilage as possible. In addition to local symptom relief, oral or topical metronidazole or ciprofloxacin may help heal fissures and ulceration by inhibiting bacterial growth, although there have been no large controlled studies to prove this [5].

Topical nitroglycerin, calcium-channel blockers, and botulinum toxin are commonly used to increase blood flow and sphincter relaxation. However, their efficacy has yet to be validated in patients with CD. For those who have not responded to medical therapy and in whom there is no evidence of active inflammation in the area, one may consider lateral sphincterotomy, although this procedure carries a risk of causing incontinence [6]. As with other perianal complications, patients with intestinal disease should be treated with the appropriate anti-inflammatory, immunomodulatory, and/or biologic therapy.

Perianal abscesses

Approximately half of patients with perianal CD will develop an anorectal abscess [7]. Anal abscesses signify complex perianal disease and are categorized according to their locations: superficial, intersphincteric, transsphincteric, ischiorectal, and supralevator. Based on a patient's presentation (i.e., pain, fever, drainage, fluctuant mass, etc.), if an abscess is suspected, the area should be promptly imaged with MRI or rectal EUS.

Perianal abscesses must be completely drained to optimize wound healing and minimize recurrence (which can be as high as 50% [6]), while avoiding damage to the sphincter. Depending on depth and whether or not an associated fistula can be identified, local incision and drainage, catheter drainage, or seton placement should be performed by an experienced surgeon in order to minimize complications.

Fistulizing disease

Fistula formation has been shown to occur in at least 20% of patients with CD [8] and is thought to occur as a track extending over time, either from fecal material forced into a site of ulceration or from a spontaneously draining anal gland abscess. In both scenarios, increased pressure is the

mechanism [9]. Fistulizing CD leads to significant morbidity, and management is accordingly aggressive.

Several different schemes have been used to classify perianal fistulizing disease, most notably the Parks and Hughes/Cardiff classifications. In 2003, the AGA Technical Review Panel proposed dividing the fistulas in two categories (simple or complex). A simple fistula begins low in the rectal canal, has a single opening on the skin, is not associated with an abscess, and does not connect to other structures. A complex fistula begins high in the canal, has multiple openings, is associated with an abscess, or connects to an adjacent structure such as the vagina or bladder. Complex fistulas increase the risk of surgical complications and reduce the chance for resolution [2].

Evaluation

Appropriate diagnostic modalities must be utilized in order to evaluate and treat fistulas accurately, thereby minimizing adverse outcomes. Diagnostic imaging is currently the preferred method used to assess perianal fistulas, as it is more sensitive and specific than DRE. To date, fistulography, CT, pelvic MRI, and anorectal EUS have all been used to diagnose and classify fistulas and abscesses. MRI and EUS are the most effective tools in delineating the perianal process of disease. Both have been shown to be comparable to examination under anesthesia (EUA), and both are substantially more accurate than CT and fistulography. Furthermore, when either MRI or EUS is combined with EUA, accuracy approaches 100% [10].

The potential for using EUS or MRI to monitor response to medical therapy is currently being evaluated and shows promise. One study revealed that 48% of patients had persistent fistula activity following seton placement that would not have been recognized by physical examination alone [11]. Another prospective study indicated that EUS-guided interventions were 80% effective in attaining long-term cessation of drainage compared to 20% in the non-EUS guided group [12].

Treatment

An array of pharmaceuticals, yielding mixed results, is currently available to treat fistulizing Crohn's, including antibiotics (e.g., metronidazole and ciprofloxacin) and immunomodulators (e.g., azathioprine or 6-mercaptopurine). Cyclosporine and tacrolimus, despite increased toxicity profiles and limited data, are newer additions to the arsenal against refractory fistulas.

While medical therapy targets the underlying inflammation, surgery remains an essential component of care. More specifically, EUA with seton placement, incision and drainage, and fistulotomy can allow for drainage and controlled healing of the fistulas. Noncutting setons are used for sphincter preservation in high fistulas, whereas flap procedures have been shown to be efficacious in low fistulas without inflammation [13]. Fibrin glue and fistula plugs have also been attempted with varied success [14,15].

Many patients demonstrate marked improvement in the severity of their illness and in their quality of life with the agents and surgeries mentioned. However, it was not until the development of anti-TNF-α antibodies that clinicians and patients could hope for complete closure of their fistulas. Both infliximab and adalimumab have proven clinically effective in reducing fistula drainage as well as maintaining fistula closure [16,17]. Seton placement and drainage prior to initiating infliximab has been shown to increase fistula closure and decrease recurrence rates [18]. The role in fistulizing disease of newer biologic agents such as certolizumab and natalizumab is unclear.

With many combinations of treatment and different levels of disease complexity, the clinician must individualize the treatment plan. The most important decision is "when to introduce biologic therapy," an issue of ongoing debate. Traditionally, a conservative approach has been taken, in which treatment incrementally progresses from the weakest agents to anti-TNF-α agents, as needed. However, because of the morbidity associated with perianal CD, treatment should begin by combining medical and surgical interventions in order to prevent further complications and achieve permanent resolution of the fistula.

Conclusions

In summary, perianal CD can manifest in a variety of ways, each requiring individualized evaluation and management. While conservative measures are usually appropriate for nonfistulizing disease, a more integrated and concerted/aggressive approach should be considered for fistulizing disease. Utilization of imaging as well as combination medical and surgical therapy has been shown to have the highest rates of healing and may prevent disease progression (e.g., avoiding a simple fistula from becoming complex). However, further studies are needed to determine the long-term success of this approach, and whether or not it outweighs the cost and toxicity.

References

1. Platell C, Mackay J, Collopy B, Fink R, Ryan P, Woods R. Anal pathology in patients with Crohn's disease. *Aust N Z J Surg* 1996; **66**(1): 5–9.

2. Sandborn WJ, Fazio VW, Feagan BG, Hanauer SB. AGA technical review on perianal Crohn's disease. *Gastroenterology* 2003; **125**: 1508–1530.

3. Linares L, Moreira LF, Andrews H, Allan RN, Alexander-Williams J, Keighley MR. Natural history and treatment of anorectal strictures complicating Crohn's disease. *Br J Surg* 1988; **75**: 653–655.

4. Buchmann P, Keighley MR, Allan RN, Thompson H, Alexander-Williams J. Natural history of perianal Crohn's disease. Ten year follow-up: a plea for conservatism. *Am J Surg* 1980; **140**: 642–644.

5. Stringer EE, Nicholson TJ, Armstrong D. Efficacy of topical metronidazole (10%) in the treatment of anorectal Crohn's disease. *Dis Colon Rectum* 2005; **48**(5): 970–974.

6. Wolkomir AF, Luchtefeld MA. Surgery for symptomatic hemorrhoids and anal fissures in Crohn's disease. *Dis Colon Rectum* 1993; **36**: 545–547.

7. Makowiec F, Ekkehard CJ, Becker HD, et al. Perianal abscess in Crohn's disease. *Dis Colon Rectum* 1997; **40**: 443.

8. Schwartz DA, Loftus EV, Tremaine WJ, et al. The natural history of fistulizing Crohn's disease in Olmsted County, Minnesota. *Gastroenterology* 2002; **122**: 875–880.

9. Hughes LE. Surgical pathology and management of anorectal Crohn's disease. *J R Soc Med* 1978; **71**: 644–651.

10. Schwartz DA, Wiersema MJ, Dudiak KM, et al. A comparison of endoscopic ultrasound, magnetic resonance imaging, and exam under anesthesia for evaluation of Crohn's perianal fistulas. *Gastroenterology* 2001; **121**: 1064.

11. Schwartz DA, White CM, Wise PE, et al. Use of endoscopic ultrasound to guide combination medical and surgical therapy for patients with Crohn's perianal fistulas. *Inflamm Bowel Dis* 2005; **11**: 727–732.

12. Spradlin NM, Wise PE, Herline AJ, et al. A randomized prospective trial of endoscopic ultrasound to guide combination medical and surgical treatment for Crohn's perianal fistulas. *Am J Gastroenterol* 2008; **103**: 2527–2535.

13. Schwartz DA, Pemberton JH, Sandborn WJ. Diagnosis and treatment of perianal fistulas in Crohn disease. *Ann Intern Med* 2001; **135**: 906–918.

14. Singer M, Cintron J, Nelson R, et al. Treatment of fistulas-in-ano with fibrin sealant in combination with intra-adhesive antibiotics and/or surgical closure of the internal fistula opening. *Dis Colon Rectum* 2005; **48**: 799–808.

15. Ky AJ, Sylla P, Steinhagen R, et al. Collagen fistula plug for the treatment of anal fistulas. *Dis Colon Rectum* 2008; **51**: 838–843.

16. Sandborn WJ, Hanauer SB, Loftus EV Jr, et al. An open-label study of the human anti-TNF monoclonal antibody adalimumab in subjects with prior loss of response or intolerance to infliximab for Crohn's disease. *Am J Gastroenterol* 2004; **99**: 1984–1989.

17. Colombel JF, Sandborn WJ, Rutgeerts P, et al. Adalimumab for maintenance of clinical response and remission in patients with Crohn's disease: the CHARM trial. *Gastroenterology* 2007; **132**: 52–65.

18. Regueiro M, Mardini H. Treatment of perianal fistulizing Crohn's disease with infliximab alone or as an adjunct to exam under anesthesia with seton placement. *Inflamm Bowel Dis* 2003; **9**: 98–103.

Does anti-TNF therapy increase the risk of complications of surgery?

Ming Valerie Lin[1], Wojciech Blonski[2,3], and Gary R. Lichtenstein[2]

[1]Department of Internal Medicine, Pennsylvania Hospital, University of Pennsylvania Health System, Philadelphia, PA, USA

[2]Division of Gastroenterology, University of Pennsylvania, Philadelphia, PA, USA

[3]Department of Gastroenterology, Medical University, Wroclaw, Poland

LEARNING POINTS

- Despite medical therapy, approximately 30% of patients with ulcerative colitis and up to 80% of patients with Crohn's disease will undergo surgery during the course of their illness.

- There are conflicting data regarding the perioperative use of infliximab and its association with the development of postoperative complications in patients with IBD.

- Evidence has suggested that use of corticosteroid and cyclosporine, and restorative proctocolectomy without use of a defunctioning ileostomy are some of the independent predictors of infectious complications.

- Although there is insufficient evidence to stop anti-TNF drugs routinely prior to surgery, patients having operations while receiving this treatment must be carefully monitored for the development of sepsis and other complications.

Introduction

The use of anti-TNF agents in the past decade has significantly reduced the need for surgery in patients with inflammatory bowel disease (IBD) [1]. Despite medical therapy, many patients with IBD will undergo surgery during the course of their illness [2,3]. The perioperative use of anti-TNF agents with its resultant effects on the immune system, combined with the need to perform surgery in patients already with risk factors known to increase the risk of surgical complications, has raised concerns about the possibility of an increased risk of postoperative complications, in particular infection. We aim to review the evidence available that focuses on the perioperative use of anti-TNF agents and the associated postoperative complications in patients with IBD.

Crohn's Disease

There have been five retrospective case-control studies [4–8] and one prospective randomized placebo-controlled study [9] assessing the relationship between perioperative use of anti-TNF and postoperative complications in patients with Crohn's disease (CD) who underwent ileo-colonic resection (Table 41.1).

A retrospective study by Brzezinski et al. evaluated the risk of postoperative complications in 35 patients with CD who received perioperative infliximab and observed no difference in the rates of postoperative complications or the length of hospitalizations between patients treated with infliximab and matched controls [4]. A group from Belgium retrospectively identified 40 patients who were pretreated with infliximab within 12 weeks prior to intestinal resection and compared them to 39 patients with CD who had never received infliximab and underwent surgery in the same period [5]. Despite greater use of corticosteroids or immunomodulators in the infliximab group (73% versus 41%, $p<0.0002$) [5], there was no significant difference between the two groups in the development of early (10 days) minor (15% versus 12.8%, $p =$ NS) or major (12.5% versus 7.7%, $p =$ NS) complications or late (3 months)

Clinical Dilemmas in Inflammatory Bowel Disease: New Challenges, Second Edition. Edited by P. Irving, C. Siegel, D. Rampton and F. Shanahan.
© 2011 Blackwell Publishing Ltd. Published 2011 by Blackwell Publishing Ltd.

minor (2.5% vs. 5.1%, $p = $ NS) or major (17.5% versus 12.8%, $p = $ NS) complications [5]. The length of hospitalization was similar in both groups (10.3 versus 9.9 days, $p = $ NS) [5]. A large retrospective study by Colombel et al. observed that 52 patients with CD who were treated with infliximab perioperatively had a similar likelihood of developing septic complications (odds ratio (OR) 0.9; 95% confidence interval (CI) 0.4–1.9) and total complications (OR 1.0; 95% CI 0.5–2.0) postoperatively when compared with 218 patients with CD who did not receive infliximab [6]. A retrospective analysis of 100 consecutive patients with CD who underwent segmental resection with primary anastomosis or strictureplasty at a tertiary referral center concluded that patients who received immunomodulator or biologic therapy within at least 8 weeks prior to surgery had fewer intra-abdominal septic complications than did those who did not receive any immunomodulator or biologic therapy (5.6% versus 25%; $p < 0.01$). Postoperative septic complications developed in 3 of 22 (13.6%) patients who received infliximab and 8 of 78 (10.3%, $p = 0.7$) patients who did not receive infliximab [7]. Of the 3 patients treated with infliximab who had postoperative septic complications, all received concomitant azathioprine or 6-MP, whereas only 1 patient received azathioprine in the non-infliximab group [7]. Finally, a recently published small randomized placebo-controlled study demonstrated the effectiveness of perioperative infliximab at preventing endoscopic and histological recurrences of CD over a 1-year period[9]. The authors randomly assigned 24 patients with CD to receive either infliximab ($n = 11$) or placebo ($n = 13$) within 4 weeks of surgery and continued for 1 year and observed that the rate of endoscopic (9.1% versus 84.6%; $p = 0.0006$) and histologic (27.3% versus 84.6%; $p = 0.01$) recurrence was significantly lower in the infliximab group. Both groups had similar adverse events during the study period (72.7% versus 84.6%, p = 0.63) [9].

Contrary to the aforementioned studies, a recently published retrospective case-control study demonstrated that patients with CD who received infliximab ($n = 60$) before surgery (ileocolonic resection) had more than twice the risk of infliximab-naïve patients ($n = 329$) of being readmitted (OR 2.33, 95% CI 1.02–5.33, $p = 0.045$) or developing sepsis (OR 2.62, 95% CI 1.12–6.13, $p = 0.027$), and a nearly six-times likelihood of developing intra-abdominal abscess (OR 5.78, 95% CI 1.69–19.7, $p = 0.005$) within 30 days post surgery [8]. Among patients treated with inflix-

imab, the incidence of sepsis was significantly lower in the presence of a diverting stoma (0% versus 27.9%, $p = 0.013$) [8]. More patients in the infliximab-exposed group had received concomitant immunomodulation (61.7% versus 16.7%, $p = 0.001$)[8]. Conversely, corticosteroid usage was significantly higher in infliximab-naïve patients than in infliximab-exposed patients (76.9% versus 65%, $p = 0.05$) [8]. Since it could be argued that patients treated with infliximab may be expected to be sicker than those not on infliximab, the authors included a comparative group of patients from the preinfliximab era who underwent surgery. In comparing those two groups, the incidence of postoperative sepsis (20% versus 5.8%, $p = 0.021$), anastomotic leak (10% versus 1.4%, $p = 0.049$) and readmission rate (20% vs. 2.9%, $p = 0.007$) remained significantly higher among infliximab-exposed patients [8].

Ulcerative colitis

There have been four retrospective case-control studies assessing the incidence of postoperative complications in patients with UC who received perioperative infliximab [10–13].

A retrospective evaluation of short-term (30 days) postoperative complications was performed in 151 patients with UC who underwent ileal pouch-anal anastomosis (IPAA) ($n = 112$) or subtotal colectomy ($n = 39$) [10] with or without perioperative infliximab treatment. Seventeen patients, who had received a median of two infliximab infusions within a median of 2 months prior to surgery, were compared with 134 infliximab-naïve patients [10]. Overall, there was no difference in the incidence of postoperative medical (6% versus 10%, $p = 0.99$), surgical (30% versus 18%, $p = 0.3$) or infectious complications (18% versus 8%, $p = 0.2$). However, patients who were treated with sequential cyclosporine and infliximab had overall significantly higher incidence of postoperative and infectious complications compared to those treated with cyclosporine alone (80% versus 29%, $p = 0.04$ and 60% versus 13%, $p = 0.03$, respectively) [10].

These data were supported by Belgian researchers who studied short-term postoperative infectious complications among 141 UC patients who underwent restorative proctocolectomy [11]. There was no significant difference in the rates of any infectious complication between patients exposed to infliximab within 12 weeks prior to surgery and infliximab-naïve patients ($n = 100$) or those who were exposed to infliximab more than 12 weeks before surgery

TABLE 41.1 Studies evaluating the development of postoperative complications in patients with IBD exposed to infliximab in a perioperative setting

Reference number	IBD type	Exposure to IFX	Duration of follow-up	Number of patients					
				Perioperative treatment		Postoperative complications		Concomitant medications in patients with postoperative complications	
				IFX	No IFX	IFX	No IFX	IFX	No IFX
[4]	CD	2 months before surgery 1 month after surgery	30 days	22 13	61	14 (64%) 0	39 (64%)	NA	NA
[5]	CD	Within 12 weeks prior to surgery	3 months	40	39	19 (47.5%)	15 (38.5%) p = NS	NA	NA
[6]	CD	Within 8 weeks prior to surgery or 4 weeks after surgery	30 days	52	218	12 (23%)	51 (23%) OR 1.0 (95% CI 0.5–2.0)	NA	NA
[7]	CD	At least 8 weeks prior to surgery	4 weeks	22	78	3 (13.6%) [a]	8 (10.3%) [a] (p = 0.7)	AZA/6MP (n = 3)	AZA (n = 1)
[8]	CD	Within 3 months before surgery	30 days	60	329	71.7%	31% p<0.0001	NA	NA
[9]	CD	Within 4 weeks of surgery	12 months	11	13	8 (72.7%)	11 (84.6%) (p = 0.63)	NA	NA
[10]	UC	1–12 months before surgery (median 2 months)	30 days	17	134	6 (35.3%)	37 (27.6%) (p = NS)	CysA (n = 4, 80%) 6-MP (n = 6, 38%)	CysA (n = 16, 29%) p = 0.04 6-MP (n = 25, 42%) p = 1.0

[11]	UC	Within 12 weeks prior to surgery	30 days	22	119	9% [b]	24% [b] (p = 0.161)	NA	NA
[12]	UC	Within 2–6 months before surgery	30 days	47	254	28 % [b]	10% [b] (OR 3.5, 95%CI 1.6–7.5)	NA	NA
[13]	UC	Median 13.5 weeks (interquartile range 4–37 weeks) before surgery	0.5–63 months for IFX 0.5–95 months for non-IFX	46	46	16 (35%) [c]	7 (15%) [c] (p = 0.027)	NA	NA
[14]	IBD	NA	30 days	41	–	11 (26.8%)	–	AZA (n = 3, 27.2%) GCS (n = 4, 36.4%) AZA and GCS (n = 2, 18.2%)	–
[15]	IBD	Within 12 weeks before surgery	30 days	101	312	16.8%	15.7% (p = 1.0)	NA	NA

NA, not available; CD, Crohn's disease; UC, ulcerative colitis; ns, not significant; AZA/6-MP, azathioprine/6-mercaptopurine; CysA, cyclosporin A; GSC, glucocorticosteroids.

[a] Intraabdominal septic complications.

[b] Infectious complications.

[c] Early postoperative complications.

($n = 19$) (9% versus 24%, $p = 0.161$) [11]. The authors concluded that moderate-to-high doses of corticosteroids and restorative proctocolectomy without defunctioning ileostomy were independent predictors of short-term infectious complications (OR 5.19, 95% CI 1.72–15.66, $p = 0.003$ and OR 6.45, 95% CI 2.12–19.64, $p = 0.001$, respectively), but not infliximab exposure[11].

However, two studies found an increased risk of postoperative complications in patients with UC who received infliximab perioperatively [12,13]. Selvasekar et al. using multivariate regression analysis demonstrated that only infliximab was significantly associated with an increased risk of infectious complications in a postoperative setting (OR 2.7; 95% CI 1.1–6.7) [12]. Similarly, Mor et al. observed in a multivariate regression model that perioperative use of infliximab was associated with a significantly increased risk of postoperative sepsis (OR 13.8, 95% CI 1.82–105), anastomotic leak (OR 7.87, 95% CI 1.55–39.8) and early (30 days) postoperative complications (OR 3.54, 95% CI 1.17–12.8) [13].

Combined cohorts

Two studies assessed the relationship between perioperative infliximab and postoperative complications in combined cohorts of CD or UC patients [14,15]. A Scandinavian multicenter retrospective analysis of infliximab-exposed patients demonstrated that among 41 patients (CD, $n = 33$; UC, $n = 8$) who underwent major surgical treatments, 11 (26.8%) experienced severe complications within 30 days postsurgery (CD, $n = 6$; UC, $n = 5$) [14]. However, 9 of these patients were also treated with azathioprine and/or corticosteroids preoperatively [14]. There were 2 deaths (4.9%) related to sepsis and pulmonary edema, and both occurred in patients who received a combination of infliximab and corticosteroids preoperatively [14]. Finally, recent data from a retrospective case-control study assessing the use of perioperative infliximab and postoperative complications found that treatment with infliximab (OR 2.5, $p = 0.14$) or corticosteroids (OR 1.2, $p = 0.74$), diagnosis of either CD (OR 0.7, $p = 0.63$) or UC (OR 0.6, $p = 0.48$), and preoperative infection (OR 1.2, $p = 0.76$) were not associated with postoperative infections [15]. However, patients exposed to infliximab ($n = 101$) had an increased duration of hospitalization compared to patients not exposed to infliximab ($n = 312$) (12.2 versus 10.2 days, $p<0.0001$) [15].

Conclusion

There are conflicting data regarding the use of perioperative infliximab and its association with postoperative complications in patients with IBD. Currently there is insufficient evidence to stop infliximab treatment prior to surgery. Further studies or large randomized trials are needed to elucidate this controversy. However, it may be appropriate to consider cessation of infliximab if medication has been ineffective and the disease has progressed while on medical therapy. This scenario would suggest that the medication has failed.

References

1. Targan SR, Hanauer SB, van Deventer SJ, et al. A short-term study of chimeric monoclonal antibody cA2 to tumor necrosis factor alpha for Crohn's disease. Crohn's disease cA2 study group. *N Engl J Med* 1997; **337**: 1029–1035.
2. Bernell O, Lapidus A, Hellers G. Risk factors for surgery and recurrence in 907 patients with primary ileocaecal Crohn's disease. *Br J Surg* 2000; **87**: 1697–1701.
3. Langholz E, Munkholm P, Davidsen M, et al. Colorectal cancer risk and mortality in patients with ulcerative colitis. *Gastroenterology* 1992; **103**: 1444–1451.
4. Brzezinski A, Armstrong L, Alvarez Del Real G, et al. Infliximab Does Not Increase the Risk of Complications in the Perioperative Period in Patients with Crohn's Disease. *Gastroenterology* 2002; **122**: A-617.
5. Marchal L, D'Haens G, Van Assche G, et al. The risk of postoperative complications associated with infliximab therapy for Crohn's disease: a controlled cohort study. *Aliment Pharmacol Ther* 2004; **19**: 749–54.
6. Colombel JF, Loftus EV, Jr., Tremaine WJ, et al. Early postoperative complications are not increased in patients with Crohn's disease treated perioperatively with infliximab or immunosuppressive therapy. *Am J Gastroenterol* 2004; **99**: 878–883.
7. Tay GS, Binion DG, Eastwood D, et al. Multivariate analysis suggests improved perioperative outcome in Crohn's disease patients receiving immunomodulator therapy after segmental resection and/or strictureplasty. *Surgery* 2003; **134**: 565–572.
8. Appau KA, Fazio VW, Shen B, et al. Use of infliximab within 3 months of ileocolonic resection is associated with adverse postoperative outcomes in Crohn's patients. *J Gastrointest Surg* 2008; **12**: 1738–1744.
9. Regueiro M, Schraut W, Baidoo L, et al. Infliximab prevents Crohn's disease recurrence after ileal resection. *Gastroenterology* 2009; **136**: 441–450.

10. Schluender SJ, Ippoliti A, Dubinsky M, et al. Does infliximab influence surgical morbidity of ileal pouch-anal anastomosis in patients with ulcerative colitis? *Dis Colon Rectum* 2007; **50**: 1747–1753.

11. Ferrante M, D'Hoore A, Vermeire S, et al. Corticosteroids but not infliximab increase short-term postoperative infectious complications in patients with ulcerative colitis. *Inflamm bowel dis* 2009; **15**: 1062–1070.

12. Selvasekar CR, Cima RR, Larson DW, et al. Effect of infliximab on short-term complications in patients undergoing operation for chronic ulcerative colitis. *J Am Coll Surg* 2007; **204**: 956–962; discussion 62–63.

13. Mor IJ, Vogel JD, da Luz Moreira A, et al. Infliximab in ulcerative colitis is associated with an increased risk of postoperative complications after restorative proctocolectomy. *Dis Colon Rectum* 2008; **51**: 1202–1207; discussion 7–10.

14. Ljung T, Karlen P, Schmidt D, et al. Infliximab in inflammatory bowel disease: clinical outcome in a population based cohort from Stockholm County. *Gut* 2004; **53**: 849–853.

15. Kunitake H, Hodin R, Shellito PC, et al. Perioperative treatment with infliximab in patients with Crohn's disease and ulcerative colitis is not associated with an increased rate of postoperative complications. *J Gastrointest Surg* 2008; **12**: 1730–1736; discussion 6–7.

42 Pouches for indeterminate colitis and Crohn's disease: act now, pay later?

Phillip Fleshner

Cedars-Sinai Medical Center, UCLA School of Medicine, Los Angeles, CA, USA

> ### LEARNING POINTS
>
> - Patients with indeterminate colitis have the same surgical outcome after ileal pouch-anal anastomosis (IPAA) as those with ulcerative colitis (UC).
>
> - Crohn's colitis patients *with* associated small bowel inflammation or anal disease should not be offered an IPAA, whereas those *without* these features may be offered an IPAA with appropriate counseling.
>
> - Patients with Crohn's disease (CD) diagnosed on the basis of features of the resected specimen appear to have the same surgical outcome after IPAA as those with UC.
>
> - Patients with CD diagnosed months or years after IPAA have more complicated disease course than those with UC and should be aggressively treated with immunomodulators or biologic agents.

Indeterminate colitis

Abdominal colectomy and ileal pouch-anal anastomosis (IPAA) has become the standard operative approach for patients with ulcerative colitis (UC) requiring colectomy for dysplasia, cancer, or medically refractory disease. In most cases, UC and Crohn's disease (CD) of the colon can be reliably distinguished from one another by careful assessment of preoperative clinical features in conjunction with pathologic assessment of the resected specimen. However, in approximately 10% of colitis patients, there are inadequate diagnostic criteria to make a definite distinction between UC and CD, especially in the setting of fulminant

colitis [1]. These patients are labeled as having indeterminate colitis (IC).

Although several large series have demonstrated good functional results and acceptable morbidity in UC patients [2], the outcome of IPAA in IC patients is controversial (Table 42.1). Although some studies have found higher rates of perineal complications, development of CD, and eventual pouch loss in IC patients [5,6], other papers have suggested that IC patients have outcomes comparable to those with UC [7–9]. These conflicting results in part arise from widespread confusion over the precise diagnosis of IC. Even though the term IC was initially applied to resection specimens, in recent years it has also been used in patients having atypical preoperative radiographic or endoscopic features, including biopsy specimens. This resulted in many studies including patients with indeterminate features preoperatively (i.e., inflammatory bowel disease-unclassified [IBDU]), postoperatively, or both. In an effort to standardize the definitions of IBDU and IC, The Working Party of the Montreal World Congress of Gastroenterology proposed that "patients with chronic IBD of the colon without *preoperative* features favoring typical UC or CD" be classified as having IBDU. Patients in whom there is no clear-cut distinction between UC and CD on the basis of findings *after* surgical resection would be classified as having IC [10]. Other factors that may account for the confusion over surgical outcomes in IC are that many studies are retrospective in design, include small patient numbers, have suboptimal patient follow-up, and are plagued with referral center bias. In addition, some authors defined pouchitis on clinical grounds alone, while others required endoscopic confirmation. The diagnosis of CD after surgery also varies

Clinical Dilemmas in Inflammatory Bowel Disease: New Challenges, Second Edition. Edited by P. Irving, C. Siegel, D. Rampton and F. Shanahan.
© 2011 Blackwell Publishing Ltd. Published 2011 by Blackwell Publishing Ltd.

TABLE 42.1 Recent studies of ileal pouch-anal anastomosis (IPAA) in indeterminate colitis

| Author [reference] | Year | Study design | Time of IC diagnosis | Clinical end point definition | | Long-term outcome (IC versus UC) |
				Pouchitis	CD	
Marcello et al. [3]	1997	R	Preop/postop	C, E	Clinical, radiographic, endoscopic, or pathologic	Increased risk of CD
Yu et al. [4]	2000	R	Postop	Not stated	Symptoms "suggestive" of CD	No difference in pouchitis; Increased risk of CD
Dayton et al. [5]	2002	P	Postop	Clinical	Not stated	No difference
Murrell et al. [11]	2009		Postop	C, E	Afferent limb inflammation or perianal disease	No difference

R, retrospective; P, prospective; C, clinical; E, endoscopic; CD, Crohn's disease.

across studies, with some authors using symptoms alone, some using serologic testing, and others using undefined clinical and subclinical criteria.

A recent prospective study specifically designed to address methodological problems associated with prior reports did not show any significant adverse clinical outcome of performing an IPAA in IC patients [11]. We recommend that future studies examining the results of IPAA in UC and IC are similarly designed, with particular attention given to precise inclusion criteria and well-defined clinical end points. Until this is done, our ability to accurately assess clinical outcomes of IPAA in these diseases will be severely hampered.

Crohn's disease

There are three different time points when patients undergoing IPAA are diagnosed with CD: (1) preoperatively, (2) perioperatively on histopathologic review of the colectomy specimen, and (3) postoperatively months or years after J-pouch reconstruction (de novo CD). The timing of the diagnosis may influence the outcome of surgery.

Preoperative colonic Crohn's disease

It has been traditionally thought that many patients with a preoperative diagnosis of IBD unclassified or CD undergoing IPAA for medically refractory disease or dysplasia/cancer have a high rate of pouch complications and ultimate pouch failure. However, emerging data has suggested that the subgroup of CD patients without anal or small bowel disease may have a more favorable surgical out-

come after IPAA. Panis et al. initially reported on IPAA in patients having isolated Crohn's colitis without anoperineal involvement and demonstrated good results at long-term follow-up [12]. However, the implication of these results has remained controversial because of the variability in pathologic criteria used for diagnosis of CD. However, this observation has recently been validated in a larger series from the Cleveland Clinic [13]. Although CD patients with small bowel inflammation and significant anal disease should not be offered an IPAA, the thoughtful use of IPAA in carefully selected Crohn's colitis patients without these sites of disease is acceptable.

Crohn's colitis diagnosed at colectomy

Histopathologic review of colectomy specimens from patients who are thought to have UC may uncover signs of CD that are not identified before surgery, including gross or microscopic transmural colonic inflammation, or discontinuous histopathologic involvement of the colon. These findings present a diagnostic dilemma, as the use of aggressive medical therapy in severe disease before surgery may result in these stigmata. Even the significance of noncaseating granulomas, a characteristic histologic finding of CD, may be unclear when they are found adjacent to a ruptured crypt. Perhaps these patients should more aptly be classified as being IC. However, as discussed above, even if labeled with IC, these patients appear to do no worse after IPAA surgery than "typical" UC patients.

Crohn's disease diagnosed after IPAA

Gastroenterologists and colorectal surgeons who manage patients with IBD regularly see patients whose diagnosis has been changed from UC to CD after IPAA. About 5–10% of patients initially believed to have UC or IC develop de novo CD [9]. Mechanisms accounting for the change in diagnosis from UC to CD are unclear. Although most likely related to the inability to accurately distinguish the two diseases before surgery, particularly in the fulminant phase [14], it is interesting to speculate that the change in diagnosis may reflect an inherent biologic behavior. In a large population study, almost 3% of nonoperated UC patients evolved into CD [15], a figure corresponding well to the incidence of CD development in the current prospectively followed patient cohort.

Patients who develop de novo CD appear to have more severe disease characteristics such as pouch-vaginal fistula, pouch stricture, and refractory pouch inflammation compared to patients who are diagnosed with CD preoperatively or after examination of the resected specimen [13]. However, this appears to be a self-fulfilling observation, as patients with active clinical disease will encourage their treating physicians to consider the possibility of de novo CD.

Prediction of patients who might develop Crohn's disease

The identification of possible predictors of de novo CD in UC, IBDU, or IC would be extremely helpful in the surgical management of these patients. A recent prospective study showed that de novo CD development after IPAA was significantly influenced by both a family history of CD and ASCA-IgA seropositivity [9]. The importance of family history has been recently validated in a separate patient cohort [16]. These data suggest that UC or IBDU patients with a family history of CD or who have seropositivity for ASCA IgA should be carefully evaluated for CD preoperatively. The role of prophylactic probiotics and/or immunomodulation in these patients is provocative but unproven.

Conclusion

The development of de novo CD has been one of the most difficult therapeutic challenges faced by both colorectal surgeons and gastroenterologists. . Older studies suggested that almost one-half of patients who developed CD in their pouch required fecal diversion for symptom control [17]. More recent studies have reported a much lower incidence of pouch failure, ranging from 16% to 28% [18,19]. One may speculate that the widespread use of biologic agents

in the management of IBD could account for this trend. It appears that immunomodulators and biologics may effectively control CD of the pouch [18].

References

1. Martland GT, Shepherd NA. Indeterminate colitis: definition, diagnosis, implications and a plea for nosological sanity. *Histopathology* 2007; **50**: 83–96.
2. Meagher AP, Farouk R, Dozois RR, Kelly KA, Pemberton JH. J ileal pouch-anal anastomosis for chronic ulcerative colitis: complications and long-term outcome in 1310 patients. *Br J Surg* 1998; **85**: 800–803.
3. Marcello PW, Schoetz DJ Jr, Roberts PL, et al. Evolutionary changes in the pathologic diagnosis after the ileoanal pouch procedure. *Dis Colon Rectum* 1997; **40**: 263–269.
4. Yu CS, Pemberton JH, Larson D. Ileal pouch-anal anastomosis in patients with indeterminate colitis. Long-term results. *Dis Colon Rectum* 2000; **43**: 1487–1496.
5. Delaney CP, Remzi FH, Gramlich T, Dadvand B, Fazio VW. Equivalent function, quality of life and pouch survival rates after ileal pouch-anal anastomosis for indeterminate and ulcerative colitis. *Ann Surg* 2002; **236**: 43–49.
6. Shen B, Fazio VW, Remzi FH, et al. Risk factors for clinical phenotypes of Crohn's disease of the ileal pouch. *Am J Gastroenterol* 2006; **101**: 2760–2768.
7. Dayton MT, Larsen KR, Christiansen DD. Similar functional results and complications after ileal pouch-anal anastomosis in patients with indeterminate colitis vs ulcerative colitis. *Arch Surg* 2002; **137**: 690–695.
8. Alexander F, Sarigol S, DiFiore J, et al. Fate of the pouch in 151 pediatric patients after ileal pouch anal anastomosis. *J Pediatr Surg* 2003; **38**: 78–82.
9. Melmed G, Fleshner PR, Bardakcioglu O, et al. Family history and serology predict Crohn's disease after ileal pouch-anal anastomosis for ulcerative colitis. *Dis Colon Rectum* 2008; **51**: 100–108.
10. Silverberg MS, Satsangi J, Ahmad T, et al. Toward an integrated clinical, molecular and serological classification of inflammatory bowel disease. Report of a Working Party of the 2005 Montreal World Congress of Gastroenterology. *Can J Gastroenterol* 2005; **19**(Suppl A): 5–36.
11. Murrell ZA, Melmed GY, Ippoliti A, et al. A prospective evaluation of the long-term outcome of ileal pouch-anal anastomosis in patients with inflammatory bowel disease-unclassified and indeterminate colitis. *Dis Colon Rectum* 2009; **52**: 872–878.
12. Panis Y, Poupard B, Nemeth J, Lavergne A, Hautefeuille P, Valleur P. Ileal pouch-anal anastomosis for Crohn's disease. *Lancet* 1996; **347**: 854–847.

13. Melton GB, Fazio VW, Kiran RP, et al. Long-term outcomes with ileal pouch-anal anastomosis and Crohn's Disease. *Ann Surg* 2008; **248**: 608–616.

14. Koltun WA, Schoetz DJ Jr., Roberts PL, et al. Indeterminate colitis predisposes to perineal complications after ileal pouch-anal anastomosis. *Dis Colon Rectum* 1991; **34**: 857–860.

15. Henriksen M, Jahnsen J, Lygren I, et al. Change of diagnosis during the first five years after onset of inflammatory bowel disease: results of a prospective follow-up study (the IBSEN study). *Scand J Gastroenterol* 2006; **41**: 1037–1043.

16. Shen B, Remzi FH, Hammel JP, et al. Family history of Crohn's disease is associated with an increased risk for Crohn's disease of the pouch. *Inflamm Bowel Dis* 2009; **15**: 163–170.

17. Sagar PM, Dozois RR, Wolff BG. Long-term results of ileal pouch-anal anastomosis in patients with Crohn's disease. *Dis Colon Rectum* 1996; **39**: 893–898.

18. Colombel J-F, Richart E, Loftus EV, et al. Management of Crohn's disease of the ileoanal pouch with infliximab. *Am J Gastroenterol* 2003; **98**: 2239–2244.

19. Shen B, Remzi FH, Brzezinski A, et al. Risk factors for pouch failure in patients with different phenotypes of Crohn's disease of the pouch. *Inflamm Bowel Dis* 2008; **14**: 942–948.

43

Dealing with pouchitis

Simon D. McLaughlin[1] and Bo Shen[2]

[1]Department of Gastroenterology, Royal Bournemouth Hospital, Bournemouth, UK
[2]Department of Gastroenterology, Cleveland Clinic Lerner College of Medicine, Case Western Reserve University, Cleveland, OH, USA

LEARNING POINTS

- Pouchitis occurs in up to 50% of patients after surgery for ulcerative colitis; risk factors include extensive ulcerative colitis, primary sclerosing cholangitis, and use of nonsteroidal anti-inflammatory drugs.

- Diagnosis should be confirmed by flexible pouchoscopy and infection with *Clostridium difficile* and other pathogens excluded.

- Asymptomatic pouch inflammation identified at surveillance pouchoscopy is common and does not require treatment.

- Acute pouchitis should be treated with ciprofloxacin, or metronidazole, or with topical budesonide.

- For patients with refractory pouchitis, before starting maintenance treatment with probiotic agents, remission should be induced with 4 weeks of treatment with ciprofloxacin and metronidazole or ciprofloxacin and rifaximin.

- Antibiotic resistant coliforms should be sought in the pouch effluent in patients who do not respond to empiric therapy.

Introduction

Pouchitis is reported to occur in 20–50% of patients following restorative proctocolectomy (RPC) for ulcerative colitis (UC). This wide variation can be explained by the different length and intensity of follow-up, practice settings, and diagnostic criteria between studies. It should be appreciated that, although pouchitis is common, the majority of patients respond to a short course of a single antibiotic and may not have a further episode or a gap of several months to years between episodes. Thus, the prevalence of chronic persisting pouchitis is around 5–10% in patients with pouchitis.

Although pouchitis is the most common long-term cause of pouch dysfunction, other inflammatory and noninflammatory conditions of the pouch can present with similar symptoms and the diagnosis should be confirmed, preferably by pouchoscopy, before starting treatment.

Risk factors for pouchitis

Extensive UC, backwash ileitis from diffuse colitis, extraintestinal manifestations (especially primary sclerosing cholangitis (PSC), taking nonsteroidal anti-inflammatory drugs, being a nonsmoker, carrying perinuclear antineutrophil cytoplasmic antibodies (pANCA), and interleukin-1 receptor antagonist gene polymorphisms are risk factors for developing pouchitis [1].

Investigation

Flexible pouchoscopy should ideally be performed in all patients with pouch dysfunction. Asymptomatic pouch inflammation is common, and it may not require treatment. Diagnosis of pouchitis relies on a triad of compatible symptoms, endoscopic, and histological findings. Sandborn's 18-point pouch disease activity index (PDAI) is a useful clinical and research tool: a score of ≥7 points is diagnostic of pouchitis. Fecal calprotectin, as well as lactoferrin, may be a useful test in those where flexible pouchoscopy cannot be arranged quickly [2], but is unlikely to be able to differentiate between pouchitis and symptoms from inflammation of

Clinical Dilemmas in Inflammatory Bowel Disease: New Challenges, Second Edition. Edited by P. Irving, C. Siegel, D. Rampton and F. Shanahan.
© 2011 Blackwell Publishing Ltd. Published 2011 by Blackwell Publishing Ltd.

retained rectal cuff (cuffitis) or Crohn's disease (CD) of the pouch. In those with treatment-resistant pouchitis or who relapse on maintenance antibiotic therapy, infection with pathogens such as *clostridium difficile*, *Cytomegalovirus*, and *Campylobacter jejuni*, should be excluded.

Treatment (see Figure 43.1 [3])

Acute (simple) pouchitis

In those taking regular nonsteroidal anti-inflammatory drugs (NSAIDs), withdrawal of these drugs alone can induce remission [4]. Antibiotics remain the mainstay of treatment and several studies have demonstrated the efficacy of ciprofloxacin and metronidazole [5,6]. Ciprofloxacin is better tolerated and probably should be considered as the first-line treatment. If available, budesonide enemas can also be considered, as one controlled study showed that the treatment was as effective as oral metronidazole [7].

There are no controlled trials of oral or topical mesalamine for treating pouchitis. As part of a study examining the efficacy of a combination of ciprofloxacin and tinidazole in patients with pouchitis, the response to mesalamine in a historical cohort was reported. Results showed that 50% of patients on mesalamine achieved clinical remission and 50% had a clinical response. Patients on mesalamine showed a significant reduction in the PDAI but no improvement in health-related quality of life score [8].

Bismuth enemas were found to be effective in an open-label study with 83% of patients entering remission after 45 days treatment [9], but a subsequent double-blind randomized trial found no difference when bismuth was compared to placebo [10]. Treatment with short-chain fatty acids (SCFAs) has been reported to be ineffective [11].

Refractory pouchitis

Patients who do not respond to a 4-week course of a single antibiotic have been classified as having

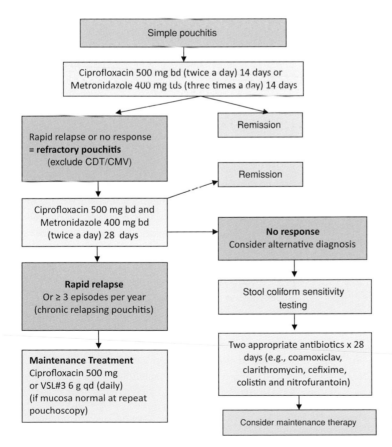

FIGURE 43.1 Algorithm for the management of pouchitis (CDT, *C. difficile* toxin; CMV, cytomegalovirus). (Adapted from [3].)

antibiotic-refractory pouchitis. Treatment options for these patients include combination antibiotic therapy and oral budesonide. Treatment with ciprofloxacin and another antibiotic (rifaximin, metronidazole, or tinidazole) is effective in up to 85% of these patients [8,12,13], and oral budesonide was effective in 75% of patients [14]. However, maintenance of remission in these patients has been challenging.

In patients who do not respond to the combination antibiotic treatment, failure appears to be due to antibiotic resistance. Fecal coliform sensitivity testing, which involves culture and antibiotic sensitivity testing of the dominant fecal organism, can be used to identify appropriate antibiotic treatment in most of these patients [15]. In addition, secondary causes for refractory pouchitis should be excluded, such as concurrent autoimmune disorders, such as Hashimoto thyroiditis and psoriasis cytomegalovirus infection, and ischemic pouchitis.

There are no studies of immunomodulators for the treatment of pouchitis. However, since pouchitis can occur in patients with PSC treated with azathioprine after orthotopic liver transplant [16], this treatment is probably not effective at preventing pouchitis.

One group has reported the outcome of pouchitis and extensive prepouch ileitis in 10 patients who were given a standard induction regimen of infliximab having previously not responded to 4 weeks treatment with ciprofloxacin. After 10 weeks, 8 of the patients had entered clinical remission with a PDAI score of ≤7. These results should be interpreted with caution since on video capsule endoscopy, the patients all had extensive jejunal as well as ileal inflammation suggestive of CD [17].

Maintenance treatment

Maintenance treatment should be considered in patients with three or more episodes of pouchitis per year or those who relapse soon after withdrawal of treatment. Maintenance treatment options include antibiotic or probiotic therapy.

The probiotic VSL#3 has been shown to be an effective maintenance agent in two randomized controlled trials (RCTs) in which it was given after induction of remission by combination antibiotic treatment [18,19]. However, in a later postmarket open-label study, less than 20% of patients were able to maintain remission. Possible reasons for these differences include the exclusion of patients who did not achieve complete or near-complete antibiotic-induced mucosal healing in the first two studies, and the use of a single antibiotic compared to combination antibiotic treatment for induction of remission in the open-label study. In addition, both RCTs included patients who had two episodes of pouchitis per year as opposed to three in the clinical study. It should be noted by those considering prescribing VSL#3 that the commercially available preparation is a lower strength than that used in the original RCTs [18,19].

Two retrospective studies have reported the outcome of antibiotic maintenance therapy. In a study using rifaximin, 58% of 51 patients remained in remission at one year; however, only 3% remained in remission after 2 years [20]. A further study that used various oral antibiotics as maintenance treatment of 25 patients, with a median follow-up of 16 months, reported that 24% developed resistance. Resistance was managed by using 2-weekly rotating antibiotics guided by fecal coliform sensitivity testing; all patients were in remission at the end of the study [21].

It is likely that long-term antibiotic therapy increases the risk of *C. difficile* infection and bacterial resistance (see below).

Preventing initial onset of pouchitis

The first study of the use of probiotics to prevent pouchitis was reported by Gosselink et al. [22]. In this controlled study, 39 patients were treated with 300 mg of *Lactobacillus* GG for 3 years after ileostomy closure. The control group consisted of 127 patients who had previously undergone RPC. The prevalence of pouchitis at 3 years was 7% in the probiotic group compared with 29% in the control group. However, importantly, there was no difference in the number of patients who developed recurrent pouchitis.

The efficacy of VSL#3 in preventing initial onset of pouchitis has also been reported. In a double-blind, placebo-controlled trial, 40 patients were randomized to VSL#3 3 g/day (900 billion bacteria) or placebo for 1 year. The prevalence of pouchitis was significantly lower in the probiotic group compared to the placebo group (10% versus 40%; $P < 0.05$)[23]. Studies with longer follow-up are required to establish whether VSL#3 reduces the risk of developing recurrent pouchitis or, more importantly, refractory pouchitis and pouch failure before its use in routine practice can be recommended.

Implications of use of antibiotics in patients with pouchitis

Chronic pouchitis is responsible for 10% of pouch failures due to failure of medical management [24]. Currently, factors that predict an increased risk for pouch failure are not known. However, it is likely that the development of antibiotic resistance is clinically important. Extended spectrum β-lactamase resistant bacteria (ESBL) are resistant to most orally available antibiotics and may be implicated in pouch failure. A recent study identified the presence of ESBL organisms in 33% of chronic pouchitis patients. Risk factors for developing ESBL were prepouch ileitis and maintenance antibiotic therapy [16]. These findings suggest that antibiotics should be used only in patients with a definite diagnosis of pouchitis and that maintenance antibiotic therapy should be avoided where possible.

References

1. Shen B, Fazio VW, Remzi FH et al. Clinical approach to diseases of ileal pouch-anal anastomosis. *Am J Gastroenterol* 2005; **100**(12): 2796–2807.
2. Johnson MW, Maestranzi S, Duffy AM et al. Faecal calprotectin: a noninvasive diagnostic tool and marker of severity in pouchitis. *Eur J Gastroenterol Hepatol* 2008; **20**(3): 174–179.
3. McLaughlin SD, Clark SK, Tekkis PP, Ciclitira PJ, Nicholls RJ. Review article: restorative proctocolectomy, indications, management of complications and follow-up: a guide for gastroenterologists. *Aliment Pharmacol Ther.* 2008;**27**(10): 895–909.
4. Shen B, Fazio VW, Remzi FH et al. Effect of Withdrawal of Nonsteroidal Anti-Inflammatory Drug Use on Ileal Pouch Disorders. *Dig Dis Sci* 2007; **52**(12): 3321–3328.
5. Madden MV, McIntyre AS, Nicholls RJ. Double-blind crossover trial of metronidazole versus placebo in chronic unremitting pouchitis. *Dig Dis Sci* 1994; **39**(6): 1193–1196.
6. Shen B, Achkar JP, Lashner BA et al. A randomized clinical trial of ciprofloxacin and metronidazole to treat acute pouchitis. *Inflamm Bowel Dis* 2001; **7**(4): 301–305.
7. Sambuelli A, Boerr L, Negreira S et al. Budesonide enema in pouchitis – a double-blind, double-dummy, controlled trial. *Aliment Pharmacol Ther* 2002; **16**(1): 27–34.
8. Shen B, Fazio VW, Remzi FH et al. Combined Ciprofloxacin and Tinidazole Therapy in the Treatment of Chronic Refractory Pouchitis. *Dis Colon Rectum* 2007; **50**(4): 498–508.
9. Gionchetti P, Rizzello F, Venturi A et al. Long-term efficacy of bismuth carbomer enemas in patients with treatment-resistant chronic pouchitis. *Aliment Pharmacol Ther* 1997; **11**(4): 673–678.
10. Tremaine WJ, Sandborn WJ, Wolff BG et al. Bismuth carbomer foam enemas for active chronic pouchitis: a randomized, double-blind, placebo-controlled trial. *Aliment Pharmacol Ther* 1997; **11**(6): 1041–1046.
11. de Silva HJ, Ireland A, Kettlewell M et al. Short-chain fatty acid irrigation in severe pouchitis. *N Engl J Med* 1989; **321**(20): 1416–1417.
12. Gionchetti P, Rizzello F, Venturi A et al. Antibiotic combination therapy in patients with chronic, treatment-resistant pouchitis. *Aliment Pharmacol Ther* 1999; **13**(6): 713–718.
13. Mimura T, Rizzello F, Helwig U et al. Four-week open-label trial of metronidazole and ciprofloxacin for the treatment of recurrent or refractory pouchitis. *Aliment Pharmacol Ther* 2002; **16**(5): 909–917.
14. Gionchetti P, Rizzello F, Poggioli G et al. Oral budesonide in the treatment of chronic refractory pouchitis. *Aliment Pharmacol Ther* 2007; **25**(10): 1231–1236.
15. McLaughlin SD, Clark SK, Shafi S et al. Fecal coliform testing to identify effective antibiotic therapies for patients with antibiotic-resistant pouchitis. *Clin Gastroenterol Hepatol* 2009; **7**(5): 545–548.
16. McLaughlin SD, Clark SK, Tekkis PP, Ciclitira PJ, Nicholls RJ. Clostridium difficile and extended spectrum beta-lactamase resistant bacteria in pouchitis patients. *Aliment Pharmacol Ther* 2010; **32**(5): 664–669.
17. Calabrese C, Gionchetti P, Rizzello F et al. Short-term treatment with infliximab in chronic refractory pouchitis and ileitis. *Aliment Pharmacol Ther* 2008; **27**(9): 759–764.
18. Gionchetti P, Rizzello F, Venturi A et al. Oral bacteriotherapy as maintenance treatment in patients with chronic pouchitis: a double-blind, placebo-controlled trial. *Gastroenterology* 2000; **119**(2): 305–309.
19. Mimura T, Rizzello F, Helwig U et al. Once daily high dose probiotic therapy (VSL#3) for maintaining remission in recurrent or refractory pouchitis. *Gut* 2004; **53**(1): 108–114.
20. Shen B, Remzi FH, Lopez AR et al. Rifaximin for maintenance therapy in antibiotic-dependent pouchitis. *BMC Gastroenterol* 2008; **8**: 26.
21. McLaughlin S.D, Clark SK, Shafi S, Tekkis PP, Ciclitira PJ., and Nicholls RJ. An open study of maintenance antibiotic therapy for chronic antibiotic dependent pouchitis; efficacy, complications and outcome. *Colorectal Dis.* 2011; **13**(4): 438–444.
22. Gosselink MP, Schouten WR, van Lieshout LM et al. Delay of the first onset of pouchitis by oral intake of the probiotic strain Lactobacillus rhamnosus GG. *Dis Colon Rectum* 2004; **47**(6): 876–884.
23. Gionchetti P, Rizzello F, Poggioli G et al. Probiotic therapy to prevent pouchitis onset. *Dis Colon Rectum* 2005; **48**(7): 1493–1494.
24. Tulchinsky H, Hawley PR, Nicholls J. Long-term failure after restorative proctocolectomy for ulcerative colitis. *Ann Surg* 2003; **238**(2): 229–234.

PART VII:
Unsolved Issues in IBD

44

Mucosal healing in IBD: does it matter?

Geert D'Haens

Academic Medical Centre, Amsterdam, The Netherlands

LEARNING POINTS

- Immunomodulatory and biologic treatments have been shown to induce mucosal healing in both Crohn's disease and ulcerative colitis.

- The disease prognosis is usually more favorable in IBD patients who can attain mucosal healing.

- New anti-inflammatory agents for IBD should be evaluated for their capacity to induce mucosal healing.

Crohn's disease

Until recently most clinical trials in the field of Crohn's disease (CD) focused on clinical outcome, using validated symptom scores such as the CD activity index (CDAI) and the Harvey–Bradshaw index (HBI). Mucosal healing was rather neglected as a goal of treatment because it was considered unimportant and virtually impossible to achieve with available treatments. Later on, an assessment tool for endoscopic appearance was designed and validated as the CD endoscopic index of severity (CDEIS) (Figure 44.1). In an initial French trial, treatment with corticosteroids for 7 weeks led to mucosal healing in 29% of the patients, whereas 9% had worsening of lesions [1].

But things gradually changed. In the 90s, it was shown that azathioprine induced endoscopic healing in postoperative recurrent ileitis and in primary Crohn's ileocolitis [2,3]. The association between mucosal healing and a more favorable disease course began to be established. Fifteen patients who underwent an ileocecal resection for their Crohn's and who subsequently developed severe recurrent ileitis were treated with azathioprine for at least

6 months after weaning off corticosteroids: complete endoscopic healing of the neoterminal ileum occurred in 6 patients, and near-complete healing with only superficial erosions in another 5. Azathioprine was proposed as the treatment of choice in severe recurrent Crohn's ileitis [2]. In another study by the same Belgian group, 20 patients with Crohn's colitis or ileocolitis in clinical remission while taking azathioprine for at least 9 months were endoscopically evaluated. Complete or near-complete healing of the mucosa was seen in 80% patients [3].

In a randomized, double-blind, controlled study investigating the effect of azathioprine withdrawal on sustained clinical remission, baseline ileocolonoscopy was performed in half of the patients in clinical remission on azathioprine for at least 42 months. Complete endoscopic remission defined as CDEIS = 0 was seen in 36% of patients [4]. In a Greek study, looking at maintenance of mucosal healing in patients who achieved clinical remission with standard steroid treatment, azathioprine was also shown to achieve and maintain endoscopic remission. After 1 year on azathioprine, complete or near complete healing was achieved in 83% of azathioprine-treated patients with mean CDEIS dropping from 7 to 0.55. Multivariate logistic regression analysis identified early initiation of azathioprine (<1 year after diagnosis) as the only factor predicting complete endoscopic healing [5].

In a pilot study on the effects of methotrexate in CD published in the late 80s, 5 of 14 patients with Crohn's colitis had mucosal healing at 12 weeks [6]. Although methotrexate proved to be an effective drug for induction and maintenance of *clinical* remission, its effect on mucosal healing has not been further investigated in CD.

Clinical Dilemmas in Inflammatory Bowel Disease: New Challenges, Second Edition. Edited by P. Irving, C. Siegel, D. Rampton and F. Shanahan.
© 2011 Blackwell Publishing Ltd. Published 2011 by Blackwell Publishing Ltd.

Several multicenter studies have examined the effects of the anti-TNF antibody infliximab on mucosal lesions in CD. "Mucosal healing," defined as disappearance of all ulcers, was seen 4 weeks after a single dose of infliximab in 74% patients in the ileum and in 96% patients in the rectum [7]. A significant correlation between the reductions in CDAI and CDEIS was observed. Later on, a substudy of the ACCENT I project compared episodic and scheduled treatment strategies with infliximab in patients with Crohn's following a single induction treatment with 5 mg/kg of infliximab [8] and demonstrated that patients randomized to "scheduled therapy" had fewer hospitalizations and surgeries and higher rates of mucosal healing, again defined as absence of ulcers. Complete mucosal healing at week 10 was seen in 31% and 0% patients with scheduled and episodic treatment, respectively. At week 54, mucosal healing was seen in 50% versus 7%, respectively. There was a direct association between the mucosal healing rates and the number of hospitalizations: no hospitalizations were needed in patients who had mucosal healing at both week 10 and week 54 [9].

In the recent SONIC trial, patients with active Crohn's who had never been exposed to biologicals or immunomodulators were randomized to treatment with azathioprine monotherapy, infliximab monotherapy, or the combination of both. All patients were colonoscoped at inclusion and at week 26. Mucosal healing (absence of ulcers) was observed in 44% of patients on combination treatment, 30% on infliximab monotherapy, and 16% on azathioprine monotherapy. The superiority of the combination was most pronounced in patients who had ulcers on the baseline endoscopy [10].

Mucosal healing has also been assessed after treatment with adalimumab and certolizumab pegol. In the EXTEND trial, 129 patients with active Crohn's received induction treatment with adalimumab 160 mg followed by 80 mg at week 2 and maintenance treatment with placebo or 40 mg adalimumab every two weeks. Endoscopies were performed at week 0, 12, and 52. At week 12, 27% of patients in the maintenance adalimumab group had complete mucosal healing versus only 13% in the placebo group ($p = 0.056$). At week 52, 24% of patients had complete healing with adalimumab versus none with placebo maintenance ($p < 0.001$) [11]. In the MUSIC study with certolizumab pegol, all ($n = 89$) patients received open-label induction with 400 mg certolizumab pegol every 2 weeks for three doses followed by 400 mg every 4 weeks, with endoscopies performed at week 0, 10, and 56. At week 10, a significant reduction in the CDEIS score was observed (42%, $p < 0.0001$). Four patients had complete absence of lesions at week 10, whereas 61% had a CDEIS response defined by a decrease in score of >5 points [12].

Ulcerative colitis

Technically, mucosal inflammation in ulcerative colitis (UC) is easier to evaluate, since the disease almost always involves the distal colon and is easily accessible for endoscopy.

In an early trial with 5-aminosalicylic acid (5-ASA) preparations, it became clear that patients with both clinical and endoscopic remission had a higher likelihood of prolonged remission than patients with only clinical remission [13]. A study in the early 90s underscored the importance of mucosal healing in the relapse rate of UC. The occurrence of flares within 1 year after an episode of active colitis was 4% in patients with clinical remission and mucosal healing versus 30% in patients with persistent mucosal lesions [14]. These findings were confirmed by an Italian trial, in which relapse rates at 1 year in patients achieving both clinical and endoscopic remission were 23% as compared to 80% in patients in clinical remission but still having endoscopic lesions [15].

In the two large ACT trials, rapid induction of mucosal healing with infliximab was associated with a 4-fold increase in clinical remission rate at week 30 [16]. Continuously inflamed mucosa probably carries an enhanced risk of dysplasia and cancer development, since there is a highly significant correlation between inflammation scores and the risk of colorectal neoplasia [17].

Given its established impact on the course of the disease, endoscopic assessment has been incorporated in the evaluation of drugs for UC. Schroeder et al. assessed the effects of oral 5-ASA at a dosage of 4.8 g/day or 1.6 g/day versus placebo for 6 weeks in mildly to moderately active UC. Flexible sigmoidoscopy showed 24% complete and 50% partial response in patients receiving 4.8 g of 5-ASA per day versus 5% complete and 13% partial response in those receiving placebo [18]. Combined analysis of two recent studies with Multi Matrix system (MMX) mesalamine revealed that approximately one-third of patients treated with up to 8 weeks of MMX mesalamine had complete mucosal healing (a sigmoidoscopy score of 0) compared with 16% of those who received placebo [19]. Similar mucosal healing effects were seen with 5-ASA enemas [20].

	Deep ulcerations *12 points*	Superficial ulcerations *6 points*	Surface of ulcerations *(0–10 cm)*	Surface of lesions *(0–10 cm)*
Ileum	0 or 12	0 or 6	0–10	0–10
Right colon	0 or 12	0 or 6	0–10	0–10
Transverse	0 or 12	0 or 6	0–10	0–10
Left colon	0 or 12	0 or 6	0–10	0–10
Rectum	0 or 12	0 or 6	0–10	0–10
TOTAL (sum of all cases)	N			
TOTAL/number of explored segments	N/1–5			
+ 3 if ulcerated stenosis	0–3			
+ 3 if nonulcerated stenosis	0–3			
CDEIS:	0 to 44			

The Mayo endoscopic score
0: normal
1: disturbed vessels, friability, granularity
2: loss of vascular pattern, mucopus, spontaneous bleeding
3: ulcers, mucopus, spontaneous bleeding

FIGURE 44.1 The Crohn's disease index of severity (CDEIS) and the Mayo endoscopic score.

A study comparing azathioprine with 5-ASA in inducing remission demonstrated that azathioprine was significantly more effective than 5-ASA. More than 50% of azathioprine-treated patients had both clinical and endoscopic remission with a therapeutic gain of approximately 35% in comparison with 5-ASA [21]. In another study in 42 patients with steroid-dependent or steroid-resistant UC, complete endoscopic remission was seen in 75% of patients tolerating azathioprine after 6 months [22].

The effects of infliximab in active UC were extensively investigated in the ACT trials. All patients in these trials underwent endoscopy. Sixty percent of patients healed their mucosa on infliximab at week 8 versus 32% on placebo ($p < 0.001$). Mucosal healing in these trials did not mean "absence of any lesion" but rather a Mayo score of 0 or 1 (Figure 44.1), allowing for milder lesions to persist. At week 30, 48–53% of patients had endoscopic healing on infliximab versus 27% on placebo ($p < 0.001$). Complete endoscopic healing with a Mayo score of 0 occurred in 25% at week 8 (versus 8% on placebo) and in 28–31% at week 30 (versus 9% on placebo) [16].

Conclusions

Accumulating data support the importance of mucosal healing in CD as well as in UC. Mucosal healing has become a reliable predictor of disease control, with evidence for fewer surgeries and higher remission rates when it is achieved in patients with CD. In UC, lower colectomy rates and longer disease control is seen in patients attaining mucosal healing. Newer therapies are efficacious in inducing complete and fast endoscopic remission. Inducing mucosal healing is not just a cosmetic exercise: it is now an essential component of clinical practice and of studies in the field of IBD.

References

1. Landi B, Anh TN, Cortot A, et al. Endoscopic monitoring of Crohn's disease treatment: a prospective, randomized clinical trial. The Groupe d'Etudes Therapeutiques des Affections Inflammatoires Digestives. *Gastroenterology* 1992; **102**: 1647–1653.

2. D'Haens G, Geboes K, Ponette E, Penninckx F, Rutgeerts P. Healing of severe recurrent ileitis with azathioprine therapy in patients with Crohn's disease. *Gastroenterology* 1997; **112**: 1475–1481.

3. D'Haens G, Geboes K, Rutgeerts P. Endoscopic and histologic healing of Crohn's (ileo-) colitis with azathioprine. *Gastrointest Endosc* 1999; **50**: 667–671.

4. Lémann M, Mary JY, Colombel JF, et al. Groupe D'Etude Thérapeutique des Affections Inflammatoires du Tube Digestif. A randomized, double-blind, controlled

withdrawal trial in Crohn's disease patients in long-term remission on azathioprine. *Gastroenterology* 2005; **128**: 1812–1818.

5. Mantzaris GJ, Christidou A, Sfakianakis M, et al. Azathioprine is superior to budesonide in achieving and maintaining mucosal healing and histologic remission in steroid-dependent Crohn's disease. *Inflamm Bowel Dis* 2009; **15**: 375–382.

6. Kozarek RA, Patterson DJ, Gelfand MD, Botoman VA, Ball TJ, Wilske KR. Methotrexate induces clinical and histologic remission in patients with refractory inflammatory bowel disease. *Ann Intern Med* 1989; **110**(5): 353–356.

7. D'Haens G, van Deventer S, van Hogezand R, et al. Endoscopic and histological healing with infliximab antitumor necrosis factor antibodies in Crohn's disease: a European multicenter trial. *Gastroenterology* 1999; **116**: 1029–1034.

8. Rutgeerts P, Feagan BG, Lichtenstein GR, et al. Comparison of scheduled and episodic treatment strategies of infliximab in Crohn's disease. *Gastroenterology* 2004; **126**: 402–413.

9. Rutgeerts P, Diamond RH, Bala M, et al. Scheduled maintenance treatment with infliximab is superior to episodic treatment for the healing of mucosal ulceration associated with Crohn's disease. *Gastrointest Endosc* 2006; **63**: 433–442.

10. Colombel JF, Rutgeerts P, Reinisch W, et al. Sonic: a randomized, double-blind, controled trial comparing infliximab and infliximab plus azathioprine to azathioprine in patients with Crohn's disease naïve to immunomodulators and biologic therapy. *N Engl J Med* 2010; **362**: 1383–1395.

11. Rutgeerts P, D'Haens GR, Van Assche G et al. Adalimumab induces and maintains mucosal healing in patients with moderate to severe ileocolonic Crohn's disease—First Results of the Extend Trial *Gastroenterology* 2009; **136** (Suppl I), A116. (Abstract).

12. Hébuterne X, Colombel J, Bouhnik Y, et al. Endoscopic improvement in patients with active Crohn's disease treated with certolizumab pegol: first results of the MUSIC trail. *Gut* 2008; **57**(Suppl II), A15. (Abstract).

13. Riley SA, Mani V, Goodman MJ, Dutt S, Herd ME. Microscopic activity in ulcerative colitis: what does it mean? *Gut* 1991; **32**: 174–178.

14. Courtney MG, Nunes DP, Bergin CF, et al. Colonoscopic appearance in remission predicts relapse of ulcerative colitis. *Gastroenterology* 1991; **100**: A205.

15. Meucci G, Fasoli R, Saibeni S, et al. Prognostic significance of endoscopic remission in patients with active ulcerative colitis treated with oral and topical mesalazine: preliminary results of a prospective, multicenter study. *Gastroenterology* 2006; **130**: A197.

16. Rutgeerts P, Sandborn WJ, Feagan BG, et al. Infliximab for induction and maintenance therapy for ulcerative colitis. *N Engl J Med* 2005; **353**: 2462–2476.

17. Rutter M, Saunders B, Wilkinson K, et al. Severity of inflammation is a risk factor for colorectal neoplasia in ulcerative colitis. *Gastroenterology* 2004; **126**: 451–459.

18. Schroeder KW, Tremaine WJ, IlstrupDM. Coated oral 5-aminosalicylic acid therapy for mildly to moderately active ulcerative colitis: a randomized study. N Engl J Med 1987; **317**: 1625–1629.

19. Sandborn WJ, Kamm MA, Lichtenstein GR, et al. MMX Multi Matrix System mesalazine for the induction of remission in patients with mild-to-moderate ulcerative colitis: a combined analysis of two randomized, double-blind, placebo-controlled trials. *Aliment Pharmacol Ther* 2007; **26**: 205–215.

20. Marteau P, Probert CS, Lindgren S, et al. Combined oral and enema treatment with Pentasa (mesalazine) is superior to oral therapy alone in patients with extensive mild/moderate active ulcerative colitis: a randomised, double blind, placebo controlled study. *Gut* 2005; **54**: 960–965.

21. Ardizzone S, Maconi G, Russo A, et al. Randomised, controlled trial, of azathioprine and 5- aminosalicylic acid for treatment of steroid-dependent ulcerative colitis. *Gut* 2006; **55**: 47–53.

22. Paoluzi OA, Pica R, Marcheggiano A, et al. Azathioprine or methotrexate in the treatment of patients with steroid-dependent or steroid-resistant ulcerative colitis: results of an open-label study on efficacy and tolerability in inducing and maintaining remission. *Aliment Pharmacol Ther* 2002; **16**: 1751–1759.

45 Vitamin D in IBD: from genetics to bone health via cancer and immunology

Helen M. Pappa and Richard J. Grand

Division of Gastroenterology and Nutrition, Center for Inflammatory Bowel Disease, Harvard Medical School, Children's Hospital Boston, Boston, MA, USA

LEARNING POINTS

- Vitamin D is a hormone.
- People with IBD are at particular risk for vitamin D deficiency.
- Vitamin D status, metabolism, and genetic variability of the vitamin D receptor may play a role in the development and course of IBD.
- Vitamin D may play a protective role against the development of dysplasia in patients with IBD.

Vitamin D In IBD: from genetics to bone health via cancer and immunology

Vitamin D–physiology and metabolism (see Figure 45.1)

Vitamin D is a steroid molecule with both hormonal and nonhormonal actions. Adequate skin exposure to solar ultraviolet B radiation can satisfy the human requirement for vitamin D. During sunlight exposure, 7-dehydrocholesterol, present in membranes of skin cells, is converted to vitamin D_3, but atmospheric conditions control cutaneous vitamin D synthesis. For example, no vitamin D_3 is produced through skin exposure to sunlight even on cloudless days in Boston, United States (42.2° N) from November through February. Ergocalciferol (vitamin D_2) and cholecalciferol (vitamin D_3) are the two forms of oral vitamin D supplements available. Vitamin D, either cutaneously synthesized or ingested, enters the circulation by binding to the plasma transport protein, vitamin D-binding protein (DBP), which delivers vitamin D first to the liver, where it undergoes 25-hydroxylation to 25-hydroxyvitamin D (25OHD), and then to the kidney where it undergoes 1-hydroxylation. 1, 25-dihydroxyvitamin D [1,25(OH)2D] is the active metabolite, and it exerts its action through activation of the vitamin D receptor (VDR) in the nucleus. Activated VDR interacts with DNA sequences affecting transcription of several genes. The VDR is present in over 30 tissues.

The most abundant metabolite in the human body is 25OHD, and its concentration in the serum is indicative of overall vitamin D status. Vitamin D deficits are defined by their consequences on bone health. The efficiency of intestinal calcium transport is maximized and serum parathyroid hormone (PTH) concentration begins to plateau when serum 25OHD concentration is ≥ 32 ng/mL (or 80 nmol/L); this is currently considered the threshold for optimal vitamin D status [1].

Hypovitaminosis D in IBD: is it really a problem?

The prevalence of hypovitaminosis D is greater among children with IBD than among healthy children serum 25OHD concentration is <15 ng/mL in up to 35% of children with IBD [1]. Similarly, serum 25OHD concentration is lower in adults with IBD than in healthy matched controls [1,2] and the prevalence of suboptimal vitamin D status (25OHD < 32 ng/mL) may be as high as 80% among adults with IBD [3]. Hypothesized mechanisms for the higher prevalence of hypovitaminosis D encountered among patients with IBD are: decreased exposure to sunlight, decreased

Clinical Dilemmas in Inflammatory Bowel Disease: New Challenges, Second Edition. Edited by P. Irving, C. Siegel, D. Rampton and F. Shanahan.
© 2011 Blackwell Publishing Ltd. Published 2011 by Blackwell Publishing Ltd.

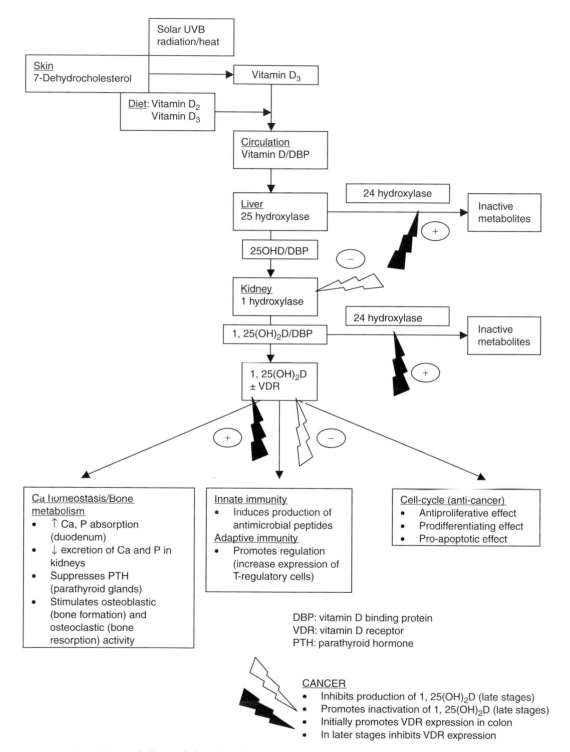

FIGURE 45.1 Vitamin D metabolism and physiology relevant to IBD.

vitamin D intake, malabsorption, and loss through the inflamed intestine.

Vitamin D and bone health

The effects of vitamin D on calcium homeostasis and bone metabolism have been well established, and include facilitation of calcium absorption in the duodenum, promotion of bone mineralization, and regulation of both osteoblastic and osteoclastic activity [1].

However, studies of the relationship between vitamin D status and bone health have yet to show a definitive connection. Several studies in adults with IBD found that serum 25OHD and vitamin D intake were not related to bone mineral density (BMD) [1]. However, a recent study found a positive such relationship not only at presentation but also between initial serum 25OHD concentration and bone gains longitudinally [3]. Although it has been reported that there is no relationship between serum 25OHD concentration and BMD in children with IBD, these reports were based on studies of children with relatively low serum 25OHD concentration [1]. Vitamin D exerts an anabolic effect on bones, which may be especially significant for the growing skeleton. Further systematic studies of the effect of vitamin D status on bone health and metabolism are needed in adults, and especially in children with IBD, to include longitudinal vitamin D interventions.

Vitamin D and treatment of IBD: a new approach to therapy and prevention?

This is an area of exciting research and great promise. Vitamin D's active metabolite, $1,25(OH)_2D$ through its interaction with the VDR, is known to induce regulatory T cells, and promote Th2 cell production and function, thereby maintaining a balanced T-cell response [4]. It is this balance that is hypothesized to be disrupted in the pathogenesis of Crohn's disease (CD). Indeed, experimental colitis in the IL-10 knockout mouse manifested itself earlier and was more severe in vitamin D deficient and in VDR-lacking mice [4]. These experiments were more recently extended to human models: in vitro at least, vitamin D derivatives act as TNF-α production suppressors in peripheral mononuclear blood cells of patients with IBD [5].

Vitamin D was lately found to affect other host defense mechanisms directly related to the development or course of IBD. Specifically, $1,25(OH)_2D$ was found to increase intestinal epithelial cell resistance to injury, reg-ulate the innate response to intraluminal gut antigens [6], and preserve mucosal integrity by enhancing intercellular junctions between gut epithelial cells [7]. These exciting discoveries underline the potential of vitamin D as an adjunct to the treatment of IBD, as well as the potential for optimal vitamin D status to be a deterrent for the future development of the disease. Recently, investigators started exploring this role of vitamin D in humans. In an epidemiologic study in France, investigators linked higher incidence rate of CD with lower sunlight exposure [8]. Although confounding by genetic background is possible, this study's importance lays in the fact that it is among the first to establish a link between vitamin D status and IBD in a relatively homogenous population. Another recent study establishes a inverse relationship between serum 25OHD concentration and disease activity in patients with IBD [9]. Although a hypothesis that vitamin D reduces disease activity in patients with IBD cannot be made without considering that inflammation itself could be contributing to the lower serum 25OHD concentration observed in patients with more active disease via malabsorption or loss of the vitamin in the inflamed intestine, the study should spearhead systematic prospective and interventional studies of the effect of vitamin D on inflammation. Vitamin D forms that are appropriate for delivery of high doses, and the serum 25OHD concentration threshold which may be protective against IBD development in susceptible hosts or exacerbation in patients with established IBD, remain to be defined.

Vitamin D, IBD and colon cancer: could it be a lifeguard?

Convincing evidence that greater sunlight exposure protects against some types of cancer led to research efforts targeting specifically the link between vitamin D status and colorectal adenocarcinoma. Indeed, a meta-analysis concluded that higher levels of vitamin D metabolites decrease the risk of colorectal cancer in women [10]. It is known that $1,25(OH)_2D$ via its interaction with the VDR, exerts an antimitotic, prodifferentiating effect on colon cancer cells in vitro [11]. Human colon cancer cell lines express both the VDR and the enzymes participating in vitamin D synthesis and catabolism [12]. The vitamin D/VDR system's role in colon cancer has been the focus of intense investigation in the last few years. It is known that in advanced stages of colon cancer, expression of 1-hydroxylase is depressed, reducing the production of the vitamin D active metabolite

[13], while 24-hydroxylase activity is enhanced increasing its degradation [14]. In addition, VDR expression is downregulated during tumor progression [15]. Long-standing ulcerative colitis (UC) increases the risk of colon adenocarcinoma, through a pathway of dysplasia [16]. A recent study reported decreased VDR expression in colon cells of patients with UC in comparison to healthy subjects and further decreased expression of VDR in colon cells of UC patients with dysplasia or adenocarcinoma [17].

Whether VDR expression patterns change over time and could be used as markers for detection of dysplasia or cancer development in patients with UC remains to be examined. In addition, it is unclear whether these changes represent a causative factor or a consequence of long-standing inflammation and cancer development and progression on vitamin D metabolism in these patients. An additional consideration is that patients with depressed colonic VDR expression may not be responsive to vitamin D or vitamin D analogues as sensitivity to these agents may be decreased due to loss of VDR.

Vitamin D receptor polymorphisms: can they predict susceptibility to IBD development and course?

Most of the genomic actions of vitamin D are exerted through the interaction between $1,25(OH)_2D$ and the VDR. The VDR gene maps at a region in chromosome 12, known as IBD-2, which is an IBD candidate gene [18], and the VDR gene exhibits several polymorphisms which could potentially result in altered vitamin D function [19] or metabolism [20]. Given the evidence that vitamin D may play a role in immune system regulation and either the development or the course of IBD, several investigators have examined the potential relationship between VDR polymorphisms and development of IBD. Indeed, European Caucasian, and Israeli Ashkenazi homozygotes for the Taq I allele were found to be more susceptible to developing CD [21] and Iranian homozygotes for the Fok I allele were more susceptible to UC [22].

These findings underline the complexity and heterogeneity of the pathogenesis of IBD. VDR genetics may contribute to the interactions between genetic and environmental factors that lead to the development of IBD. Further study of VDR receptor polymorphisms and their effect on vitamin D functions, especially those related to immune system regulation, may shed light on the pathogenesis of IBD and offer therapeutic alternatives.

Conclusion

Circumstances related to their disease render IBD patients particularly prone to vitamin D deficiency. On the other hand, this hormone may be of particular importance to patients with IBD. The importance extends to several aspects of the disease: (a) compromised bone health, where vitamin D can act as an anabolic agent, (b) immune dysregulation, where vitamin D could enhance and promote innate gut immunity, (c) IBD genetics, where vitamin D receptor polymorphisms may contribute to the pathogenesis of IBD, (d) development of dysplasia, where vitamin D might offer anticancer effects. Many of these effects of vitamin D are still under investigation. Presently, clinicians taking care of patients with IBD should be aware that these patients are at increased risk for deficiency of this hormone, and they should aim for the establishment of serum 25OHD concentration greater than 32 ng/mL through monitoring and adequate supplementation.

References

1. Pappa HM, Bern E, Kamin D, Grand RJ. Vitamin D status in gastrointestinal and liver disease. *Curr Opin Gastroenterol* 2008; **24**(2): 176–183.
2. Joseph AJ, George B, Pulimood AB, Seshadri MS, Chacko A. 25 (OH) vitamin D level in Crohn's disease: association with sun exposure & disease activity. *Indian J Med Res* 2009; **130**(2): 133–137.
3. Leslie WD, Miller N, Rogala L, Bernstein CN. Vitamin D status and bone density in recently diagnosed inflammatory bowel disease: the Manitoba IBD Cohort Study. *Am J Gastroenterol* 2008; **103**(6): 1451–1459.
4. Froicu M, Weaver V, Wynn TA, McDowell MA, Welsh JE, Cantorna MT. A crucial role for the vitamin D receptor in experimental inflammatory bowel diseases. *Mol Endocrinol* 2003; **17**(12): 2386–2392.
5. Stio M, Treves C, Martinesi M, Bonanomi AG. Biochemical effects of KH 1060 and anti-TNF monoclonal antibody on human peripheral blood mononuclear cells. *Int Immunopharmacol* 2005; **5**(4): 649–659.
6. Froicu M, Cantorna MT. Vitamin D and the vitamin D receptor are critical for control of the innate immune response to colonic injury. *BMC Immunol* 2007; **8**: 5.

7. Kong J, Zhang Z, Musch MW, et al. Novel role of the vitamin D receptor in maintaining the integrity of the intestinal mucosal barrier. *Am J Physiol Gastrointest Liver Physiol* 2008; **294**(1): G208–216.

8. Neriche V, Monnet, E, Boutron-Ruault, MC, Alemmand, H, Weill, A, Carbonnel, F. Geographic distribution of inflammatory bowel disease (IBD) in France and sunlight exposure. *Gastroenterology* 2009; **136**(5, Suppl 1): A-21.

9. Bosworth B, Iroku, U, Cohen, M, et al. Serologic vitamin D levels correlate with IBD disease activity. *Gastroenterology* 2009; **136**(5, Suppl 1): A-670.

10. Feskanich D, Ma J, Fuchs CS, et al. Plasma vitamin D metabolites and risk of colorectal cancer in women. *Cancer Epidemiol Biomarkers Prev* 2004; **13**(9): 1502–1508.

11. Cross HS, Huber C, Peterlik M. Antiproliferative effect of 1, 25-dihydroxyvitamin D3 and its analogs on human colon adenocarcinoma cells (CaCo-2): influence of extracellular calcium. *Biochem Biophys Res Commun* 1991; **179**(1): 57–62.

12. Cross HS, Bareis P, Hofer H, et al. 25-Hydroxyvitamin D(3)-1alpha-hydroxylase and vitamin D receptor gene expression in human colonic mucosa is elevated during early cancerogenesis. *Steroids* 2001; **66**(3–5): 287–292.

13. Bises G, Kallay E, Weiland T, et al. 25-hydroxyvitamin D3-1alpha-hydroxylase expression in normal and malignant human colon. *J Histochem Cytochem* 2004; **52**(7): 985–989.

14. Matusiak D, Benya RV. CYP27A1 and CYP24 expression as a function of malignant transformation in the colon. *J Histochem Cytochem* 2007; **55**(12): 1257–1264.

15. Matusiak D, Murillo G, Carroll RE, Mehta RG, Benya RV. Expression of vitamin D receptor and 25-hydroxyvitamin D3-1{alpha}-hydroxylase in normal and malignant human colon. *Cancer Epidemiol Biomarkers Prev* 2005; **14**(10): 2370–2376.

16. Eaden JA, Abrams KR, Mayberry JF. The risk of colorectal cancer in ulcerative colitis: a meta-analysis. *Gut* 2001; **48**(4): 526–535.

17. Wada K, Tanaka H, Maeda K, et al. Vitamin D receptor expression is associated with colon cancer in ulcerative colitis. *Oncol Rep* 2009; **22**(5): 1021–1025.

18. Curran ME, Lau KF, Hampe J, et al. Genetic analysis of inflammatory bowel disease in a large European cohort supports linkage to chromosomes 12 and 16. *Gastroenterology* 1998; **115**(5): 1066–1071.

19. Whitfield GK, Remus LS, Jurutka PW, et al. Functionally relevant polymorphisms in the human nuclear vitamin D receptor gene. *Mol Cell Endocrinol* 2001; **177**(1–2): 145–159.

20. Smolders J, Damoiseaux J, Menheere P, Tervaert JW, Hupperts R. Fok-I vitamin D receptor gene polymorphism (rs10735810) and vitamin D metabolism in multiple sclerosis. *J Neuroimmunol* 2009; **207**(1–2): 117–121.

21. Simmons JD, Mullighan C, Welsh KI, Jewell DP. Vitamin D receptor gene polymorphism: association with Crohn's disease susceptibility. *Gut* 2000; **47**(2): 211–214.

22. Naderi N, Farnood A, Habibi M, et al. Association of vitamin D receptor gene polymorphisms in Iranian patients with inflammatory bowel disease. *J Gastroenterol Hepatol* 2008; **23**(12): 1816–1822.

Got milk? Medication use and nursing in women with IBD

Sunanda Kane

Mayo Clinic College of Medicine, Rochester, MN, USA

LEARNING POINTS

- Women with Crohn's disease in the United States are less likely to breastfeed than those with ulcerative colitis or the general population.

- Mesalamine and steroids are safe in nursing mothers.

- Thiopurines appear safe for nursing; warnings appear outdated.

- Adalimumab has been found at very low concentrations in breast milk; infliximab and certolizumab have not been found in breast milk.

Introduction

The advantages and benefits of breastfeeding for the neonate are well established, but its effect on the course of IBD is uncertain. Some work has suggested that breastfeeding is protective [1,2], but this association has not been well characterized. Unfortunately, most recommendations regarding breastfeeding are made by obstetricians, pediatricians, or lactation consultants and treating gastroenterologists usually have no role in this decision.

Effect of nursing on course of IBD

Work in rheumatoid arthritis (RA) suggests an adverse effect of nursing on disease activity in the mother [3,4]. In two human observational studies, women with RA had an apparent increased risk for disease activity with breastfeeding [5,6]. In the study by Barrett et al. [5], disease activity in nonbreastfeeders was compared with first-time and repeat breastfeeders. First-time breastfeeders had increased disease activity 6 months postpartum, based on subjective and objective criteria, after adjusting for medication use. Of the women with severe RA, 46% had breastfed for more than 6 months prior to disease onset, compared with just 26% of those with mild disease. Breastfeeding more than three children increased the risk of poor disease prognosis by nearly 4-fold (odds ratio (OR) 3.7, 95% confidence interval (CI) 1.04–13.22).

In one review [6], breastfeeding was associated with an increased risk of developing RA, particularly after the first pregnancy. The authors discussed the available data for the risk of disease relapse, in which breastfeeding was one possible factor, medications and nutritional interventions were also reviewed. These findings were also postulated for women with both RA and multiple sclerosis.

In a study of women with IBD, the association between breastfeeding and postpartum disease activity was assessed [7]. Of the 122 women surveyed, over half did not breastfeed their infants. Interestingly, the majority were women with Crohn's disease (CD) rather than ulcerative colitis (UC). The national rate for breastfeeding in the United States is approximately 60%, with active initiations by the US government to increase this number [8]. The proportion of women with UC who breastfed was higher than the national average, while the proportion of CD patients was significantly lower (29%). The reason cited by most women for not breastfeeding was fear of medication interactions, but it is unclear if this is the entire explanation for such a low percentage of breastfeeders among the CD patients. The medications most often discontinued were mesalamine and the antimetabolites, 6-MP, and azathioprine. No patients were

---

Clinical Dilemmas in Inflammatory Bowel Disease: New Challenges, Second Edition. Edited by P. Irving, C. Siegel, D. Rampton and F. Shanahan.
© 2011 Blackwell Publishing Ltd. Published 2011 by Blackwell Publishing Ltd.

TABLE 46.1 Safety of IBD medications during breastfeeding

Low risk to use when indicated	Limited data but appear low risk	Contraindicated
Oral mesalamine	Olsalazine	Methotrexate
Topical mesalamine	Azathioprine	Thalidomide
Sulfasalazine	6-mercaptopurine	Cyclosporine
Corticosteroids	Infliximab	Ciprofloxacin
(<20 mg)		
Loperamide		Metronidazole

taking infliximab in this series. Most women discussed the decision to stop IBD-related medications with their obstetrician and/or pediatrician, but not their gastroenterologist. Of the 54 women who breastfed, 23 (43%) experienced a postpartum disease flare. The unadjusted OR for disease activity with a history of breastfeeding was 2.2 (95% CI 1.2–3.9; $p = 0.004$). When stratified by disease type, the OR for UC was 0.89 (95% CI 0.29–2.7; $p > 0.05$) and 3.8 for CD (95% CI 1.9–7.4; $p < 0.05$). When adjusted for medication cessation, the OR became nonsignificant.

Medication safety during breastfeeding

Table 46.1 summarizes safety data regarding medications and their use during breastfeeding.

Mesalamine

Diarrhea in a nursing infant, apparently as a result of the rectal administration of mesalamine, has been reported [9]. The mother had ulcerative proctitis and, 6 weeks after childbirth, treatment was initiated for disease activity with 500 mg suppositories twice daily. Her infant developed watery diarrhea 1 hour after the first dose. Four additional challenges of breastfeeding, following suppository administration, produced the same results. Plasma and milk concentrations of mesalamine were not obtained at that time. On the basis of this single report, the American Academy of Pediatrics classified mesalamine as a drug that has produced adverse effects in a nursing infant and should be used with caution during breastfeeding.

However, in a subsequent study, low concentrations of mesalamine and its metabolites were found in the breast milk of a woman taking 1 g orally, three times a day [10]. Maternal serum levels determined at 7 and 11 days' postpartum were 0.6 and 1.1 mcg/mL, representing milk–plasma ratios for mesalamine of 0.17 and 0.09, respectively. The

corresponding ratios for the mesalamine and metabolites were 16.5 and 6.8, respectively. The estimated daily intake of mesalamine and metabolites by the infant was 0.065 mg (0.015 mg/kg) and 10 mg (2.3 mg/kg), respectively, considered to be negligible amounts. On the basis of these data I recommend continuation of mesalamine during nursing, as the benefit of continued therapy and disease remission outweighs the small risk of infant drug exposure.

Corticosteroids

Prednisone is found in trace amounts in breast milk at doses as low as 5 mg/day. At doses higher than 40 mg/day, waiting at least for 4 hours after a dose before nursing is recommended.

Thiopurines

Currently, there are few data available regarding antimetabolite milk:plasma ratios. A case report documents negligible amounts of 6-MP in a single sample from a woman taking 6-MP after renal transplantation, who was tested using high performance liquid chromatography [11]. Two other case series also failed to find significant metabolite levels in milk samples [12,13]. Recently a study by Christensen et al. demonstrated negligible amounts in serial milk samples [14]. On the basis of their data, the recommendation is to have women take their medication at night then "pump and dump" their first milk of the morning, which has a higher concentration of metabolites than throughout the day.

Infliximab

A case report of maternal use of infliximab failed to demonstrate any antibody in breast milk [15]. A second case series corroborated this finding: in 4 mothers nursing while receiving infliximab, no antibody was detected in the milk samples [16]. Based on these findings, and the knowledge that as an antibody infliximab would be susceptible to infant gastric acid if ingested, I recommend continued infliximab use during nursing. Adalimumab has been detected in breast milk at levels of less than 1% of those found in the serum [17]. A small study with mothers receiving certolizumab pegol does not demonstrate any significant amounts of this agent in breast milk [18].

Other drugs

Other medications that are known to be safe for breastfeeding include loperamide and steroids at doses of ≤20 mg.

Mothers planning on nursing should discontinue the use of metronidazole, ciprofloxacin, and methotrexate.

Other commonly used medications that are safe for use during pregnancy include acetaminophen (paracetamol) and metoclopramide. Of the antidepressants, amitriptyline and sertraline are known to be safe, while doxepin, citalopram, and fluoxetine are not, as the levels of these drugs found in the breast milk are high.

Herbal supplements

Some commonly used herbal supplements can also affect maternal health. For instance, fenugreek (*Trigonella foenum-graecum*), a herb that is readily available in nutritional and herbal stores, has been used for centuries to potentiate milk production. However, one potential side effect is an increased risk of bleeding, and there are anecdotes of women who experienced significant rectal bleeding attributed to the use of this herb. Women with IBD should be careful when using this supplement. Another preparation to be used with caution is St. John's wort, where there is no definitive data regarding breastfeeding. Chamomile and ginger, used for general gastrointestinal symptoms, are considered safe in breastfeeding.

Problems and unresolved issues

The decision to breastfeed involves several factors including maternal health and current medications. Gastroenterologists are not historically consulted when nursing issues arise. Large studies with breast milk are lacking and recommendations are based on small numbers of patients, which can make some new mothers nervous. Further, work in milk analysis will help all healthcare professionals make educated recommendations.

References

1. Bergstrand O, Hellers G. Breastfeeding during infancy in patients who later develop Crohn's disease. *Scand J Gastroenterol* 1983; **18**: 903–906.
2. Whorwell PJ, Holdstak G, Whorwell GM, et al. Bottle feeding, early gastroenteritis, and inflammatory bowel disease. *BMJ* 1979; **1**: 382–384.
3. Jorgensen C, Picot MC, Bologna C, et al. Oral contraception, parity, breastfeeding and severity of rheumatoid arthritis. *Ann Rheum Dis* 1996; **55**: 94–98.
4. Chikanza IC, Petrou P, Chrousos G, et al. Excessive and dysregulated secretion of prolactin in rheumatoid arthritis: immunopathogenic and therapeutic implications. *Br J Rheumatol* 1993; **32**: 445–448.
5. Barrett JH, Brennan P, Fiddler M, et al. Breastfeeding and postpartum relapse in women with rheumatoid and inflammatory arthritis. *Arhtritis Rheum* 2000; **43**: 1010–1015.
6. Hampl JS, Papa DJ. Breastfeeding related onset, flare and relapse of rheumatoid arthritis. *Nutr Rev* 2001; **59**: 264–268.
7. Kane SV, Lemieux N. The role of breastfeeding and disease activity in inflammatory bowel disease. *Am J Gastroenterol* 2005; **100**(1): 102–105.
8. Ryan AS. The resurgence of breastfeeding in the United States. *Pediatrics* 1997; **99**: E12.
9. Neils GF. Diarrhoea due to 5-aminosalicylic acid in breast milk. *Lancet* 1989; **1**: 383.
10. Klotz U, Harings-Kaim A. Negligible excretion of 5-aminosalicylic acid in breast milk. *Lancet* 1993; **342**: 618–619.
11. Fagerholm MI, Coulam CB, Moyer TP. Breastfeeding after renal transplantation: 6-mercaptopurine content in human breast milk. *Surg Forum* 1980; **10**: 447–449.
12. Gardiner SJ, Gearry RB, Roberts RL, et al. Exposure to thiopurine drugs through breast milk is low based on metabolite concentrations in mother-infant pairs. *Br J Clin Pharmacol* 2006 Oct; **62**(4): 453–456.
13. Moretti ME, Verjee Z, Ito S, Koren G. Breast-feeding during maternal use of azathioprine. *Ann Pharmacother* 2006; **40**(12): 2269–2272.
14. Christensen LA, Dahlerup JF, Nielsen MJ, Fallingborg JF, Schmiegelow K. Azathioprine treatment during lactation. *Aliment Pharmacol Ther* 2008; **28**(10): 1209–1213.
15. Vasiliauskas EA, Church JA, Silverman N, et al. Case report: evidence for transplacental transfer of maternally administered infliximab to the newborn. *Clin Gastroenterol Hepatol* 2006; **4**(10): 1255–1258.
16. Kane S, Ford J, Cohen R, Wagner C. Absence of infliximab in infants and breast milk from nursing mothers receiving therapy for Crohn's disease before and after delivery. *J Clin Gastroenterol* 2009; **43**(7): 613–616.
17. Ben-Horin S, Yavzori MI, Katz LI, et al. Adalimumab level in breast milk of a nursing mother. *Clin Gastroenterol Hepatol* 2010; **8**(5): 475–476.
18. Mahadevan U and Abreu M. Certolizumab use in pregnancy: low levels detected in cord blood. *Gastroenterol* 2009; **134**(Suppl 1): A960.

47 Does stress matter?

Robert G. Maunder

Mount Sinai Hospital and University of Toronto, Toronto, ON, Canada

LEARNING POINTS

- There are plausible mechanisms by which stress can trigger relapse in IBD.
- Stress may trigger relapse in ulcerative colitis; on the other hand, depressive symptoms may increase inflammation in Crohn's disease.
- Stress and depressive symptoms contribute to disease course in some people with IBD but not in all.
- Depression and anxiety increase the burden and cost of IBD.
- Psychological factors influence the severity of symptoms reported by patients.
- Treatments of mood disorders and stress management may improve quality of life in patients with IBD.

Introduction

Psychological stress is the result of experiences that threaten to overwhelm an individual's capacity to respond effectively. Stress is a ubiquitous aspect of life, and there is much evidence that stress in its many forms (e.g., major life events, daily hassles, personal perceptions of feeling stressed) contributes to the occurrence, severity, and burden of many diseases. The idea that stress contributes to Crohn's disease (CD) and ulcerative colitis (UC) has a long history, but has only relatively recently acquired a substantial basis in evidence. The conclusions that can be drawn from well-designed studies suggest a somewhat more complex situation than a simple answer of "yes" or "no" to the question posed in the title of this chapter. This chapter reviews some

clinically useful highlights of that literature and broadens its scope to other psychological factors, such as depression and anxiety when they are relevant.

Plausible mechanisms by which stress can increase gut inflammation

Animal models have confirmed that stress can precipitate colitis in predisposed individuals [1]. Furthermore, both animal and human studies have identified plausible mechanisms by which psychological stress could be translated into gut inflammation. The potential range of mechanisms is wide, since there is evidence that responses to psychological stress influence the regulation of many molecules that may have a role in the pathophysiology of IBD. These molecules include tumor necrosis factor α, glucocorticoids, the glucocorticoid receptor, substance P, vasoactive intestinal peptide, oxidant molecules, and heat shock proteins [2]. Because mucosal barrier function is hypothesized to play a role in the pathophysiology of IBD, it is of particular interest that stress increases intestinal permeability, even in healthy animals [3].

The role of stress and other psychological factors is probably different in Crohn's disease than in ulcerative colitis

Stress does not cause IBD in healthy persons. However, among people who have IBD, stress *may* trigger recurrence of active disease after a period of remission, at least for some people. The epidemiological evidence suggests that psychological stress can trigger relapse in UC, whereas depressive symptoms seem to be a more potent trigger of relapse in CD [4].

Clinical Dilemmas in Inflammatory Bowel Disease: New Challenges, Second Edition. Edited by P. Irving, C. Siegel, D. Rampton and F. Shanahan.
© 2011 Blackwell Publishing Ltd. Published 2011 by Blackwell Publishing Ltd.

In UC, increased risk of relapse from remission has been associated with both the occurrence of major life events (hazards ratio 1.26/life event, 95% confidence interval (CI) 1.04–1.53) [5] and the subjective perception of feeling chronically stressed (hazards ratio 2.8 over 45 months, 95% CI 1.1–7.2)[6].

The link between depressive symptoms and CD is complicated and circular because it is likely that having CD *causes* symptoms of depression for some people, and it is also true that in time-lag studies the presence of depressive symptoms predicts worsening of CD [7]. Furthermore, the presence of major depression predicts lower likelihood of achieving remission with infliximab [8]. There is emerging evidence that psychological treatments can improve not only psychological well-being but also disease course in IBD[9].

Stress matters for some people with IBD but not for all

Although the evidence that there is a genuine link between stress, depression, and the course of IBD is persuasive, the small effect sizes and the inconsistency in this literature suggest that psychological factors are more relevant to some people with IBD than to others. How does a clinician determine if stress is a relevant contributor to disease for a particular patient? There is less evidence to guide responses to this question. One common sense approach is to take a full history and be aware that a past history of major depression or of an anxiety disorder may increase the likelihood that stress and other psychological factors will contribute to the burden of an individual's disease. In addition, particular patients may have a strong intuition that their course of disease has been either quite sensitive to life stresses or that stress has had no role at all. Since the scientific literature at present supports both of those possibilities, it makes sense to respect the patient's self-knowledge until proven otherwise. Recent studies suggest that there are both biological and psychological determinants of individual differences in vulnerability to stress and depression in IBD [10,11]. While psychological responses to stress occur along a continuous spectrum that depends on the magnitude of the stressor, the effectiveness of coping, and other variables, these studies suggest that the link between stress and the biology of IBD may reside in biological and psychological traits that are present in some IBD patients and not in others. While the evidence on this distinction is in its infancy, there is

hope that in the future we may be better able to determine objectively which patients are more susceptible to stress.

Stress and other psychological factors have a substantial impact on the management of IBD, whether or not they influence its course

Perhaps the most important links between psychological factors and IBD have nothing to do with the risk of relapse. In IBD, as in virtually every other chronic illness, depression, anxiety, and chronic stress can add dramatically to the burden of disease, increasing symptoms and medical costs and reducing quality of life. Since IBD increases the risk of major depression [12] and anxiety disorders [13], a vicious cycle often develops in which illness increases anxiety, stress, or depressive symptoms, which, in turn, increase the burden of disease. As a result, gastroenterologists and other clinicians treating patients with IBD should be attuned to emerging psychological symptoms in order to initiate assessment and treatment of comorbid psychiatric illnesses if they occur. When it comes to identifying major depression, the depressive symptoms that do not overlap with the systemic effects of IBD are the best clue: withdrawal from relationships, lack of pleasure in usually enjoyable activities, attitudes of helplessness, hopelessness or worthlessness, suicidal thoughts, and impairment of social and occupational activities that seems out of proportion to physical impairment.

Another way in which psychological factors influence the management of IBD is that they influence how patients experience and report symptoms. Since much of a clinician's ability to monitor the course of disease depends on the symptoms that patients report, individual differences in reporting style are important. Comparing self-reported symptoms of UC to endoscopic findings, a group at our hospital found that patients who experience strong health anxiety and no visible signs of inflammation at endoscopy had self-reported symptom scores that were elevated to the same level as patients with a more typical reporting style and obviously inflamed mucosa. On the other hand, patients with a repressive (minimizing) style of expressing themselves had very low symptom scores, whether they had visible mucosal inflammation or not [14]. It is no surprise to experienced clinicians that patients differ in how dramatically they report symptoms; however, these findings emphasize the importance of continuity of care. A gastroenterologist who knows his or her patients well is better equipped to recognize whether today's symptoms indicate the emergence of a new disease activity or not than a clinician working in a clinic where patients see a different doctor each time.

Once mood or anxiety disorders are identified effective treatments are available, including both pharmacological options and psychotherapy. Implementing psychiatric treatment is beyond the scope of practice of most gastroenterologists, but a well-timed referral to a psychiatrist or communication to a family doctor is valuable. Open communication with the physician treating the mood or anxiety disorder is often important because the course of IBD and its treatments (such as corticosteroids) may have a substantial influence on the course of depression or anxiety, and vice versa. Furthermore, the selection of psychiatric medications depends in part on their gastrointestinal side effects (such as the risk of cholinergic drugs in patients who are prone to bowel obstruction, or the risk of GI bleeding associated with selective serotonin reuptake inhibitors).

Beyond the treatment of psychiatric illness, there is a wide array of interventions to reduce the impact of life stress, ranging from learning relaxation and coping skills to developing a practice of mindfulness meditation [15]. These interventions may provide welcome psychological benefits, but there is little evidence so far that they reliably alter the course of IBD.

Conclusion

And so the answer to the question, "Does stress matter?" is "Yes, definitely, but not for everyone with UC and CD and not in the same way for everyone." Nonetheless, careful attention to the role of stress and other psychological factors in the lives of patients with UC and CD may provide substantial benefits both for the quality of patients' lives and in some cases for maintenance of remission and reducing inflammation.

References

1. Collins SM. Stress and the Gastrointestinal Tract IV. Modulation of intestinal inflammation by stress: basic mechanisms and clinical relevance. *Am J Physiol Gastrointest Liver Physiol* 2001; **280**(3): G315–G318.
2. Maunder R. Mediators of stress effects in inflammatory bowel disease: Not the usual suspects. *J Psychosom Res* 2000; **48**: 569–577.
3. Meddings JB, Swain MG. Environmental stress-induced gastrointestinal permeability is mediated by endogenous glucocorticoids in the rat. *Gastroenterology* 2000; **119**(4): 1019–1028.
4. Maunder RG, Levenstein S. The role of stress in the development and clinical course of inflammatory bowel disease: epidemiological evidence. *Curr Mol Med* 2008; **8**(4): 247–252.
5. Bitton A, Sewitch MJ, Peppercorn MA, deB Edwardes MD, Shah S, Ransil B et al. Psychosocial determinants of relapse in ulcerative colitis: a longitudinal study. *Am J Gastroenterol* 2003; **98**(10): 2203–2208.
6. Levenstein S, Prantera C, Varvo V, Scribano M, Andreoli A, Luzi C et al. Stress and exacerbation in ulcerative colitis: A prospective study of patients enrolled in remission. *Am J Gastroenterol* 2000; **95**: 1213–1220.
7. Mardini HE, Kip KE, Wilson JW. Crohn's disease: a two-year prospective study of the association between psychological distress and disease activity. *Dig Dis Sci* 2004; **49**(3): 492–497.
8. Persoons P, Vermeire S, Demyttenaere K, Fischler B, Vandenberghe J, Van Oudenhove L et al. The impact of major depressive disorder on the short- and long-term outcome of Crohn's disease treatment with infliximab. *Aliment Pharmacol Ther* 2005; **22**(2): 101–110.
9. Wahed M, Corser M, Goodhand JR, Rampton DS. Does psychological counseling alter the natural history of inflammatory bowel disease? *Inflamm Bowel Dis* 2009; **16**(4): 664–669.
10. Maunder RG, Greenberg GR, Hunter JJ, Lancee WJ, Steinhart AH, Silverberg MS. (2006) Psychobiological subtypes of ulcerative colitis: pANCA status moderates the relationship between disease activity and psychological distress. *Am J Gastroenterol* 2006; **101**(11): 2546–2551.
11. Maunder RG, Lancee WJ, Hunter JJ, Greenberg GR, Steinhart AH. Attachment insecurity moderates the relationship between disease activity and depressive symptoms in ulcerative colitis. *Inflamm Bowel Dis* 2005; **11**(10): 919–926.
12. Fuller-Thomson E, Sulman J. Depression and inflammatory bowel disease: findings from two nationally representative Canadian surveys. *Inflamm Bowel Dis* 2006; **12**(8): 697–707.
13. Maunder RG. Panic disorder associated with gastrointestinal disease: review and hypotheses. *J Psychosom Res* 1997; **44**(1): 91–105.
14. Maunder RG, Greenberg GR. Comparison of a disease activity index and patients' self-reported symptom severity in ulcerative colitis. *Inflamm Bowel Dis* 2004; **10**(5): 632–636.
15. Lehrer PM, Woolkfold RL, Sime WE, eds. *Principles and Practice of Stress Management*, 3rd Ed. New York: Guilford Press; 2007.

IBS is common in IBD: fact or fallacy?

James Goodhand and David S. Rampton

Centre for Digestive Diseases, Barts and The London School of Medicine and Dentistry, London, UK

LEARNING POINTS

- Symptoms resembling those of irritable bowel syndrome (IBS) are common in IBD, particularly Crohn's disease.

- Careful investigation shows that in many patients with IBD, IBS symptoms indicate occult inflammation or noninflammatory complications of IBD such as fibrotic strictures, bacterial overgrowth, or bile salt malabsorption.

- Failure to recognize the frequency with which IBS symptoms occur in patients with IBD may lead to a failure to offer appropriate anti-inflammatory treatment or other interventions in patients with established IBD.

- Conversely, underdiagnosis of true IBS can result in inappropriate escalation of their therapy to potentially toxic and expensive drugs.

Introduction

The seriousness of its therapeutic implications makes this question an important one to answer. Thus, overdiagnosis of irritable bowel syndrome (IBS) risks underutilization of effective anti-inflammatory or other specific interventions in patients with IBD. Conversely, underdiagnosing IBS in IBD patients can lead to inappropriate prescription of potentially toxic as well as expensive therapies, a problem that has been encountered in clinical trials of anti-TNF and other biological therapies [1].

The first step in assessing the incidence or prevalence of IBS in patients with IBD is to establish a clear definition of IBS.

What is IBS?

IBS is defined by its symptoms, which, according to the Rome III criteria comprise abdominal pain relieved by defecation, and/or associated with a change in the form or frequency of stool, for at least 3 days a month for at least 3 months in the absence of alarming symptoms [2]. The prevalence of IBS in the general population is 10–20%, with a clear female predominance [3]. The overlap of some of the symptoms of IBS with a number of other gastrointestinal symptom complexes, including chronic constipation, functional dyspepsia, and functional diarrhea, suggests that it is not a discrete entity; indeed, personality type, coping mechanisms, and illness behavior may influence not only the prevalence but also the heterogeneity of IBS, as they may in other disorders that rely on symptom clusters to establish a diagnosis [4,5]. Other potential pathogenic factors in IBS include not only diet [6] but also infection [7,8], although it is not yet clear how these factors lead to abnormal gastrointestinal motility, visceral hypersensitivity, and other features of IBS. In recent years, it has become apparent, too, that many patients with IBS, particularly of the postinfectious type, show an increase in mucosal permeability [9], infiltration of the lamina propria with activated immune (particularly mast) cells [10], and in at least study a one limited response to 5-aminosalicylates [11]. Indeed, it has been proposed that IBS may lie at the benign end of a spectrum of IBD that, at its most severe, includes Crohn's disease (CD) and ulcerative colitis (UC) [12]. The association of IBS with both psychological disturbance and subtle mucosal inflammation is a potential source of confusion when efforts are made to determine whether symptoms

Clinical Dilemmas in Inflammatory Bowel Disease: New Challenges, Second Edition. Edited by P. Irving, C. Siegel, D. Rampton and F. Shanahan.
© 2011 Blackwell Publishing Ltd. Published 2011 by Blackwell Publishing Ltd.

in patients with IBD are due to IBS, since both disorders are frequently accompanied by mood disorders as well as inflammation [13,14].

What is the prevalence of IBS in IBD?

IBS and IBD are not mutually exclusive and can coexist by chance (IBS–IBD). Studying the overlap between IBS and IBD is difficult because symptoms of active IBD, especially those of CD, can resemble those of IBS. There have been eight cross-sectional studies reporting the prevalence of IBS in IBD [15–22]. In most of these reports, functional symptoms appear to be more common in IBD than in the general population, reportedly affecting 11–57% patients with apparently inactive CD, and 9–33% patients with inactive UC, the results obtained depending in part on the definition of IBS used (see Table 48.1).

Definition of IBD activity

A criticism of all but three of these studies [15,21,22] is that disease activity was not accurately defined by endoscopy or other objective criteria, instead reliance being placed on disease activity-defining symptom scores that may overlap with those of functional syndromes and may be influenced by mood and personality. The two studies that have used fecal biomarkers to define disease activity have shown that Crohn's patients with apparently inactive disease who report IBS symptoms frequently have raised calprotectin levels [21,22]. When these patients were excluded, the prevalence of true IBS in our study was 11% [21], similar to that of the general population [3].

IBS symptoms in relation to noninflammatory complications of IBD

IBS symptoms in patients with IBD may not only be due to inflammation, but also due to noninflammatory

TABLE 48.1 Cross-sectional studies reporting the prevalence of irritable bowel syndrome (IBS) in inflammatory bowel disease

Study [reference]	Patient sample	Inclusion criteria	Disease activity	IBS criteria	Prevalence of IBS symptoms
Isgar et al. 1983 [15]	98 UC 98 HC	Remission (equivalent Baron score ≤1)	Endoscopy	Manning	33% UC 7% HC
Simren et al. 2002 [16]	43 UC 40 CD	Remission (no relapse in prior year)	Retrospective case Note review	GISRS	33% UC 57% CD
Minderhoud et al. 2004 [17]	73 UC 34 CD 66 HC	Remission (CAI <10 (UC) or CDAI <150 (CD) and steroid free for 3 months)	CAI (UC) CDAI (CD)	Rome II	32% UC 42% CD 8% HC
Barrett et al. 2005 [18]	88 UC 76 CD	All-comers	MCDAI, HBI BRFUCI	Manning	38% UC 43% CD
Farrokhyer et al. 2006 [19]	44 UC 105 CD	Remission (no change in medications in last year)	DAI	Rome II	9% UC 26% CD
Keohane et al. 2010 [22]	44 UC 62 CD	Remission UCDAI < or equal to 3 (UC), CDAI<150 and CRP <10 (CD)	UCDAI, CDAI FCP and CRP	Rome II	39% UC 60% CD
Mikocka-Walus et al. 2008 [20]	61 IBD (30UC: 31CD)	All-comers	CDAI (CD) SCCAI (UC)	Rome III	31% IBD
Goodhand et al. 2009 [21]	80 CD	Remission (CDAI < 150)	CDAI FCP and CRP	Rome III	11% CD

UC, ulcerative colitis; CD, Crohn's disease; HC, Healthy control; IBD, inflammatory bowel disease; CAI, colitis activity index; CDAI, Crohn's disease activity index; MCDAI, modified Crohn's disease activity index; HBI, Harvey Bradshaw Index; BRFUCI, Birmingham/Royal Free ulcerative colitis index; DAI, disease activity index; UCDAI, ulcerative colitis disease activity index; SCCAI, simple clinical colitis activity index; GISRS, gastrointestinal symptom rating scale.

complications of IBD, in particular in CD. For example, noninflammatory strictures in CD can produce pain or diarrhea because of small bowel bacterial overgrowth, the symptoms of which could be mistaken for IBS. Diarrhea because of bile salt malabsorption is another common complication of CD, in the presence or absence of ileal resection, which can lead to an errant diagnosis of IBS.

IBS is common in IBD: fact or fallacy?

Indeed, it is true that IBS symptoms are common in IBD, but data from recent studies suggest that to interpret them as indicating the frequent coexistence of true IBS with IBD is a fallacy. Thus, while many IBD patients have IBS symptoms, they can usually be accounted for by occult inflammation or by noninflammatory complications of the disease. Accordingly, IBD patients with IBS symptoms should be carefully investigated to look for active disease or noninflammatory complications, specific treatment of which may improve quality of life and disease course. Conversely, patients in whom investigation shows them to have true IBS, in association with their IBD, require an entirely different therapeutic approach. Indeed, care should be taken to avoid escalation of such patients' treatment to potentially toxic and expensive anti-inflammatory or immunomodulatory drugs.

To end at the beginning, it is to be hoped that wider recognition of the frequency with which patients with IBD have symptoms consistent with, but not due to IBS, will shorten the lengthy delay faced by many in getting their real diagnosis made [23].

References

1. Sands BE, Abreu MT, Ferry GD, Griffiths AM, Hanauer SB, Isaacs KL, et al. Design issues and outcomes in IBD clinical trials. *Inflamm Bowel Dis* 2005 Nov; **11**(Suppl 1): S22–S28.

2. Longstreth GF, Thompson WG, Chey WD, Houghton LA, Mearin F, Spiller RC. Functional bowel disorders. *Gastroenterology* 2006; **130**(5): 1480–1491.

3. Spiegel BM. The burden of IBS: looking at metrics. *Curr Gastroenterol Rep* 2009; **11**(4): 265–269.

4. Paine P, Kishor J, Worthen SF, Gregory LJ, Aziz Q. Exploring relationships for visceral and somatic pain with autonomic control and personality. *Pain* 2009; **144**(3): 236–244.

5. Taylor SE, Stanton AL. Coping resources, coping processes, and mental health. *Annu Rev Clin Psychol* 2007; **3**: 377–401.

6. Morcos A, Dinan T, Quigley EM. Irritable bowel syndrome: role of food in pathogenesis and management. *Journal of Digestive Diseases* 2009; **10**(4): 237–246.

7. Marshall JK, Thabane M, Garg AX, Clark WF, Salvadori M, Collins SM. Incidence and epidemiology of irritable bowel syndrome after a large waterborne outbreak of bacterial dysentery. *Gastroenterology* 2006; **131**(2): 445–450.

8. Neal KR, Hebden J, Spiller R. Prevalence of gastrointestinal symptoms six months after bacterial gastroenteritis and risk factors for development of the irritable bowel syndrome: postal survey of patients. *BMJ* 1997; **314**(7083): 779–782.

9. Piche T, Barbara G, Aubert P, et al. Impaired intestinal barrier integrity in the colon of patients with irritable bowel syndrome: involvement of soluble mediators. *Gut* 2009; **58**(2): 196–201.

10. Cremon C, Gargano L, Morselli-Labate AM, et al. Mucosal immune activation in irritable bowel syndrome: gender-dependence and association with digestive symptoms. *Am J Gastroenterol* 2009; **104**(2): 392–400.

11. Corinaldesi R, Stanghellini V, Cremon C, et al. Effect of mesalazine on mucosal immune biomarkers in irritable bowel syndrome: a randomized controlled proof-of-concept study. *Aliment Pharmacol Ther* 2009; **30**(3): 245–252.

12. Grover M, Herfarth H, Drossman DA. The functional-organic dichotomy: postinfectious irritable bowel syndrome and inflammatory bowel disease-irritable bowel syndrome. *Clin Gastroenterol Hepatol* 2009; **7**(1): 48–53.

13. Graff LA, Walker JR, Bernstein CN. Depression and anxiety in inflammatory bowel disease: A review of comorbidity and management. *Inflamm Bowel Dis* 2009; **15**(7): 1105–1118.

14. Whitehead WE, Palsson OS, Levy RR, Feld AD, Turner M, Von Korff M. Comorbidity in irritable bowel syndrome. *Am J Gastroenterol* 2007; **102**(12): 2767–2776.

15. Isgar B, Harman M, Kaye MD, Whorwell PJ. Symptoms of irritable bowel syndrome in ulcerative colitis in remission. *Gut* 1983; **24**(3): 190–192.

16. Simren M, Axelsson J, Gillberg R, Abrahamsson H, Svedlund J, Bjornsson ES. Quality of life in inflammatory bowel disease in remission: the impact of IBS-like symptoms and associated psychological factors. *Am J Gastroenterol* 2002; **97**(2): 389–396.

17. Minderhoud IM, Oldenburg B, Wismeijer JA, van Berge Henegouwen GP, Smout AJ. IBS-like symptoms in patients with inflammatory bowel disease in remission; relationships with quality of life and coping behavior. *Dig Dis Sci* 2004; **49**(3): 469–474.

18. Barratt HS, Kalantzis C, Polymeros D, Forbes A. Functional symptoms in inflammatory bowel disease and their potential influence in misclassification of clinical status. *Aliment Pharmacol Ther* 2005; **21**(2): 141–147.

19. Farrokhyar F, Marshall JK, Easterbrook B, Irvine EJ. Functional gastrointestinal disorders and mood disorders in patients with inactive inflammatory bowel disease: preva-

lence and impact on health. *Inflamm Bowel Dis* 2006; **12**(1): 38–46.

20. Mikocka-Walus AA, Turnbull DA, Andrews JM, Moulding NT, Holtmann GJ. The effect of functional gastrointestinal disorders on psychological comorbidity and quality of life in patients with inflammatory bowel disease. *Aliment Pharmacol Ther* 2008; **28**(4): 475–483.

21. Goodhand JR, Wahed M, Lindsay JO, Rampton DS. True IBS is uncommon in Crohn's disease: IBS symptoms imply active disease. *Gut* 2009; **58**(suppl II): A320.

22. Keohane J, O'Mahony C, O'Mahony L, O'Mahony S, Quigley EM, Shanahan F. Irritable bowel syndrome-type symptoms in patients with inflammatory bowel disease: a real association or a reflection of occult inflammation? *Am J Gastroenterol* 2010; **105**(8):1789–1794.

23. Burgmann T, Clara I, Graff L, et al. The Manitoba Inflammatory Bowel Disease Cohort Study: prolonged symptoms before diagnosis–how much is irritable bowel syndrome? *Clin Gastroenterol Hepatol* 2006; **4**(5): 614–620.

49 So where is all the cancer?

Judith E. Baars[1,2] and C. Janneke van der Woude[2]

[1]Erasmus University, Rotterdam, The Netherlands
[2]Department of Gastroenterology and Hepatology, Erasmus MC Hospital, Rotterdam, The Netherlands

LEARNING POINTS

- IBD patients are at increased risk for developing colorectal cancer (CRC).

- IBD-related CRC accounts for 10–15% of all deaths in IBD patients.

- Recent population-based studies demonstrated a lower risk of CRC than was initially reported, suggesting a range from 1/500 to 1/1600 patients annually.

- Risk factors for CRC include extensive disease and long duration of IBD, severity of inflammation, concomitant PSC, pseudopolyps, and a family history of CRC.

- Identification of patients at special risk is needed, if we are to improve the prevention and management of IBD-related CRC.

Colorectal cancer in IBD remains an unsolved issue

IBD patients are at an increased risk of developing colorectal cancer (CRC): CRC causes 10–15% of all deaths in IBD patients. Due to this risk, surveillance colonoscopy with multiple biopsies is currently recommended for detection of dysplasia or asymptomatic early CRC [1] (see Chapter 13). Because recent studies indicate a much lower risk of CRC than was previously reported, it is debatable whether this invasive strategy is necessary for all IBD patients. This chapter will give an overview and critical appraisal of current knowledge about the epidemiology of IBD-related CRC.

What do we know?

Epidemiology

A frequently cited meta-analysis from 2001 estimated the cumulative incidence of CRC in ulcerative colitis (UC) patients to be 2% after 10 years of disease, 8% after 20 years, and 18% after 30 years of disease [2]. The relative CRC-risk in Crohn's disease (CD) patients has been estimated at approximately 5.6 and should therefore raise the same concerns as in UC [3]. More recent population-based studies suggest that the data from 2001 overestimate the actual IBD-related CRC risk and lean toward more conservative risk estimates ranging from 1/500 to 1/1600 patients annually [4, 5].

Risk factors

The CRC risk is increased in patients with extensive and long-standing colitis. Additional risk factors include the presence of primary sclerosing cholangitis (PSC), pseudopolyps, chronic mucosal inflammation, and a family history of sporadic CRC [3,6]. The risk also varies with geography, incidence rates for CRC being higher in the United States and the United Kingdom as compared to Scandinavian and other countries [2].

Have we been overestimating the true risk of IBD-related CRC?

Controversies in published data

The exact magnitude of the CRC-risk has remained controversial because of various biases and methodological differences in published studies. Initial reports were mainly based on data from referral centers during an era with

Clinical Dilemmas in Inflammatory Bowel Disease: New Challenges, Second Edition. Edited by P. Irving, C. Siegel, D. Rampton and F. Shanahan.
© 2011 Blackwell Publishing Ltd. Published 2011 by Blackwell Publishing Ltd.

different medical and surgical options than are available today for IBD. Therefore, the high risk reported may have been a consequence of referral bias and overinterpretation because of the high percentage of extensive and chronically active cases in these cohorts. Nowadays, better methods of surveillance and more widespread use of medicines that control inflammation are likely to influence the CRC risk in IBD patients. Recent population-based studies have demonstrated a much lower risk (Table 49.1). Although this could be an effect of improved medical and surgical therapies, these population-based studies probably included more patients with limited and less severe disease, and therefore may have underestimated the CRC risk.

A critical appraisal of recent studies

Of the recent population-based studies, the largest two originate from Copenhagen, Denmark and Manitoba, Canada [7–9]. The Danish study reported a standardized morbidity ratio of 1.05 (95% confidence interval (CI) 0.6–1.8) and a cumulative probability of CRC of only 2.1% at 30 years of disease. However, there was a high rate of surgery and long-term use of 5-ASA maintenance therapy in this cohort that could explain the low CRC incidence rates. In the Canadian study, a somewhat higher incidence rate ratio (RR) of 2.75 (95% CI 1.9–4.0) for colon cancer and 1.9 (95% CI 1.1–3.4) for rectal cancer was reported. Despite the large population-based cohort, there was a relatively short follow-up period, so the authors suspect that in time there will be higher rates of CRC in these patients.

Two smaller studies from Italy and Olmsted County with only 12 cases each revealed no significantly increased CRC risk [10,11]. However, Minnesota is comparable to Denmark with a high surgery rate and also advocates maintenance-treatment with 5-ASA. Surprisingly, CD-patients with small bowel involvement only were at higher risk for developing CRC than those with colonic involvement only [11]. The relatively small number of patients and low frequencies of events observed may have masked differences in risk between subsets of patients.

Another recent population-based study originates from the United Kingdom [12] and also demonstrated a low RR for CRC in UC patients (RR-colon 2.2; 95% CI 1.7–2.8). Although this was a relatively large study, the mean follow-up time per patient was only 8.5 years. To avoid short-term misdiagnosis or ascertainment bias, this report excluded cancer cases that occurred within 1 year of the first recorded IBD-admission, which accounted for 39% of all UC cases and 48% of CD cases. Therefore, calculated cancer rates may have been artefactually lower than they really were. The existence of asymptomatic colitis may have put a patient at risk without the patient or physician being aware: in our opinion these patients should have been included, with a resultant estimated increase in RRs of 0.5–1.2 points. The most recent population-based study originates from The Netherlands [4]. In this nation-wide case-control study we identified a low incidence rate of CRC in both academic and non-academic medical centers. Although it was limited by a retrospective study design, the strength of this large cohort was the long follow-up time of 15.5 years and the inclusion of 78 different general hospitals all over the country. Moreover, all data were confirmed by clinical chart review, including endoscopy- and pathology reports.

A recent Hungarian population-based study revealed a relatively high cumulative incidence (7.5% at 30 years of disease), despite the fact that most patients in this cohort received sulfasalazine or 5-ASA for maintenance treatment and that colonoscopic surveillance was performed in all compliant patients [13]. However, the percentage of patients with non-CRC-related colectomies was below than that reported in Western European countries. Fewer colectomies likely results in longer standing refractory inflammatory disease, which may have contributed to the relatively high CRC risk reported [13].

An increased CRC risk is also demonstrated in an American case-control study [14]. In this study, IBD diagnosis was associated with a 6- to 7-fold increase in CRC-risk. However, this study analyzed administrative claims data only and the IBD diagnostic codes were not verified by independent investigators. Therefore, the strong association found between CRC and IBD may have been secondary to diagnostic misclassification. Moreover, there was the potential for confounding, especially by variables not captured using medical claims data, such as family history of CRC and duration, extent and severity of colonic involvement with IBD.

Conclusion

In conclusion, it remains unclear whether we are over- or underestimating the actual IBD-related CRC risk.

TABLE 49.1 Risk of colorectal cancer (CRC) in recent (population-based) studies

Study [reference]	Location	Observed period	Total IBD	Cohort size		Follow-up Person-years		Number of cases		Crude incidence per year (%)		Risk expressed in relative terms (95% CI)			Cumulative incidence UC (%)**		
				UC	CD	UC	CD	UC	CD	UC	CD	Term	UC	CD	10 years	20 years	30 years
Baars et al. [4]*	The Netherlands	1990–2006	26,855	–	–	416252.5		163			0.04	–	–	–	–	–	–
Winther et al. [7]+ Jess et al. [8]	Copenhagen, Denmark	1962–1987	1534	1160	374	22,290	6569	13	4	0.06	0.06	SMR	1.05 (0.6–1.8)	1.64 (0.2–5.9)	0.4	1.1	2.1
Bernstein et al. [9]	Manitoba, Canada	1984–1997	5529	2672	2857	19,665	21,340	36	24	0.18	0.11	IRR Colon	2.75 (1.9–4.0)	2.6 (1.7–4.1)	–	–	–
								13	5	0.07	0.02	IRR rectum	1.90 (1.1–3.4)	1.08 (0.4–2.7)			
Palli et al. [10]	Florence, Italy	1978–1992	920	689	231	7877	2716	10	2	0.13	0.07	SIR	1.79 (0.9–3.3)	1.43 (0.2–5.3)	–	–	–
Jess et al. [11]	Olmsted, MN, USA	1940–2001	692	378	314	5567	4908	6	6	0.11	0.12	SIR	1.1 (0.4–2.4)	1.9 (0.7–4.1)	***	***	***
Lakatos et al. [13]	Veszprem, Hungary	1974–2004	–	723	0	8564	–	13	–	0.15	–		–	–	0.6	5.4	7.5
Goldacre et al. [12]	Oxford, UK	1963–1999	12,117	6990	5127	59,415	51,270	68	28	0.11	0.06	RR Colon	2.2 (1.7–2.8)**	1.6 (1.1–2.4)**	–	–	–
								35	11	0.06	0.02	RR rectum	1.8 (1.3–2.6)**	1.2 (0.6–2.15)**			
Terdiman et al.**** [14]	USA	2001–2003	1172	695	476	–	–	231	177	–	–	Crude OR	6.72 (5.8–7.0)	6.6 (5.6–7.8)	–	–	–

SMR, standardized mortality ratio; IRR, incidence rate ratio; RR, rate ratio; OR, odds ratio

*UC and CD patients were taken together in this cohort

**Cases that occurred within the first year of IBD admission were excluded. When including these cases, the SIR for colon would be (UC colon 3.2 (95% CI 2.6–3.6) / CD colon 2.8 (95% CI 2.1–3.6)/UC rectum 2.3 (95% CI 1.7–3.1)/ CD rectum 2.0 (95% CI 1.2–3.1)

***The cumulative incidence in the study from olmsted, MN was reported at 5 years (0% for UC, 0.3% for CD), at 15 years (0.4 % for UC, 1.6% for CD) and at 25 years (2% for UC and 2.4% for CD)

****Not a population-based study. The cohort consisted of CRC cases from two large administrative claims databases

Geographical differences as well as differences in local treatment policies and methodological differences compromise interpretation of published studies. Moreover, the recently reported lower incidence rates might result from successful treatment strategies, including 5-ASA maintenance therapy and dysplasia surveillance programs. The latter is supported by a 30-year analysis of a colonoscopic surveillance program in a British referral center, which suggests that the CRC rate in IBD patients is approximately half of what had initially been reported in 2001 [15].

A glance into the future

CRC is among the most feared long-term complications of IBD. Therefore, a sound knowledge of the overall epidemiology of CRC in IBD patients is important if we are to improve clinical practice and strengthen the basis of surveillance guidelines to decrease CRC-related morbidity and mortality. Surveillance colonoscopy is used as the foundation of a prevention strategy, with colectomy being reserved for patients in whom dysplasia or CRC are discovered. However, if the IBD-related CRC risk is indeed low, we should question whether we should continue performing surveillance in all IBD patients, bearing in mind its invasive nature and cost. Factors that influence time to CRC in both referral and nonreferral centers need to be determined to identify patients in need of an earlier start of surveillance. Consequently, a risk-prediction tool should be developed for individually tailored CRC surveillance. To facilitate such an approach, further research on the epidemiology of IBD-related CRC is essential.

References

1. Mpofu C, Watson AJ, Rhodes JM. Strategies for detecting colon cancer and/or dysplasia in patients with inflammatory bowel disease. *Cochrane Database Syst Rev* 2004; CD000279.
2. Eaden JA, Abrams KR, Mayberry JF. The risk of colorectal cancer in ulcerative colitis: a meta-analysis. *Gut* 2001; **48**: 526–535.
3. Jess T, Gamborg M, Matzen P, Munkholm P, Sorensen TI. Increased risk of intestinal cancer in Crohn's disease: a meta-analysis of population-based cohort studies. *Am J Gastroenterol* 2005; **100**: 2724–2729.
4. Baars JE, Looman CWN, Steyerberg EW, et al. The risk of inflammatory bowel disease-related colorectal carcinoma is limited: results form a nationwide nested case-control study. *Am J Gastroenterol* 2011; **106**:319–328.
5. Lakatos PL, Lakatos L. Risk for colorectal cancer in ulcerative colitis: changes, causes and management strategies. *World J Gastroenterol* 2008; **14**: 3937–3947.
6. Velayos FS, Loftus EV, Jr., Jess T, et al. Predictive and protective factors associated with colorectal cancer in ulcerative colitis: a case-control study. *Gastroenterology* 2006; **130**: 1941–1949.
7. Winther KV, Jess T, Langholz E, Munkholm P, Binder V. Long-term risk of cancer in ulcerative colitis: a population-based cohort study from Copenhagen County. *Clin Gastroenterol Hepatol* 2004; **2**: 1088–1095.
8. Jess T, Winther KV, Munkholm P, Langholz E, Binder V. Intestinal and extra-intestinal cancer in Crohn's disease: follow-up of a population-based cohort in Copenhagen County, Denmark. *Aliment Pharmacol Ther* 2004; **19**: 287–293.
9. Bernstein CN, Blanchard JF, Kliewer E, Wajda A. Cancer risk in patients with inflammatory bowel disease: a population-based study. *Cancer* 2001; **91**: 854–862.
10. Palli D, Trallori G, Bagnoli S, et al. Hodgkin's disease risk is increased in patients with ulcerative colitis. *Gastroenterology* 2000; **119**: 647–653.
11. Jess T, Loftus EV, Jr., Velayos FS, et al. Risk of intestinal cancer in inflammatory bowel disease: a population-based study from olmsted county, Minnesota. *Gastroenterology* 2006; **130**: 1039–1046.
12. Goldacre MJ, Wotton CJ, Yeates D, Seagroatt V, Jewell D. Cancer in patients with ulcerative colitis, Crohn's disease and coeliac disease: record linkage study. *Eur J Gastroenterol Hepatol* 2008; **20**: 297–304.
13. Lakatos L, Mester G, Erdelyi Z, et al. Risk factors for ulcerative colitis-associated colorectal cancer in a Hungarian cohort of patients with ulcerative colitis: results of a population-based study. *Inflamm Bowel Dis* 2006; **12**: 205–211.
14. Terdiman JP, Steinbuch M, Blumentals WA, Ullman TA, Rubin DT. 5-Aminosalicylic acid therapy and the risk of colorectal cancer among patients with inflammatory bowel disease. *Inflamm Bowel Dis* 2007; **13**: 367–371.
15. Rutter MD, Saunders BP, Wilkinson KH, et al. Thirty-year analysis of a colonoscopic surveillance program for neoplasia in ulcerative colitis. *Gastroenterology* 2006; **130**: 1030–1038.

PART VIII:
Nutrition in IBD

50 What should patients with IBD eat?

Emile Richman[1], Keith Leiper[2], and Jonathan M. Rhodes[3]

[1] Department of Nutrition and Dietetics, Royal Liverpool University Hospital, Liverpool, UK
[2] Royal Liverpool University Hospital, Liverpool, UK
[3] Division of Gastroenterology, School of Clinical Sciences, University of Liverpooland Royal Liverpool University Hospital, Liverpool, UK

LEARNING POINTS

- Both Crohn's disease (CD) and ulcerative colitis (UC) are statistically linked with a westernized diet and high meat and animal fat intakes.

- The evidence base for specific dietary modifications other than full enteral liquid feeding (CD) is weak.

- It is reasonable to advise patients with CD to limit their intake of animal fat, fibrous fruit and vegetables, and processed foods, while encouraging a balanced and nutritious diet.

- Some patients with UC may benefit from cow's milk exclusion.

- Further research is urgently needed to clarify which dietary components are harmful/beneficial, particularly in CD.

- Replacement of normal diet by enteral feeding is an effective therapy for CD, but not for ulcerative colitis.

- Some enteral feeds work better than others and further research is needed to determine why

Although there are many similarities between Crohn's disease (CD) and ulcerative colitis (UC), the response to dietary manipulation has proved strikingly different, with impressive responses, including mucosal healing, to replacement of normal food by specialized enteral feeds in CD but not UC. It is not yet clear whether this effect of enteral feeding is due to avoidance of harmful factors in the normal diet or presence of a beneficial factor in the enteral feed.

Interventional studies are needed to prove or disprove dietary factors in IBD pathogenesis. We have previously shown in an intensive case study in CD that the diet needed to induce remission might need to be much more restricted than the diet to maintain remission, possibly because ulcerated small intestinal mucosa is associated with a much greater likelihood of food intolerance (Figure 50.1) [1]. Therefore, the studies will require very careful design and will be difficult, but it may prove to be an important area for future research.

Diet in IBD causation

The marked increase in IBD over the past 50 years in Western and westernized countries can only be due to changes in environmental factors. Late twentieth century changes in diet are a plausible explanation. Possible factors include increased calorie intake and associated obesity, a more specific increase in animal fat, and increased intake of food additives in processed foods, including emulsifiers and particles.

Epidemiology

The relationship between diet and IBD is probably complex and the evidence base is poor for several reasons: paucity of prospective trials, poor recall of pre-illness diet, and underpowered studies. However, there are some consistent findings. IBD is more common in "westernized" countries and "westernization" is associated with increased incidence of IBD.

Studies of pre-illness diet have consistently associated an increased risk of IBD with increased intake of refined

Clinical Dilemmas in Inflammatory Bowel Disease: New Challenges, Second Edition. Edited by P. Irving, C. Siegel, D. Rampton and F. Shanahan.
© 2011 Blackwell Publishing Ltd. Published 2011 by Blackwell Publishing Ltd.

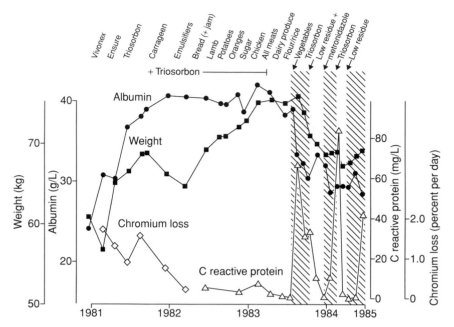

FIGURE 50.1 Effects of dietary interventions on an adult patient with multiple small bowel strictures due to Crohn's disease (CD). Inflammation was assessed initially by fecal chromium loss and later by serum C-reactive protein (CRP). Remission was induced by enteral feeding with an amino-acid-based feed (Vivonex) and then maintained with a whole-protein (casein) feed (Trisorbon) while various dietary challenges were undertaken. Relapse (clinical—denoted by cross hatching—and with raised CRP) occurred when green vegetables were introduced, remission was then reobtained with a return to enteral feeding but on two occasions reintroduction of the low-residue diet that had been previously well tolerated was associated with relapse. The conclusion is that once inflammation (and probably mucosal ulceration) is present the diet used to induce remission needs to be stricter (i.e., full enteral feeding) than the diet that can be tolerated once the mucosa has healed. This necessitates very careful design of interventional dietary studies. (Adapted from [1].)

sugar, fat, and fast foods, and decreased risk with increased vegetable and fiber intake [3]. Data from pediatric studies are consistent with adult studies showing increased risk of CD with a higher n-6/n-3 fatty acid ratio and protection against CD with a high vegetable, fruit, fish, and fiber diet.

Several studies have correlated increased meat intake with UC risk. The European Prospective Investigation into Cancer and Nutrition (EPIC) study showed that the highest quartile for linoleic acid intake was associated with an odds ratio (OR) for UC of 2.49 (95% CI 1.23–5.07) [4]. Linoleic acid is an n-6 polyunsaturated fatty acid (PUFA) and is present in red meat, cooking oils, and margarine. Relapse of established UC has also been associated with increased red or processed meat intake (highest tertile of intake OR 5.19 [95% CI 2.1–12.9]) [5]. Surprisingly, there are no data on risk of UC in vegetarians.

Intervention studies

(i) Enteral nutrition

Relatively few large-scale prospective dietary intervention studies have been performed. Greatest efficacy has been seen with the use of exclusive enteral nutrition (EEN) in inducing remission in CD. Some studies have shown remission rates in excess of 80% [6]. Although a meta-analysis has favored corticosteroids over enteral feeding, it seems likely that not all enteral feeds are equally effective. An inverse relationship has been reported between efficacy of enteral feeding and the proportion of calories given as long chain triglyceride [7]. Whole protein feeds generally have similar efficacy to amino-acid-based "elemental" feeds [1]. In children, EEN has been shown to be at least as effective as steroid treatment with significantly fewer side effects and better growth. About two-thirds of patients will tolerate enteral nutrition, suitably flavored, by mouth for up to 3 weeks.

Important questions about EEN remain, including its mode of action and its efficacy in colonic versus ileal CD. No clear benefit has been demonstrated for modified enteral formulae (e.g., tumor growth factor (TGF) beta, omega-3, or glutamine enriched) [8]. At present, it seems plausible that much of the beneficial effect of enteral feeding might be the result of the minimal residue and its impact on the intestinal microbiota. Neither EEN nor complete bowel rest, with intravenous feeding, have been shown to induce remission in UC.

(ii) Dietary modification

Unfortunately, about 50% of Crohn's patients who enter remission with enteral feeding will relapse within 6 months of return to a normal diet. There is no clear evidence that dietary modification can reduce this relapse rate. A large trial of the combination of low-refined sugar and high fiber intake showed no benefit [9]. Avoidance of refined sugar [10] and of fiber [11] also proved ineffective in separate studies. An intriguing hypothesis has been based on the possibility that microparticles in the diet, for example due to the white pigment, titanium oxide, might act as haptens and enhance the inflammatory response to bacterial lipopolysaccharide. However, a controlled trial of particle exclusion was negative [12]. Emulsifiers are another common modern food additive and there are theoretical reasons why these might increase gut permeability and thus be harmful but, as yet, no intervention studies have tested this hypothesis.

In UC, there is even less evidence to support dietary modification. A controlled trial has shown benefit in about 1 in 5 patients as a result of excluding cow's milk [13], but further trials are clearly needed.

Prebiotics and synbiotics are covered in Chapter 8.

Malnutrition in IBD

It has been reported that 14% of outpatients with CD and 6% of those with UC are malnourished [14]. Inpatient surveys have shown malnutrition in up to 80% of the patients with IBD, with a higher prevalence among CD than UC. Anxiety about possible harmful dietary factors should not be allowed to result in undernutrition.

Dietary treatment should be aimed at increasing overall nutrition orally then, if nutritional requirements are still not met, nasogastric feeding should be considered. Micronutrient deficiency is common in IBD; however, there is little evidence for clinical benefit from supplementation. Nevertheless, specific supplements including multivitamins and more specifically vitamins C, D, folate, and iron (see Chapter 52) will commonly be required, particularly in CD, and patients with significant distal ileal disease or resection (>20 cm) are likely to need regular vitamin B_{12} injection [2]. Calcium and vitamin D supplementation is recommended in people with IBD taking corticosteroids [15].

"Best current advice"

Any advice should be given with the caveat that supporting evidence is generally weak. Strongest evidence exists for the role of specialized enteral feeds as sole nutrition, e.g., for 3 weeks, in induction of remission in CD. They are probably also effective in maintenance of remission but inconvenience usually precludes this, although there is some evidence to support partial enteral feeding, e.g., 50% of caloric intake [16]. Marked variation in response has been reported with different enteral feeds, so it is preferable to use feeds with proven efficacy in clinical trials.

Further advice is speculative but the "best bet" current advice for patients with CD arguably includes a low intake of animal fat, avoidance of obviously fibrous fruit and vegetables, particularly in those with stricturing disease, and avoidance of processed foods. In children with oral Crohn's or orofacial granulomatosis, there is some evidence to support avoidance of carbonated drinks containing cinnamon or benzoates [17]. In patients with persistent watery diarrhea, a trial of exclusion of fructose polymers and oligosaccharides (the fermentable oligo-, di-, monosaccharides, and polyols [FODMAP] diet) may be considered [18].

In UC, it should be emphasized that the advice is even more speculative. Based solely on epidemiological studies, a low intake of red meat and low intake of foods that are high in n-6 fatty acids might be reasonable. Exclusion of cow's milk may help some patients [13].

Need for future work

There is now compelling evidence that sole nutrition with selected enteral feeds can achieve remission in patients with active CD. This should be built upon with further interventional studies to test specific hypotheses. Studies would be relatively straightforward for food additives and therefore it might be reasonable to tackle these first. In UC a different approach is needed. Initial studies might usefully focus on whether or not there is reduced risk in vegetarians and then be followed by maintenance trials of low meat or meat avoidance.

References

1. Raouf AH, V Hildrey, J Daniel et al. Enteral feeding as sole therapy for Crohn's disease: A controlled trial of whole protein versus amino-acid based feed and a case study of dietary challenge. *Gut* 1991; **32**: 702–707.

2. Duerksen DR, Fallows G, Bernstein CN. Vitamin B12 malabsorption in patients with limited ileal resection. *Nutrition* 2006; **22**: 1210–1213.

3. Chapman-Kiddell CA, Davies PS, Gillen L, Radford-Smith GL. Role of diet in the development of inflammatory bowel disease. *Inflamm Bowel Dis* 2009; **16**(1): 137–151. [Epub ahead of print]

4. IBD in EPIC Study Investigators, Tjonneland A, Overvad K, et al. Linoleic Acid, a dietary n-6 polyunsaturated fatty acid, and the aetiology of ulcerative colitis—a nested case-control study within a European prospective cohort study. *Gut* 2009; **58**(12): 1606–1611. [Epub ahead of print]

5. Jowett SL, Seal CJ, Pearce MS, et al. Influence of dietary factors on the clinical course of ulcerative colitis: a prospective cohort study. *Gut* 2004; **53**: 1479–1484.

6. Zachos M, Tondeur M, Griffiths A. Enteral nutritional therapy for induction of remission in Crohn's disease. *Cochrane Database Syst Rev* 2007; **1**: CD000542.

7. Middleton SJ, Rucker JT, Kirby GA, Riordan AM, Hunter JO. Long-chain triglycerides reduce the efficacy of enteral feeds in patients with active Crohn's disease. *Clin Nutr* 1995; **14**: 229–236.

8. Lochs H, Dejong C, Hammarqvist, X et al. ESPEN Guidelines on Enteral Nutrition: Gastroenterology. *Clin Nutr* 2006; **25**: 260–274.

9. Ritchie JK, Wadsworth J, Lennard-Jones JE, Rogers E. Controlled multicentre therapeutic trial of an unrefined carbohydrate, fibre rich diet in Crohn's disease. *Br Med J* 1987; **295**: 517–520.

10. Brandes JW, Lorenz-Meyer H. Sugar free diet: a new perspective in the treatment of Crohn disease? Randomized, control study. *Z Gastroenterol* 1981; **19**: 1–12.

11. Levenstein S, Prantera C, Luzi C, D'Ubaldi A. Low residue or normal diet in Crohn's disease: a prospective controlled study in Italian patients. *Gut* 1985; **26**: 989–993.

12. Lomer MC, Grainger SL, Ede R, et al. Lack of efficacy of a reduced microparticle diet in a multi-centred trial of patients with active Crohn's disease. *Eur J Gastroenterol Hepatol* 2005; **17**: 377–384.

13. Wright R, Truelove SC. A controlled therapeutic trial of various diets in ulcerative colitis. *Br Med J* 1965; **2**: 138–141.

14. Rocha R, Santana GO, Almeida N et al. Analysis of fat and muscle mass in patients with inflammatory bowel disease during remission and active phase. *Br J Nut* 2009; **101**: 676–679.

15. British Society of Gastroenterology Guidelines for osteoporosis in inflammatory bowel disease and coeliac disease. [Online]; 2007 Available from: www.bsg.org.uk.

16. Akobeng AK, Thomas AG. Enteral nutrition for maintenance of remission in Crohn's disease. *Cochrane Database Syst Rev* 2007; (3): CD005984.

17. White A, Nunes C, Escudier M, et al. Improvement in orofacial granulomatosis on a cinnamon- and benzoate-free diet. *Inflamm Bowel Dis* 2006; **12**: 508–14.

18. Gearry RB, Irving PM, Barret JS et al. Reduction of dietary poorly absorbed short-chain carbohydrates (FODMAPs) improves abdominal symptoms in patients with inflammatory bowel disease—a pilot study. *J Crohns Colitis* 2009; **3**: 8–14.

51 Enteral nutrition in Crohn's—who for, when, how and which formula?

Raanan Shamir[1,2] and Ernest G. Seidman[3]

[1] Institute for Gastroenterology, Nutrition, and Liver Diseases, Schneider Children's Medical Center, Petach-Tikva, Israel
[2] Sackler Faculty of Medicine, Tel-Aviv University, Tel-Aviv, Israel
[3] Division of Gastroenterology, McGill University Health Center, Faculty of Medicine, McGill University, Montreal, QC, Canada

---

LEARNING POINTS

- Enteral nutrition (EN) induces remission in patients with Crohn's disease (CD).

- EN is also used to reverse malnutrition in CD and ulcerative colitis.

- EN is as good as steroids to induce remission in children with CD, but is less effective than steroids in adults.

- Available evidence suggests that EN has a role in maintaining remission in pediatric and adult patients with CD.

Diet and risk of IBD

Two meta-analyses suggested that breastfeeding is protective against later development of ulcerative colitis (UC) and Crohn's disease (CD). In the first, the highest quality studies (four each for CD and UC) observed a pooled odds ratio (OR) for developing CD of 0.45 (0.26–0.79) and UC of 0.56 (0.38–0.81) [1]. However, methodological limitations included the reporting of studies that were heterogeneous and retrospective, and which contained selection bias and confounding factors. The second meta-analysis examined the effect of breastfeeding on the overall development of IBD in the pediatric age group [2] Analysis of seven studies showed that breast milk had an overall protective effect (OR 0.69; 95% confidence interval (CI) 0.51–0.94; $p = .02$) for early-onset IBD. However, nonsignificant differences were found for UC and CD, individually.

Several dietary factors have been studied for association with risk of developing IBD. A review [3] noted that several small studies suggest that certain dietary constituents such as fats, refined sugar, fruit, vegetables, and fiber affect the likelihood of IBD. However, insufficient data or methodological limitations compromise the ability to implicate any specific nutrient in the risk for IBD. In a large European study with dietary data available for 203,193 participants, and a median follow-up of 4 years, a diagnosis of UC was made in 126 subjects. Individuals with the highest quartile of intake of linoleic acid had an increased risk of UC (OR = 2.49, 95%, CI = 1.23 to 5.07, $p = 0.01$) [4]. It was recently suggested [5] that genetic polymorphisms play a role in the risk attributable to fat intake (saturated, monounsaturated, and the ration of n-3 to n-6 polyunsaturated fat), providing an explanation for the inconsistent results previously observed.

IBD and malnutrition

Malnutrition is prevalent in IBD patients, especially in active CD [6], with weight loss identified in up to 80% of patients [7]. Mechanisms involved include decreased food intake due to anorexia, limited food intake due to elicited pain, and iatrogenic limitations (fasting for diagnostic procedures, directives to avoid certain foods, malabsorption of nutrients, increased nutrient losses, increased energy requirements (usually due to fever), and interactions between drugs and nutrients (such as sulfasalazine and folic acid). Iron deficiency, particularly common in IBD, may be due to intestinal blood loss, malabsorption,

---

Clinical Dilemmas in Inflammatory Bowel Disease: New Challenges, Second Edition. Edited by P. Irving, C. Siegel, D. Rampton and F. Shanahan.
© 2011 Blackwell Publishing Ltd. Published 2011 by Blackwell Publishing Ltd.

and limited intake (see Chapter 52). Although almost any nutrient may be deficient in IBD, studies have revealed that the most frequently reported deficiencies other than iron include folic acid, zinc, magnesium, calcium, and vitamins A, B_{12}, D, E, and K [8]. Vitamin D status is particularly important to ascertain due to the low bone mineral density and increased fracture risk seen in IBD (reviewed in Chapter 52).

One of the consequences of chronic malnutrition and inflammation in children with IBD is growth failure [9]. Growth failure and delayed puberty are less common in UC than CD. Up to 40% of children continue to have significant linear growth retardation over time, and final height is commonly affected in CD children with early onset of symptoms [6,7,9].

Nutrition as primary therapy for CD

Parenteral nutrition

The safety and efficacy of parenteral nutrition (PN) for active CD was first documented over 4 decades ago. It was subsequently realized that although PN can induce clinical remission and fistula healing, the benefits are usually short lived [6]. Moreover, since enteral nutrition (EN) is at least as beneficial, less costly, and safer, PN is recommended only for high-output fistulas and intestinal obstruction.

Enteral nutrition

Induction of remission. EN induces remission in patients with CD, while in UC it is used to reverse malnutrition. In addition to improving nutritional status, EN induces mucosal healing, and decreases serum concentrations of proinflammatory cytokines and inflammatory markers in patients with CD [10,11]. Suggested mechanisms include improvement of nutritional status, the anti-inflammatory effects of EN, promotion of epithelial healing, decreased gut permeability, decreased antigenic load to the gut, bowel rest, and modification of gut microbes [6]. Although EN is generally safe, refeeding syndrome may rarely ensue in extremely malnourished patients when it is started.

Recent meta-analyses and Cochrane reviews examined the efficacy of EN compared to corticosteroids in CD, concluding that steroids are superior to EN in achieving clinical remission. In the most recent Cochrane review, the pooled OR in favor of steroids was 0.33 (95% CI, 0.21–0.53) [12]. In contrast to studies in adults, 2 meta-analyses in pedi-

atric patients with CD showed that the use of EN induces remission in up to 85% of patients and is as effective as steroids [13,14]. Furthermore, the growth enhancing ability of EN provides an advantage over corticosteroids in young patients [6,7,9]. Dissimilar results between adult and pediatric studies based on intent to treat analysis are explained in part by children being more compliant with EN.

The type of protein in a particular formula (polymeric versus oligopeptide versus amino acid based) has not been demonstrated to affect remission rates in adult [12] or pediatric studies [14]. Notably however, the trials were underpowered to detect a difference. Although the fat content of EN was not found consistently to affect the remission rate, a double-blind trial revealed that a formula with a high oleic acid content had an inferior outcome [15]. In children, the use of partial EN (PEN), providing only 50% of calories yielded remission in only 15% compared with 42% in those receiving exclusive EN [16]. The duration of therapy is somewhat controversial, as studies examined the response to regimens varying from 4 to 8 weeks' duration of treatment. Many clinicians suggest exclusive EN for 6 weeks to induce remission.

It is still not clear whether the location of bowel involvement influences outcomes to EN therapy for CD. One study suggested that pediatric patients with colonic involvement alone do not respond as well to EN as when the ileum is also involved. [17] In another retrospective study, no effect of disease location on remission rate was observed. [18] In a more recent publication [19], exclusive EN for 8 weeks ($n = 114$) yielded an overall 80% remission rate. However, a significantly lower remission rate was observed in children with isolated terminal ileal disease ($n = 4$, $p = 0.02$). Nevertheless, the authors concluded that, "disease phenotype should not influence clinicians when commencing patients on exclusive EN" [19].

Exclusive EN can be administered orally in highly motivated children who have supportive families. In our experience, compliance is achieved in most cases when the patient and parents are given the choice to select the appropriate product and route of administration. When oral feeding is not tolerated, nasogastric tube feeding can be employed with success. Gastrostomy tubes can be used safely in children with CD [20]. However, this is justified only if EN is to be used long term, to maintain remission and/or to support growth.

The question as to whether intake other than clear liquids is permissible during EN treatment has not been systematically studied. Moreover, studies on how to reintroduce food items after EN treatment are lacking. Nevertheless, common sense dictates that foods should be introduced gradually, since an adverse response to specific food items is largely unpredictable.

Maintenance of remission. Only 2 studies met the inclusion criteria in the recent Cochrane review [21] examining the potential role of EN in maintaining remission in CD. In one, patients who received half of their daily caloric requirements as elemental EN had a significantly lower relapse rate compared to those allowed unrestricted intake (9 of 26 versus 16 of 25; OR 0.3, 95% CI 0.09–0.94). In the other, elemental and polymeric formulas (providing between 35% and 50% of caloric needs) were equally effective in maintaining remission and withdrawing steroids (8 of 19 versus 6 of 14; OR 0.97, 95% CI 0.24–3.92) [18]. Long-term partial EN in patients with quiescent CD had significant beneficial effects on clinical activity, endoscopic findings, and mucosal inflammatory cytokine levels [10].

Conclusions

Nutrition plays multiple roles in IBD, including pathogenesis, manifestations (malnutrition and nutrient deficiencies) as well as in its management. EN is effective to induce and maintain remission of CD. Nutritional rehabilitation of malnutrition is fundamental to patient care in IBD. A complete nutritional evaluation and a nutrition plan are mandatory for these patients regardless of whether EN is used.

References

1. Klement E, Cohen RV, Boxman J, et al. Breastfeeding and risk of inflammatory bowel disease: a systematic review with meta-analysis. *Am J Clin Nutr* 2004; **80**: 1342–52.
2. Barclay AR, Russel RK, Wilson ML, et al. Systematic review: the role of breast feeding in the development of pediatric inflammatory bowel disease. *J Pediatr* 2009; **155**: 421–426.
3. Yamamoto T, Nakahigashi M, Saniabadi AR. Review article: diet and inflammatory bowel disease-epidemiology and treatment. *Aliment Pharmacol Ther* 2009; **30**: 99–112.
4. Tjonneland A, Overvad K, Bergmann MM, et al. Linoleic acid, a dietary n-6 polyunsaturated fatty acid, and the aetiology of ulcerative colitis: a nested case-control study within a European prospective cohort study. *Gut* 2009; **58**: 1606–1611.
5. Guerreiro CS, Ferreira P, Tavares L, et al. Fatty acids, IL6, and TNFα polymorphisms: An example of nutigenetics in Crohn's disease. *Am J Gastroenterol* 2009; **104**: 2241–2249.
6. Hartman C, Eliakim R, Shamir R. Nutritional status and nutritional therapy in inflammatory bowel diseases. *World J Gastroenterol* 2009; **15**: 2570–2578.
7. Ruemmele F, Roy CC, Levy E, Seidman EG. Nutrition as primary therapy in pediatric Crohn's disease: Fact or fantasy? *J Pediatr* 2000; **136**: 285–291.
8. Filippi J, Al-Jaouni R, Wiroth JP, et al. Nutritional deficiencies in patients with Crohn's disease in remission. *Inflamm Bowel Dis* 2006; **12**: 185–191.
9. Shamir R, Phillip M, Levine A. Growth retardation in pediatric Crohn's disease: pathogenesis and interventions. *Inflamm Bowel Dis* 2007; **13**: 620–628.
10. Yamamoto T, Nakahigashi M, Saniabadi AR, et al. Impacts of long-term enteral nutrition on clinical and endoscopic disease activities and mucosal cytokines during remission in patients with Crohn's disease: a prospective study. *Inflamm Bowel Dis* 2007; **13**: 1493–1501.
11. Bannerjee K, Camacho-Hübner C, Babinska K, et al. Anti-inflammatory and growth-stimulating effects precede nutritional restitution during enteral feeding in Crohn's disease. *J Pediatr Gastroenterol Nut* 2004; **38**: 270–275.
12. Zachos M, Tondeur M, Griffiths AM. Enteral nutritional therapy for induction of remission in Crohn's disease. *Cochrane Database Syst Rev* 2007; (1): CD000542.
13. Heuschkel RB, Menache CC, Megerian JT, et al. Enteral nutrition and corticosteroids in the treatment of acute Crohn's disease in children. *J Pediatr Gastroenterol Nutr* 2000; **31**: 8–15.
14. Dziechciarz P, Horvath A, Shamir R, et al. Meta-analysis: enteral nutrition in active Crohn's disease in children. *Aliment Pharmacol Ther* 2007; **26**: 795–806.
15. Gassull MA, Fernández-Bañares F, Cabré E, et al. European Group on Enteral Nutrition in Crohn's Disease. Fat composition may be a clue to explain the primary therapeutic effect of enteral nutrition in CD: results of a double blind randomized multicentre European trial. *Gut* 2002; **51**: 164–168.
16. Johnson T, Macdonald S, Hill SM, Thomas A, Murphy MS. Treatment of active Crohn's disease in children using partial enteral nutrition with liquid formula: a randomized controlled trial. *Gut* 2006; **55**: 356–361.
17. Afzal NA, Davies S, Paintin M, et al. Colonic Crohn's disease in children does not respond well to treatment with enteral

nutrition if the ileum is not involved. *Dig Dis Sci* 2005; **50**: 1471–1475.

18. Knight C, El-Matary W, Spray C, et al. Long-term outcome of nutritional therapy in pediatric Crohn's disease. *Clin Nutr* 2005; **24**: 775–779.

19. Buchanan E, Gaunt WW, Cardigan T, et al. The use of exclusive enteral nutrition for induction of remission in children with Crohn's disease demonstrates that disease phenotype does not influence clinical remission. *Aliment Pharmacol Ther* 2009; **30**: 501–507.

20. Anstee QM, Forbes A. The safe use of percutaneous gastrostomy for enteral nutrition in patients with Crohn's disease. *Eur J Gastroenterol Hepatol* 2000; **12**: 1089–1093.

21. Akobeng AK, Thomas AG. Enteral nutrition for maintenance of remission in Crohn's disease. *Cochrane Database Syst Rev* 2007; (3): CD005984.

52 Optimizing treatment of iron deficiency anemia

Hermann Schulze and Axel Dignass

Department of Medicine I, Markus Hospital, Frankfurt/Main, Germany

---

LEARNING POINTS

- Despite regular blood tests, the importance of anemia is frequently overlooked in patients with IBD.

- The serum ferritin cutoff levels for diagnosis of iron deficiency are dependent on the inflammatory disease activity.

- All patients with anemia should be considered for treatment.

- Intravenous iron supplementation is the treatment of choice for IBD patients with severe iron deficiency anemia or who are intolerant of, or nonresponsive to oral iron.

- New formulations of intravenous iron have replaced iron dextran and are much safer.

- Erythropoietin treatment can be considered in patients that are not responding to parenteral iron supplementation.

Introduction

Anemia is one of the most common systemic manifestations of ulcerative colitis (UC) and Crohn's disease (CD), affecting at least one-third of all patients [1]. Symptoms associated with anemia may substantially affect the quality of life of IBD patients who can get significant benefit from appropriate treatment. The most common causes of anemia in IBD patients are iron deficiency and anemia of chronic disease. There has been controversy in the past about the optimal route and dosing of iron supplementation, and in this chapter we shall discuss oral and intravenous iron replacement and the use of erythropoietin.

Anemia in IBD

According to the guidelines of the World Health Organization, anemia is best defined by hemoglobin thresholds of 12 mg/dL in nonpregnant women and 13 mg/dL in men [2]. Severe anemia is usually defined by hemoglobin of <10 mg/dL. These definitions are generally applicable in IBD patients.

Anemia is one of the most common complications in IBD. The prevalence of anemia in IBD was estimated in a systematic review to be between 8.8% and 73.7% and varies between subpopulations [3]. Anemia in IBD is considered to be a multifactorial and complex condition resulting from different causes and thus a systematic diagnostic approach is essential to find the appropriate therapy. Among all potential causes of anemia, iron deficiency is the most prevalent in IBD patients. It is caused by intestinal blood loss, deficient dietary iron intake, or malabsorption due to disease activity. In active IBD, iron deficiency anemia and the anemia of chronic disease (related to inflammation) overlap. Proinflammatory cytokines affect the absorption, transport, and distribution of iron, erythropoietin production, and erythropoiesis itself [4]. Other types of anemia in IBD patients, including vitamin B_{12} or folic acid deficiency and drug-associated anemia (for example, due to azathioprine,

Clinical Dilemmas in Inflammatory Bowel Disease: New Challenges, Second Edition. Edited by P. Irving, C. Siegel, D. Rampton and F. Shanahan.
© 2011 Blackwell Publishing Ltd. Published 2011 by Blackwell Publishing Ltd.

6-mercaptopurine, or sulfasalazine), are also commonly seen. Hemoglobinopathies, hemolysis, and other diseases impairing erythropoiesis are rarely seen in IBD patients.

Screening

All IBD patients should undergo screening for anemia on a regular basis. Patients in remission or with a mild course of disease should be examined every 6 to 12 months, whereas nonhospitalized patients with active disease should be examined every 3 months. Vitamin B_{12} and folic acid serum levels should be measured annually in all patients at risk due to small bowel disease or after resection. Macrocytosis may be related to vitamin B_{12} and/or folic acid deficiency, azathioprine or 6-mercaptopurine use, hemolysis, or other causes such as concomitant medications and alcohol use. On the other hand, microcytosis and a low mean corpuscular volume is normally indicative of iron deficiency.

Diagnostics

If the hemoglobin level has fallen below the lower limit of normal, the following diagnostic steps should be initiated: serum ferritin, transferrin, transferrin saturation, and C-reactive protein. A low ferritin concentration and low transferrin saturation in combination with increased transferrin levels indicate iron deficiency anemia. Low iron levels confirm the diagnosis. The cutoff levels are dependent on inflammatory disease activity [5]. In the absence of clinical or biochemical signs of inflammation, a serum ferritin <30 μg/L or a transferrin saturation <16% indicates iron deficiency. In patients with active disease, i.e., with clinical or biochemical signs of inflammation, iron deficiency anemia is indicated by a serum ferritin <100 μg/L. Oral as well as intravenous iron supplementation affect transferrin saturation and ferritin levels. The plasma concentration of the soluble form of the transferrin receptor is an excellent indicator of iron deficiency and is especially useful for the distinction between iron deficiency anemia and anemia of chronic disease, but its limited availability and high cost restrict its routine use. If the cause of anemia is not detected by the above mentioned tests, vitamin B_{12}, folic acid, haptoglobin, lactate dehydrogenase, creatinine, blood urea nitrogen, and differential blood cell count (including reticulocytes) should be checked.

Therapy

All patients presenting with symptoms of anemia (chronic fatigue, dyspnea, impaired physical fitness, elevated heart rate, palpitations, etc.) should be considered for treatment. Further factors such as etiology, severity, speed of development, comorbidity, and the expected spectrum of adverse effects of iron therapy have to be considered as well, and may influence the treatment decision.

In all patients with iron deficiency anemia, iron supplementation should be started. When iron deficiency becomes apparent without anemia, the treatment options and possible adverse effects should be discussed with the patient. Treatment goals are the improvement of quality of life, an elevation of hemoglobin level, and normalization of serum ferritin and transferrin saturation. Early and adequate treatment will reduce the need for blood transfusions. An increase of the hemoglobin level of 2g/dL in 2–4 weeks is possible by using intravenous iron supplementation. Continuous and close treatment surveillance should be provided. A transferrin saturation (iron/TIBC) higher than 50% suggests iron overload. The total iron deficit (ID) can be estimated using Ganzoni's formula (ID = weight (kg) × (target Hb – actual Hb)(g/dL) × 2.4 + iron depot). The iron depot that has to be refilled is usually considered to be 500–1000 mg (e.g., 70 (kg) × (12 (g/dL) – 10 (g/dL)) × 2.4 + 1000 mg = 1336 mg [6]).

There are two different options for iron administration: oral and intravenous, both are safe and effective. Oral iron supplementation is less invasive and easy to manage but only a small proportion of oral iron intake (<20%) can be absorbed, while the remaining iron will pass through the GI tract and may, at least in animal models, cause mucosal injury. The nonabsorbed iron load may worsen inflammatory disease activity and could theoretically cause disease exacerbations by generation of reactive oxygen species. However, increased ROS generation after administration of oral iron in patients with IBD has not been reported [7]. Since not more than 10–20 mg/day of oral iron can be absorbed, irrespective of total oral iron intake, there is in fact no need for oral doses higher than 100 mg/d, and a total iron deficit of 1000 mg can be compensated by oral supplementation in 50–100 days. Oral supplementation induces significantly more nonspecific side effects than intravenous administration, for example, abdominal pain, diarrhea, constipation, bloating, dark stools, nausea, and vomiting [8,9]. However, oral iron usually provides a safe,

TABLE 52.1 Characteristics of selected intravenous iron compounds

	High-molecular-weight iron dexteran	Low-molecular-weight iron dextran	Iron gluconate	Iron sucrose	Ferric carboxymaltose
Chemical properties					
Complex stability	High	High	Low	Moderate	High
Dosing					
Max. dose, mg iron per week	1000	1000	62.5–125	500	1000
Min.infusion time, min	360	360	60	30–210	15
Max. bolus dose, mg iron	100	100	125	200	200
Min. injection time, min	2	2	10	10	Bolus push
Safety profile					
Risk of dextran-induced anaphylxis	Yes	Yes	No	No	No
Relative risk of serious adverse events	High	Moderate	Low	Lowest	Very low

cheap, and effective means of restoring iron deficiency. Iron is not absorbed in the stomach and is absorbed best from the duodenum and proximal jejunum. Thus, enteric-coated or sustained-release iron capsules are less efficient sources of iron. Iron salts should not be given with food because phosphates, phytates, and tannates in food bind the iron and impair its absorption. In addition, the absorption of iron salts is impaired by antacids, certain antibiotics (e.g., quinolones, tetracycline), and the ingestion of iron along with cereals, dietary fiber, tea, coffee, eggs, or milk. Iron should be given 2 hours before, or 4 hours after, ingestion of antacids. Iron is best absorbed as the ferrous (Fe^{2+}) salt in a mildly acidic medium. The most appropriate oral iron formulations include: ferrous fumarate (106 mg elemental iron/tablet), ferrous sulfate (65 mg elemental iron/tablet), and ferrous gluconate (28–36 mg iron/tablet). There is no evidence that one iron preparation is more effective than another. The main advantages of oral iron supplementation lie in its convenience and cost, but a substantial minority of IBD patients will not tolerate its side effects and will need to terminate the treatment [10].

Intravenous iron supplementation

Intravenous therapy enables fast and efficient replenishment of iron stores. It is better tolerated, more effective, and improves quality of life more rapidly than when iron is given orally [5,7,9]. All these advantages make intravenous iron supplementation the preferred option in IBD patients with significant anemia due to iron deficiency; it is also of course indicated in patients who are intolerant of or do not respond to oral iron.

Four different intravenous iron preparations are available: sodium ferric gluconate complex, iron sucrose, iron dextran, and ferric carboxymaltose (Table 52.1). The sodium ferric gluconate complex is degraded quickly after intravenous administration and can oversaturate the transferrin binding capacity with the consequence of severe side effects. The recommended maximum dose for sodium ferric gluconate is 62.5 mg per day in order to minimize the risk of side effects.

Iron sucrose seems to be the safest of the parenteral iron preparations [11,12]. Infusions of up to 7 mg/kg bodyweight, or a total dose of 500 mg of iron over 3.5 hours once a week seem to be safe.

Iron dextrans may cause dextran-induced anaphylactic reactions. These reactions have been frequently observed when using high molecular weight iron dextran, and this preparation is now considered to be obsolete. However, low molecular weight iron dextran seems to be safer [13].

Ferric carboxymaltose is one of the stable iron complexes and allows the administration of up to 1000 mg iron in a single infusion (once a week) or up to 200 mg in a single injection (one per day) [14].

Further therapy options

Since iron deficiency anemia and anemia of chronic disease overlap in most IBD patients, in some patients iron supplementation alone will not be sufficient. The response rate to iron supplementation in IBD patients is generally higher than 70%. If iron supplementation fails after 4 weeks of treatment and the hemoglobin level is <10 g/dL, erythropoietin treatment should be considered [15]. All available erythropoietin derivatives (i.e., epoetin alfa, epoetin beta, darbepoetin alfa) are effective and should be combined with iron supplementation according to the specific prescription information of the individual products.

Conclusion

Iron deficiency is common in patients with IBD and, if mild, is best treated with oral iron. The evolution of better tolerated preparations of intravenous iron has resulted in an increase in their use in patients with marked deficiency or who are intolerant of oral iron. It is generally safe and rapidly effective. Where iron supplementation fails, consideration should be given to the use of erythropoietin.

References

1. Gasche C. Anemia in IBD: the overlooked villain. *Inflamm Bowel Dis* 2000; **6**(2): 142–150.
2. World Health Organization *Iron deficiency anaemia: assessment, prevention, and control. A guide for programme managers.* Geneva; 2001, (WHO/NHD/01.3).
3. Wilson A, Reyes E, Ofman J. Prevalence and outcomes of anemia in inflammatory bowel disease: a systematic review of the literature. *Am J Med* 2004; **116**(Suppl 7A): 44S–49S.
4. Weiss G, Goodnough LT. Anemia of chronic disease. *N Eng. J Med* 2005; **352**(10): 1011–1023.
5. Gasche C, Berstad A, Befrits R, et al. Guidelines on the diagnosis and management of iron deficiency and anemia in inflammatory bowel diseases. *Inflamm Bowel Dis* 2007; **13**(12): 1545–1553.
6. Ganzoni AM. Intravenous iron-dextran: therapeutic and experimental possibilities. *Schweiz Med Wochenschr* 1970; **100**(7): 301–303.
7. Erichsen K, Ulvik RJ, Nysaeter G, et al. Oral ferrous fumarate or intravenous iron sucrose for patients with inflammatory bowel disease. *Scand J Gastroenterol* 2005; **40**(9): 1058–1065.
8. de Silva AD, Tsironi E, Feakins RM, Rampton DS. Efficacy and tolerability of oral iron therapy in inflammatory bowel disease: a prospective, comparative trial. *Aliment Pharmacol Ther* 2005; **22**(11–12): 1097–1105.
9. Schröder O, Mickisch O, Seidler U, et al. Intravenous iron sucrose versus oral iron supplementation for the treatment of iron deficiency anemia in patients with inflammatory bowel disease–a randomized, controlled, open-label, multicenter study. *Am J Gastroenterol* 2005; **100**(11): 2503–2509.
10. Kulnigg S, Gasche C. Systematic review: managing anaemia in Crohn's disease. *Aliment Pharmacol Ther* 2006; **24**(11–12): 1507–1523.
11. Chertow GM, Mason PD, Vaage-Nilsen O, Ahlmén J. Update on adverse drug events associated with parenteral iron. *Nephrol Dial Transplant* 2006; **21**(2): 378–382.
12. Lindgren S, Wikman O, Befrits R, et al. Intravenous iron sucrose is superior to oral iron sulphate for correcting anaemia and restoring iron stores in IBD patients: A randomized, controlled, evaluator-blind, multicentre study. *Scand J Gastroenterol* 2009; **44**(7): 838–845.
13. Koutroubakis IE, Oustamanolakis P, Karakoidas C, Mantzaris GJ, Kouroumalis EA. Safety and efficacy of total-dose infusion of low molecular weight iron dextran for iron deficiency anemia in patients with inflammatory bowel disease. *Dig. Dis. Sci* 2010; **55**(8): 2327–2331.
14. Kulnigg S, Stoinov S, Simanenkov V, et al. A novel intravenous iron formulation for treatment of anemia in inflammatory bowel disease: the ferric carboxymaltose (FERINJECT) randomized controlled trial. *Am J Gastroenterol* 2008; **103**(5): 1182–1192.
15. Koutroubakis IE, Karmiris K, Makreas S, et al. Effectiveness of darbepoetin-alfa in combination with intravenous iron sucrose in patients with inflammatory bowel disease and refractory anaemia: a pilot study. *Eur J Gastroenterol Hepatol* 2006; **18**(4): 421–425.

PART IX:
Management Process

Michael D. Kappelman

Division of Pediatric Gastroenterology, Department of Pediatrics, University of North Carolina Chapel Hill, Chapel Hill, NC, USA

LEARNING POINTS

- Abundant evidence suggests that the quality of care delivered to patients with a range of diseases in Western countries is suboptimal.

- Limited evidence suggests that IBD-related care may be similarly deficient.

- The first step in measuring and improving the care and outcomes for patients with IBD is the development of IBD standards/quality metrics.

- Quality metrics generally cover three domains of care: (1) structure, (2) process, and (3) outcomes, with advantages and limitations in each of these.

- Several groups have recently completed or are actively engaged in developing IBD standards.

- In addition to developing standards, improvements in patient care will require strategies for their dissemination, implementation, and process improvement.

Quality of care: an overview

Healthcare quality is defined by the Institute of Medicine as "the degree to which health services for individuals and populations increase the likelihood of desired health outcomes and are consistent with current professional knowledge" [1]. Quality measurement began with Earnest Codman's "end-result" system of tracking patient outcomes over 100 years ago [2], and was reborn in the 1970s with the pioneering work of John Wennberg and Alan Gittelsohn, who described small-area variations in healthcare utilization [3]. Variation in care, generally attributed to underuse, overuse, or misuse of diagnostic and therapeutic services, is often an indicator of "serious and widespread quality problems" [4]. Examples include failure to prescribe β-blockers following acute myocardial infarction [5] or controller medications for children with asthma [6] (underuse), antibiotic prescribing for viral infections [7] (overuse), and preventable adverse drug events [8] (misuse).

Two reports published by the Institute of Medicine galvanized the quality of care movement. *To Err is Human* [9] reported that "tens of thousands of Americans die each year from errors in their care, and hundreds of thousands suffer or barely escape non-fatal injuries." *Crossing the Quality Chasm* [10] concluded that "between the health care we have and the care we could have lies not just a gap but a chasm." These two reports were a call to action—demanding accountability from the healthcare system and implying that system-wide changes were necessary to substantially improve care.

Subsequent studies published over the last 5 years have reinforced the findings of the IOM reports. McGlynn and colleagues demonstrated that adults receive only 54.9% of recommended outpatient care [11]. Similarly, in a study of inpatient care, Jha et al. observed significant performance gaps across a number of diseases including acute myocardial infarction, congestive heart failure, and pneumonia [12]. Many additional studies provide further evidence of these and other deficiencies in inpatient, outpatient, and pediatric care.

Clinical Dilemmas in Inflammatory Bowel Disease: New Challenges, Second Edition. Edited by P. Irving, C. Siegel, D. Rampton and F. Shanahan.
© 2011 Blackwell Publishing Ltd. Published 2011 by Blackwell Publishing Ltd.

Quality of IBD care

Quality of care research is less robust for IBD than for other chronic illnesses, owing largely to the lack of established IBD-specific quality metrics. However, limited literature suggests that the quality gap may be just as significant.

A multicenter pediatric study reported substantial intercenter variation in the use of corticosteroids, 5-aminosalicylates (ASA), immunomodulators, and antibiotics, even after controlling for factors such as patient age, disease severity, and disease location [13]. Further evidence of a gap in IBD quality comes from a retrospective study of 67 adult IBD patients referred to a tertiary care center. Sixty-four percent were inadequately dosed with 5-ASA medications, 60% receiving chronic steroids had not initiated steroid-sparing medications, and 82% of patients treated with immunomodulators received suboptimal dosages. Surveillance for colorectal dysplasia and osteopenia/osteoporosis management in steroid-exposed patients were also deficient. [14]. In the United Kingdom, Mawdsley et al. demonstrated performance gaps in monitoring patients initiated on immunosuppressive therapy, bone protection at times of steroid use, and surveillance colonoscopy [15]. Further quality deficits were observed in a nationwide UK audit of inpatient and outpatient IBD management [16].

Taken together, the above studies suggest that quality of care for IBD is no different from chronic illnesses: a gap exists between ideal IBD care and actual patient care. Given the costs, resource utilization, and morbidity associated with IBD, efforts to define IBD standards, measure performance, and address gaps are of utmost importance.

Defining IBD standards: structure, process, and outcomes

Quality of care is typically measured across three dimensions: structure, process, and outcomes [17,18]. *Structural Measures* are characteristics of the setting in which care is delivered. In terms of IBD care, this could include practice volume, teaching status, use of health information technology, and the qualifications and ratios of personnel involved in care delivery (Table 53.1). Although structural measures are efficient to monitor and, from a policy perspective, can drive change at the practice level (adoption of electronic medical records and patient registries, etc), such practice-level measures do not reflect the care delivered to, or outcomes experienced by, individual patients. Nevertheless, carefully selected structural measures may be useful components of an overall package of IBD quality indicators.

Process measures indicate the steps taken by healthcare providers in the care of an individual patient. Examples in IBD care could include smoking cessation counseling, immunization practices, and strategies for monitoring disease activity, complications, and drug safety. Although process measures are generally easy to measure and may be related to patient outcomes (a prerequisite for a valid process measure), the development of widely accepted process measures has been impeded by a lack of strong evidence-based practices. In other words, defining optimal IBD care is challenging.

Outcome measures describe what happens to patients as the result of the care they receive. These are intrinsically appealing because they describe what matters the most to patients—their state of health. IBD-specific outcome measures may include disease activity/remission rates, surgery, hospitalization, steroid exposure, quality of life, disease complications, and anthropometric measurements. However, some outcomes occur over a period of many years, hindering the ability to obtain immediate measurement of quality over short time intervals. Additionally, factors outside the control of the healthcare provider (e.g., severity, phenotype, comorbidity, adherence, etc.) also contribute to patient outcomes. Thus, the relationship between process measures (*i.e., doing the right thing*) and outcome measures (*i.e., having the desired result*) is not always linear.

Compared to outcome measures, process measures are more sensitive and responsive to change and less susceptible to bias from imperfect risk-adjustment strategies. For these reasons, most efforts to measure quality of care initially focus on process measures.

Current efforts to define IBD standards

Several groups have recently completed or are currently engaged in developing IBD-specific quality indicators. The American Gastroenterological Association is completing a set of process measures to be submitted to the Center for Medicare & Medicaid Services' Physician Quality Reporting Initiative, a pay-for-performance (P4P) program. The Crohn's and Colitis Foundation of America has also recently formed a Quality of Care Initiative, which is currently undertaking an extensive literature review and developing candidate process and outcome measures for future

TABLE 53.1 Methods of measuring healthcare quality

	Structure	Process	Outcome
Definition	Characteristics of the setting in which the care is delivered	Steps taken by healthcare providers in the care of an individual patient	Change in a patient's current/ future health status that can be attributed to antecedent healthcare
Examples in IBD	1. Practice volume 2. Qualifications and ratios of personnel involved in care delivery 3. Use of health information technology	1. Steroid-sparing maintenance strategies 2. Monitoring of disease status and complications 3. Bone density in appropriate patients 4. Drug-safety monitoring 5. Immunization practices 6. Smoking cessation	1. Disease activity/remission rates 2. Hospitalization 3. Surgery 4. Health-related quality of life 5. Disability 6. Growth and development 7. Steroid exposure
Advantages	1. Easiest to measure 2. Reflect attributes of the health system as an entire unit 3. Indicate opportunities for system redesign	1. Direct measure of care at the patient level 2. Can reflect evidence-based care 3. Measurable in a timely manner 4. May influence actual practice (P4P as example)	1. Intrinsically the most meaningful quality indicator (to patients and providers)
Disadvantages	1. Do not measure care at the level of the individual patient 2. Relatively weak association with patient outcomes	1. Costly to develop and collect 2. Limited number of broadly applicable evidence-based practices for IBD care 3. Often do not reflect comprehensive care 4. May encourage overutilization 5. Rely on documentation of services performed; however, clinical records often incomplete	1. Factors outside of the provider's control may influence outcomes; risk adjustment remains problematic 2. Often a long time must elapse before outcomes occur

dissemination. In the United Kingdom, seven professional societies have recently launched the Inflammatory Bowel Disease Standards Group, which aims to "ensure that IBD patients receive consistent, high-quality care and that IBD services throughout the United Kingdom are knowledge-based, engaged in local and national networking, based on modern IT, and meet specific minimum standards": their conclusions have recently been published [19]. In the pediatric arena, an IBD improvement collaborative was formed in 2007 by eight participating practices. Over the last 3 years, this initiative has grown to include over 22 academic, non-profit, and private practices and has recently announced a partnership with the North American Society for Pediatric Gastroenterology, Hepatology, and Nutrition. The collaboration has developed a series of core process and outcome measures, and is using continuous quality improve-

ment methods to track and improve patient care and outcomes.

Future directions: using quality measures to enhance care

Establishing IBD standards (quality measures) is a challenging but necessary first step in quality improvement. However, measuring development alone does little to enhance patient care. Carefully selected and appropriately targeted strategies for dissemination, implementation, and process improvement will be required in order to improve IBD care and outcomes. Approaches used in other chronic illnesses include P4P programs, enhancements in health information technology, formation of improvement collaboratives, and the plan-do-study-act model for process improvement. Ultimately, future work incorporating these and other methods into IBD care should lead to meaningful and sustainable changes in the way healthcare is delivered and the outcomes are achieved.

References

1. Lohr KN. *Medicare: A Strategy for Quality Assurance*, in Variation: IOM publication: National Academy Press; 1990.
2. A journey through the history of the joint commission. [Online]; 2008 Available from: http://www. jointcommission.org/AboutUs/joint_commission_history.htm
3. Wennberg J, Gittelsohn A. Small area variations in health care delivery. *Science* 1973; **182**(117): 1102–1108.
4. Chassin MR, Galvin RW. The urgent need to improve health care quality: institute of medicine national roundtable on health care quality. *JAMA* 1998; **280**(11): 1000–1005.
5. Soumerai SB, McLaughlin TJ, Spiegelman D, Hertzmark E, Thibault G, Goldman L. Adverse outcomes of underuse of beta-blockers in elderly survivors of acute myocardial infarction. *JAMA* 1997; **277**(2): 115–121.
6. Finkelstein, JA, Lozano P, Farber HJ, Miroshnik I, Lieu TA. Underuse of controller medications among Medicaid-insured children with asthma. *Arch Pediatr Adolesc Med* 2002; **156**(6): 562–567.
7. Gonzales R, Steiner JF, and Sande MA. Antibiotic prescribing for adults with colds, upper respiratory tract infections, and bronchitis by ambulatory care physicians. *JAMA* 1997; **278**(11): 901–904.
8. Bates DW, Cullen DJ, Laird N, et al. Incidence of adverse drug events and potential adverse drug events. Implications for prevention. ADE Prevention Study Group. *JAMA* 1995; **274**(1): 29–34.
9. Kohn LT, Corrigan JM, Donaldson MS, eds. *To Err is Human : Building a Safer Health System*. Washington, DC: National Academy Press; 2000.
10. Institute of Medicine. *Crossing the Quality Chasm : A New Health System for the 21st Century*. Washington, DC: National Academy Press; 2001. Available from: http://www.nap.edu/openbook.php?isbn=0309072808.
11. McGlynn EA, Asch SM, Adams J, et al. The quality of health care delivered to adults in the United States. *N Engl J Med* 2003; **348**(26): 2635–2645.
12. Jha AK, Li Z, Orav EJ, Epstein AM. Care in U.S. Hospitals – The hospital quality alliance program. *N Engl J Med* 2005; **353**(3): 265–274.
13. Kappelman MD, Bousvaros A, Hyams J, et al. Intercenter variation in initial management of children with Crohn's disease. *Inflamm Bowel Dis* 2007; **13**(7): 890–895.
14. Reddy SI, Friedman S, Telford JJ, Strate L, Ookubo R, Banks PA. Are patients with inflammatory bowel disease receiving optimal care? *Am J Gastroenterol* 2005; **100**(6): 1357–1361.
15. Mawdsley JE, Irving PM, Makins RJ, Rampton DS. Optimizing quality of outpatient care for patients with inflammatory bowel disease: the importance of specialist clinics. *Eur J Gastroenterol Hepatol* 2006; **18**(3): 249–253.
16. Down C. Clincal Effectiveness and Evaluation Unit-IBD Audit. [Online]; 2008. Available from: http://www.rcplondon.ac.uk/clinical-standards/ceeu/Current-work/Pages/UK-IBD-Audit.aspx.
17. Donabedian A. The role of outcomes in quality assessment and assurance. *QRB Qual Rev Bull* 1992; **18**(11): p. 356–360.
18. Brook RH, McGlynn EA, Cleary PD. Measuring quality of care—part two of six. *N Engl J Med* 1996; **335**(13): p. 966–970.
19. IBD Standards Group; 2009. Available from: http://www.ibdstandards.org.uk/ibd-standards.cfm.

54 Your treatment will not work if the patient does not take it

Rob Horne

Centre for Behavioural Medicine, The School of Pharmacy, University of London, London, UK

LEARNING POINTS

- Nonadherence to drug therapy is common in IBD, but it should not be seen as the patient's problem. It represents a failure of the healthcare system to negotiate treatments and support optimal adherence.

- Nonadherence is best understood as a variable behavior with intentional and unintentional causes. Unintentional nonadherence is linked to limitations in capacity or resources that reduce the ability to adhere to the treatment, while intentional nonadherence is the product of beliefs, emotions, and preferences.

- Adherence is influenced by patients' beliefs about medicines, in particular how they judge their need for them (necessity beliefs) relative to their concerns about adverse effects. These evaluations are informed by their beliefs about the illness and by social representations of pharmaceuticals (which are often viewed with suspicion).

- Adherence support should be tailored to the needs of the individual. This can be achieved by addressing both the perceptual barriers (e.g., beliefs and emotions) affecting motivation to start and continue taking medication, and the practical barriers (e.g., capacity and resources) influencing ability to adhere to treatment.

Introduction

The efficacy of treatment to prevent relapse in IBD is compromised by nonadherence [1,2]. This chapter summarizes our current understanding of the reasons for nonadherence and discusses its implications for clinical care. It draws on recent research into patients' perspectives of IBD and its treatment, and the psychology of medicines usage and will outline the perceptions and practicalities approach (PPA) to supporting adherence.

Nonadherence to maintenance treatment in IBD

Most studies of nonadherence to oral maintenance treatment for IBD report that 30–45% patients do not adhere to treatment, increasing the risk of relapse and healthcare costs [3]. Despite the high costs of nonadherence to patients and the healthcare system, effective interventions to improve adherence remain elusive [4,5] due to limitations in the way interventions have been designed and tested [6].

The four myths of nonadherence

The development of effective ways for supporting adherence has been hampered by misconceptions and myths about the causes of nonadherence.

Myth 1: Adherence rates are higher in more severe diseases

Nonadherence is not explained by the type or severity of the disease with rates of 25%–30% noted across 17 studies [7].

Myth 2: The nonadherent patient

There are no clear, consistent links between nonadherence and sociodemographic variables in adults, across illnesses [8]. Although some studies have found nonadherence to be higher among young men with IBD, a recent systematic review concluded that this was not a consistent finding [3]. In fact, adherence rates vary, not just between individuals,

Clinical Dilemmas in Inflammatory Bowel Disease: New Challenges, Second Edition. Edited by P. Irving, C. Siegel, D. Rampton and F. Shanahan.
© 2011 Blackwell Publishing Ltd. Published 2011 by Blackwell Publishing Ltd.

but within the same individual, over time and across treatments: we are all nonadherent some of the time.

Myth 3: "Once a day" treatments solve the problem

Simplifying the regimen can be helpful for many patients but nonadherence also occurs with *once daily* treatments. We need to think beyond formulation and dosage regimens.

Myth 4: Providing clear instructions is enough:

Providing clear instructions, although essential, is not enough to guarantee adherence. In order to change behavior, information has to either concur with patients' beliefs or change them.

The perceptions and practicalities approach (PPA) [9]

The PPA provides a theoretical framework for moving beyond the myths of adherence to developing effective, patient-centered solutions. Following are the central tenets of PPA:

1. The many causes of nonadherence fall into two overlapping categories: intentional and unintentional.
2. Unintentional nonadherence occurs when the patient wants to take the medicine but is prevented from doing so by barriers beyond their control, such as poor recall or comprehension of instructions, difficulties in administering the treatment, simply forgetting, or because they cannot afford it. Deliberate or intentional nonadherence arises when the patient decides not to follow the treatment recommendations.
3. Unintentional nonadherence results from limitations in capacity and resources that reduce the person's ability to adhere. These are *practical* barriers. Intentional nonadherence can be understood in terms of the beliefs and preferences influencing the person's motivation to start and continue with treatment. These are *perceptual* barriers.
4. To understand nonadherence and facilitate adherence, we need to consider following two issues: (1) motivation and (2) ability (resources). There is a degree of overlap between intentional and unintentional nonadherence. Motivation may overcome resource barriers and resource barriers may reduce motivation.

5. Each individual has a unique mix of perceptual and practical barriers to adherence, and interventions should be tailored to meet the needs of individuals by first assessing the specific barriers and then selecting appropriate techniques to address each.
6. Perceptual and practical barriers require different types of interventions. For example, perceptual barriers might be addressed by cognitive behavioral techniques or motivational interviewing, whereas practical barriers might be overcome by interventions that increase capacity or improve ability (e.g., reminder systems to reduce forgetting).
7. The perceptual and practical barriers for each individual will be affected by sociodemographic, cultural and economic factors, and trait characteristics. However, the effect of these variables will vary among individuals. For this reason, the assessment of the specific perceptual and practical barriers for each individual should be the starting point for adherence interventions. One size does not fit all.

The PPA explains the limited efficacy of interventions to improve adherence through information provision or "education." In order for information to change behavior, it must be consistent with patients' underlying beliefs or change them. But, what are the key beliefs influencing uptake and adherence to medication?

How patients evaluate prescribed medication: necessity beliefs and concerns

Patients' motivation to start and continue with prescribed medication is influenced by the way in which they judge their personal need for medication (necessity beliefs), relative to their concerns about potential adverse effects. Studies spanning long-term conditions [10], including IBD [11,12] show that nonadherence is related to doubts about personal need for the treatment and concerns about side effects.

Medication necessity beliefs

To arrive at a necessity belief, we ask the question, "How much do I need this treatment?" Perceived necessity is not a form of efficacy belief. We might believe that a treatment will be effective but not that we need it. Necessity beliefs are influenced by perceptions of the condition being treated as well as by symptom expectations and experiences [13].

People do not blindly follow treatment advice even from respected clinicians. Rather, we evaluate the advice and decide whether it is a good idea for us, based on our understanding of the illness and treatment. This is where an adherence problem often begins. In order to be convinced of a personal need for ongoing medication, we must first perceive a good fit between the problem (the illness or condition) and the solution (the medication) [11].

Patients' common-sense perceptions of illness influence their beliefs about the necessity of medication. Symptom perceptions relative to expectations are key. Until we experience a chronic condition, most of our experience of illness is symptomatic and acute. However, for many long-term conditions the medical rationale for maintenance treatment is based on a prophylaxis model. The benefits of treatment are often silent and long-term. This may be in stark contrast to our intuitive common-sense model of "no symptoms, no problem." [14]. Moreover, missing doses may not lead to an immediate deterioration in symptoms, so reinforcing the (erroneous) perception that high adherence to the medication may not be necessary. Related to this is the fact that people often stop taking treatment when they judge that the condition has improved. These judgments are often based on potentially misleading symptom perceptions rather than on objective clinical indicators of disease severity [15].

Medication concerns

One obvious source of concern is the experience of symptoms as medication "side effects" and the disruptive effects of medication on daily living, but this is not the whole picture. Many patients receiving regular medication who have not experienced adverse effects are still worried about possible problems in the future. In a survey of over 1800 patients in the United Kingdom, 35% reported that their maintenance treatment caused unpleasant side effects. However, more patients were concerned about long-term effects (73%), or that taking medication regularly would make it less effective (57%) or cause dependence (52%) [11]. Concerns about prescribed medication are often related to suspicions of pharmaceuticals as a class of treatments [11]. Many people are suspicious of pharmaceuticals and the pharmaceutical industry, seeing medicines as intrinsically harmful, addictive poisons that are overused by physicians and the healthcare system.

Implications for practice

The PPA has informed NICE (National Institute of Health and Clinical Excellence) adherence guidelines in the United Kingdom [1], developed to help health professionals support patients in making informed choices about and adhering to prescribed medication. The principle is to identify the specific perceptual and practical barriers to adherence for each individual and apply specific interventions to address the unique mix of perceptual and/or practical barriers for each patient. This can be summarized in three steps as follows:

1. Communicate a "common-sense" rationale for why the treatment is needed. Patients need to perceive a close fit between the problem (IBD) and the proposed solution (e.g., regular use of maintenance treatment), and to provide a convincing "story" for why medication is still necessary, even when symptoms are not present or when symptom resolution is delayed.

2. Elicit and address patient concerns about the medication, help the patient to make treatment choices that are informed by an understanding of the likely risks and benefits, rather than by potentially erroneous beliefs or misconceptions about the condition and treatment. It is important to understand this from the patient's perspective. For example, the patient may be worried about subjective side effects that clinicians may perceive to be clinically insignificant.

3. Identify and address potential, practical barriers and make the regimen as convenient and easy to take as possible.

It is important to take a "no-blame approach" that facilitates honest disclosure of nonadherence and encourages patients to express doubts and concerns. Many are reluctant to do this because they believe that clinicians will perceive doubts about treatment as a doubt about themselves.

Adherence support should occur, not just at the start of treatment, but also during treatment review as perceptions, abilities and adherence can change over time. This requires a team approach involving clinicians, nurses, and pharmacists who can contribute through medication counseling and reviewing [16].

Conclusion

Nonadherence prevents many patients from getting the best from IBD treatment. We need to develop more effective ways of supporting optimal adherence to appropriately prescribed treatments. This might be achieved by applying the PPA to tailor support to meet the needs and preferences of the individual. This takes a no-blame approach to identify and address not just the practical barriers (such as poor comprehension or regimen complexity) that affect patients' ability to follow treatment recommendations but also the perceptual barriers (such as beliefs, preferences and emotions) influencing their motivation to start and continue with treatment. Although this approach represents a challenge in relation to the time and resources it requires to be implemented, benefits in terms of patient outcome in the medium- and long-term are likely to be substantial.

References

1. Nunes V, Neilson J, O'Flynn N, et al. *Clinical Guidelines and Evidence Review for Medicines Adherence: Involving Patients in Decisions about Prescribed Medicines and Supporting Adherence.* London: National Collaborating Centre for Primary Care and Royal College of General Practitioners; 2009.

2. Higgins PDR, Rubin DT, Kaulback K, et al. Systematic review: impact of non-adherence to 5-aminosalicylic acid products on the frequency and cost of ulcerative colitis flares. *Aliment Pharmacol Ther* 2009; **29**(3): 247–257.

3. Jackson CA, Clatworthy J, Robinson A, et al. Factors associated with non-adherence to oral medication for inflammatory bowel disease: a systematic review. *Am J Gastroenterol* 2010; **105**(3): 525–539.

4. Haynes RB, Ackloo E, Sahota N, et al. Interventions for enhancing medication adherence. *Cochrane Database Syst Rev.* 2008 (2): CD000011.

5. Haynes RB, McDonald HP, Garg AX. Helping patients follow prescribed treatment: clinical applications. *JAMA* 2002; **288**(22): 2880–2883.

6. Horne R, Kellar I. Chapter 6: Interventions to Facilitate Adherence. In: Horne R, Weinman J, Barber N, et al., eds. *Concordance, Adherence and Compliance in Medicine Taking: A conceptual map and research priorities.* London: National Institute for Health Research (NIHR) Service Delivery and Organisation (SDO) Programme; 2005. Available from: http://www.sdo.nihr.ac.uk/sdo762004.html.

7. DiMatteo MR. Variations in patients' adherence to medical recommendations: a quantitative review of 50 years of research. *Med Care* 2004; **42**(3): 200–209.

8. Horne R, Weinman J, Barber N, et al. *Concordance, adherence and compliance in medicine taking: a conceptual map and research priorities.* London: National Co-ordinating Centre for NHS Service Delivery and Organisation NCCSDO 2006.

9. Horne R. Compliance, adherence and concordance. In: Taylor K, Harding G, eds. *Pharmacy Practice.* London: Taylor and Francis; 2001. p. 165–184.

10. Horne R. Adherence to treatment. In: Ayers S, Baum A, McManus C, et al., eds. *Cambridge Handbook of Psychology, Health & Medicine* 2nd Ed. Cambridge: Cambridge University Press; 2007. pp. 417–421.

11. Horne R, Parham R, Driscoll R, et al. Patients' attitudes to medicines and adherence to maintenance treatment in inflammatory bowel disease. *Inflamm Bowel Dis* 2009; **15**(6): 837–844. Online pre-publication(December).

12. Moshkovska T, Stone M, Baker R, et al. Qualitative investigation of patient adherence to 5-aminosalicylic acid therapy in patients with ulcerative colitis. *Inflamm Bowel Dis* 2008; **14**(6): 763–768.

13. Cooper V, Gellaitry G, Horne R. Treatment perceptions and self-regulation in adherence to HAART. *Int J Behav Med* 2004; **11**(Suppl): 81.

14. Halm EA, Mora P, Leventhal H. No symptoms, no asthma: the acute episodic disease belief is associated with poor self-management among inner-city adults with persistent asthma. *Chest* 2006; **129**(3): 573–580.

15. Horne R, Cooper V, Gellaitry G, et al. Patients' perceptions of highly active antiretroviral therapy in relation to treatment uptake and adherence: the utility of the necessity-concerns framework. *J Acquir Immune Defic Syndr* 2007; **45**(3): 334–341.

16. Clifford S, Barber N, Elliott R, et al. Patient centred advice is effective in improving adherence to medicines. *Pharm World Sci* 2006; **28**(3): 165–170.

Louise Langmead

Endoscopy Unit, Barts and the London NHS Trust, The Royal London Hospital, London, UK

LEARNING POINTS

- True emergencies in IBD are uncommon
- Dialogue between the patients and their IBD team can often avert a visit to the emergency department (ED)
- IBD patients should be provided with written details about their illness and treatment to be taken to the ED, should the need arise. ED physicians should be aware of common pitfalls in the acute management of IBD such as:
  - unnecessary use of ionizing radiation imaging;
  - failure to look for infection and sepsis; and
  - inappropriate initiation of corticosteroid therapy.
- It is often best to delay specific treatment until an IBD specialist has been consulted.

Introduction

Every IBD specialist will recognize the scenario of a patient receiving an inappropriate course of corticosteroids started during an attendance in the emergency department (ED). At best this can be frustrating and at worst dangerous. There are many other potential pitfalls in the emergency care of patients with IBD. At the outset, it should be emphasized that inadequacies in the management of IBD in the ED are usually attributable to the inexperience of the nonspecialist emergency clinicians working there and inappropriate attendances at ED by IBD patients who cannot easily access their specialist team. The purpose of this chapter is to highlight contexts in which suboptimal management of IBD may occur in the ED and to suggest ways of improving their outcome.

The scale of the problem

IBD patients attend the ED more frequently than do the general population. The rate of IBD-related ED visits in a recent study was 26/100,000 population, which equated to 26 ED visits/1000 ambulatory IBD visits. In the same study, younger patients, those who were uninsured and those with Crohn's disease (CD) were disproportionately represented in the ED attendances [1].

Reasons for ER attendance

Patients usually attend the ED because they cannot access care urgently elsewhere. This may be due to a true emergency but it is often because of an inability to achieve a specialist review for milder symptoms. IBD is a complex disease that is unpredictable and beset with complications. Associated conditions can also flare up or appear suddenly making patients need treatment in emergency departments. For this reason, ED teams will see not only "true IBD emergencies" such as acute severe ulcerative colitis (UC) or small bowel obstruction, but also a mixture of subacute and chronic IBD-related problems (Table 55.1).

Approach to the patient with IBD presenting as an emergency

Doctors in the ED are trained to make quick decisions, but even experienced IBD specialists may need time to evaluate patients presenting acutely. Jumping to the wrong

---

Clinical Dilemmas in Inflammatory Bowel Disease: New Challenges, Second Edition. Edited by P. Irving, C. Siegel, D. Rampton and F. Shanahan.
© 2011 Blackwell Publishing Ltd. Published 2011 by Blackwell Publishing Ltd.

TABLE 55.1 Complications of IBD which may present to ED teams

Bowel disease related	Abscess	
	Perianal	
	Intra-abdominal	
	Bowel perforation	
	GI hemorrhage	
	Symptomatic anemia	
	Vitamin B_{12} deficiency	
	Electrolyte disturbances and dehydration due to diarrhea or high stoma output	
Thromboembolic	Deep venous thrombosis	
	Pulmonary embolus	
	Sagittal sinus thrombosis	
	Arterial thrombosis	
	Myocardial infarction	
	Limb ischemia	
Other	Fractures secondary to osteoporosis (not necessarily steroid related)	
	Renal stones	
Extraintestinal manifestations	Erythema nodosum	
	Pyoderma gangrenosum	
	Acute arthritis	
	Acute red eye	
Drug-related		
Idiosyncratic	Acute pancreatitis	Azathioprine, 6-mercaptopurine, 5-ASA rarely
	Leukopenia, thrombocytopenia	5-ASA, sulfasalazine
	Interstitial nephritis	5-ASA, sulfasalazine
Immunosuppression related	Neutropenia	Thiopurines, cyclosporine, methotrexate, tacrolimus, biologics (infliximab, adalimumab, certolizumab pegol)
	Opportunistic infections	Same drugs and corticosteroids,
Allergic/hypersensitivity reactions		Biologics (infliximab, adalimumab, certolizumab pegol) Sulfasalazine
Toxicity	Cushing's syndrome, diabetes, Osteoporosis	Corticosteroids
	Hypertension, renal impairment	Cyclosporine
	Neuropathy	Long-term metronidazole, thalidomide
	Hepatotoxicity	Methotrexate, antibiotics, thiopurines

conclusion can lead to bad management, and it is worth remembering that it is very unusual for IBD to present with emergencies that need immediate decisions. Much more commonly, supportive treatment, simple investigations, and initiation of specialist referral is all that is required in the first 12 hours.

History

It is important to get an accurate history of both the presenting complaint and the background of IBD. Details of previous surgery can help to provide a picture of a patient's bowel anatomy. A history of travel and potential exposure to infections is vital; a bowel pathogen can be identified in up to 20% of flares of IBD [2]. A drug history including doses, regimens, allergies, and intolerances is necessary.

Examination

All patients should undergo a thorough physical examination: complications of IBD can affect any organ or system. An assessment of hydration and nutritional status is valuable as patients with diarrhea or an ileostomy may be fluid depleted.

Careful inspection for perianal disease, including description of site and appearance of fistulation or abscesses, should be made. Digital rectal examination may be helpful but is not essential if it is very painful, since the patient may need to have an examination under anaesthetic, and/or a flexible endoscopy later.

Investigations
Blood and stool
Most patients need a minimum set of blood tests including blood count, urea and electrolytes, liver function tests, C-reactive protein, calcium, magnesium, and serum amylase. It is essential to send stool for culture, *Clostridium difficile* toxin [3] and microscopy; steroids may be lethal in the presence of amebiasis. A septic screen including blood cultures should be undertaken in febrile patients.

Imaging
Patients with IBD, especially CD, are frequently exposed to diagnostic radiation during the course of their disease (see Chapter 12) and it is important to minimize its use in the ED.

Plain X-rays are justifiable in some acute presentations of IBD. For example, a plain abdominal film is appropriate to diagnose toxic dilatation or small bowel obstruction and an erect chest radiograph may diagnose intestinal perforation. Chest X-ray is also indicated in patients on biologics presenting with fever to look for tuberculosis or other infections.

Abdominal CT scanning is overused in the ED in patients with CD. In a recent study of children with IBD, ED attendance more than doubled the chance of moderate radiation exposure, levels reached resembling those of patients undergoing surgery for IBD [4]. As discussed in Chapter 12, nonionizing imaging is the preferred way of assessing CD. In the rare situation where an emergency laparotomy is needed, urgent CT is clearly reasonable. If imaging is needed only to distinguish between intra-abdominal sepsis and bowel wall inflammation, then it is usually safe to provide supportive treatment while awaiting specialist nonionizing imaging services.

Treatment
Supportive treatment with oral or IV fluids as well as symptomatic treatment for pain, nausea, or vomiting should be instigated. Specific treatment for IBD or other complications is usually most safely delayed until a specialist opinion has been given, preferably by the patient's usual gastroenterologist.

- **Initiation of corticosteroid therapy:** It is *almost never* necessary to start corticosteroid therapy in IBD patients as an emergency. Many patients with Crohn's presenting with abdominal pain or diarrhea have septic or noninflammatory causes for their symptoms for which use of steroids will be unhelpful or even detrimental [5]. In patients with UC presenting with severe symptoms, if there is a history of foreign travel to a country where amebic dysentery is prevalent, it is safest to wait a few hours while infection is excluded before initiating steroid therapy. In patients without foreign travel there is no advantage in the addition of antibiotic therapy unless specifically indicated by a positive stool sample; and it is probably safe to start treatment with steroids while awaiting these results. However, supportive treatment is equally, if not more, important in the first few hours after admission.

- **Fluid depletion:** In patients with watery diarrhea or an increased ileostomy output, dehydration is secondary to salt loss. Drinking hypoosmotic fluids, such as water, makes it worse. Patients need to *reduce oral water intake* and increase salt intake. In the ED, intravenous normal saline (0.9% sodium chloride), should be administered.

- **Perianal disease:** Patients with CD who present with perianal pain or discharge need careful clinical examination and assessment by a colorectal surgeon. They should not simply be prescribed antibiotics and sent home with an appointment for review in the outpatient department.

- **Venous thromboembolism (VTE) prophylaxis:** Patients with IBD are at high risk of VTE [6] and should have low molecular weight heparin initiated if they need hospital admission.

Non-IBD related attendances to ER

Patients with IBD can, of course, suffer the usual illnesses and accidents that require ED attendances. A few points mentioned below are worth remembering:

- **Analgesia:** Selection of an analgesic for use in IBD patients is difficult. Usually the most effective treatment for the situation is appropriate. Nonsteroidal anti-inflammatory drugs (NSAIDs) should be avoided if possible [7], as should opiates in patients with acute colitis because of their propensity to induce megacolon [8].

- **Anticoagulation, antiplatelet agents and VTE prophylaxis:** It is important to recognize that a history of rectal bleeding in IBD does not preclude use of anticoagulants. Similarly, aspirin and antiplatelet agents should be used according to the guidelines for the condition that the patient presents with (e.g., myocardial infarction or stroke). The risk of serious bleeding in IBD is extremely low, and the benefit of treatment normally outweighs the risk. All patients with IBD should have VTE prophylaxis.
- **Adrenal suppression:** Patients who are already taking corticosteroids may need an increase in dose, temporarily, when they present to the ED with an intercurrent illness. Furthermore, symptoms of steroid withdrawal syndrome (e.g., diarrhea, fatigue, abdominal pain) can be difficult to distinguish from a disease flare in patients recently decreasing their steroid dose.

How to improve emergency care for patients with IBD

The IBD team

Ideally, an IBD specialist opinion would be available in every ED 24/7. However, while the majority of hospitals will not see enough IBD emergencies to justify an instant on-the-spot service, it should be possible to arrange immediate telephone access, at least during working hours, to a member of the IBD team.

Educating and supporting the IBD patient

Patients need to know when to attend the ED and what to expect when they get there. Education of patients about their disease is important. They need to be able to access urgent specialist care, by provision of contact information for the IBD team, so as to avoid attending EDs inappropriately. The IBD team should provide patients with written details about their illness and its treatment, for presentation to doctors in the ED. Patients must be encouraged not to attend EDs just because they have run out of prescription medications.

Training ED staff

Education of colleagues in the ED about common presentations and pitfalls of IBD care is essential. Guidelines and protocols may be of some benefit. However, because of the complexity of IBD, comprehensive guidance to cover all eventualities is impossible, and the most important message to ED staff is that they contact the IBD team promptly.

References

1. Ananthakrishnan AN, McGinley EL, Saeian K, et al. Trends in ambulatory and emergency room visits for inflammatory bowel diseases in the United States: 1994–2005. *Am J Gastroenterol* 2009; **105**(2): 363–370.
2. Mylonaki M, Langmead L, Pantes A, et al. Enteric infection in relapse of inflammatory bowel disease: importance of microbiological examination of stool. *Eur J Gastroenterol Hepatol* 2004; **16**: 775–778.
3. Issa M, Ananthakrishnan AN, Binion DG. Clostridium difficile and inflammatory bowel disease. *Inflamm Bowel Dis* 2008; 1432–1442.
4. Palmer L, Herfarth H, Porter CQ, et al. Diagnostic ionizing radiation exposure in a population-based sample of children with inflammatory bowel diseases. *Am J Gastroenterol* 2009; **104**: 2816–2823.
5. Lichtenstein GR, Feagan BG, Cohen RD, et al. Serious infections and mortality in association with therapies for Crohn's disease: TREAT registry. *Clin Gastroenterol Hepatol* 2006; **4**: 621–630.
6. Twig G, Zandman-Goddard G, Szyper-Kravitz M, Shoenfeld Y. Systemic thromboembolism in inflammatory bowel disease: mechanisms and clinical applications. *Ann N Y Acad Sci* 2005; **1051**: 166–173.
7. Kefalakes H, Stylianides TJ, Amanakis G, Kolios G. Exacerbation of inflammatory bowel diseases associated with the use of nonsteroidal anti-inflammatory drugs: myth or reality? *Eur J Clin Pharmacol* 2009; **65**: 963–970.
8. Hartong WA, Arvanitakis C, Skibba RM, Klotz AP. Treatment of toxic megacolon. A comparative review of 29 patients. *Am J Dig Dis* 1977; **22**: 195–200.

Transitioning from pediatric
to adult care

Elizabeth J. Hait and Laurie N. Fishman

Center for Inflammatory Bowel Disease, Division of Gastroenterology and Nutrition, Children's Hospital Boston,
Harvard Medical School, Boston, MA, USA

LEARNING POINTS

- Start the transition process from a pediatric to an adult gastroenterologist early.

- Establish a clear timeline for transfer of care.

- Ensure clear communication between the pediatric and adult provider.

- Discuss potential barriers of smooth transition openly.

- Prepare for a new medical "culture" with the adult gastroenterologist.

Introduction

It is generally agreed that adolescent patients should make the transition from pediatric to adult specialty care in a smooth, developmentally appropriate way. The actual age of transfer varies, depending on the insurance (where relevant) and general medical culture. The topic of transition often engenders negative feelings on the part of patients, families, and providers, leading to delay in discussions of transition. A structured approach, with the patient gradually assuming more personal responsibility for self-management and being given a clear timeline for the transition, works best. Combined pediatric–adult clinics (transition clinics) or meeting adult providers before transfer can be extremely helpful in calming the fears of a young patient and their family.

Barriers

Resistance to transition is noted universally among patients with a chronic disease that has onset in childhood. For some congenital diseases such as sickle cell disease or cystic fibrosis, there is a fear that the adult providers will not have sufficient knowledge of their condition. Fortunately, IBD providers in the adult healthcare setting are experienced and skilled in managing these conditions. The benefits of receiving age-appropriate care become clear to patients after transfer, but having pediatric providers enumerate these benefits beforehand can be very helpful to patients.

Often the patient and family have a long-standing relationship with the pediatric provider. Leaving this relationship can induce sadness in the provider as well as the patient and family. In addition, starting a new relationship takes effort. Often young adults and family members do not want to "start all over again." It is important to discuss these feelings openly and give time for the closure process.

Having a clear timeline is crucial to avoid denial on the part of the patient and the provider. Patients need to know when they will need to move from the pediatric setting, and this expectation can be set in terms of age or development stage, such as graduation from high school. It allows patients time to adjust and develop any skills that will be needed in the new setting. An abrupt or unexpected transfer will exacerbate feelings of anger and abandonment, and creates an inauspicious start for the adult provider.

Clinical Dilemmas in Inflammatory Bowel Disease: New Challenges, Second Edition. Edited by P. Irving, C. Siegel, D. Rampton and F. Shanahan.
© 2011 Blackwell Publishing Ltd. Published 2011 by Blackwell Publishing Ltd.

Fear of the unknown often plays a role in the resistance of patients and families. Many patients have become very familiar with the physical setting of their pediatric care and feel in control by knowing what to expect there. Changing providers is often accompanied by a change in office or clinic location. There may be new procedures for registration, contacting the office or clinic, insurance forms (where necessary), and obtaining laboratory work. All of these changes can provoke significant anxiety. Touring the new facility, meeting new providers early, and discussing exactly how the adult facility functions will alleviate many concerns.

The differences between the subcultures of adult medical care and pediatric medical care are often underestimated. Pediatric care is family-centered and values nurturing. Adult care is patient-centered and values patient autonomy. Providers on both sides may misinterpret the other culture and view it as suboptimal. They can undermine patient's confidence by inability to praise the other culture. Communication between these groups needs to flow in both directions. Pediatric providers need to provide timely medical information with important social and psychological issues noted. Adult providers should send follow-up notes for a set period of time to keep a connection with the pediatric providers.

Patients need to understand the new role they will play in their own medical care and feel confident about their knowledge and skills. This is a long process toward self-management and is best started many years before the actual transfer.

Parents may have a dramatic change in their role as patients go through transition. It is not easy for parents to balance the competing demands of adherence with adolescent's autonomy. Parents may worry that without their input, the patient will deteriorate medically. In some cases, this is an accurate assessment and in others it represents an overprotective response to the disease. Parents may feel ignored when the new provider focuses on the patient and may feel offended if the provider will not talk alone with them. As patients move toward self-management, parents need to practice taking a supportive but less involved role.

The transition process

Practitioners must approach the transition process within a developmental framework, starting as soon as the patient is capable of abstract thinking and future orientation. We propose the following timeline, but emphasize that the transition course must be tailored to the developmental abilities of the individual patient.

Ages 11–13
The patient should be able to do the following:

- Name his or her medications, including dosages and side effects
- Identify strategies to take their medications
- Express the impact of IBD on daily life

The medical team should introduce the idea of future independent visits. Ideally, parents should leave the exam room for a portion of the visit. Anticipatory guidance on fitness, sexuality, and substance use can be initiated.

Ages 14–16
Patients should be able to do the following tasks:

- Name procedures and understand their purpose
- Relate their medical history
- Explain risks of nonadherence, illicit drugs and alcohol

The provider should direct questions and explanations to the patient, not the parent. Ensure that the physician asks the patient for input first, and then solicit feedback from the parent. Address the family's apprehensions about the patient taking on a primary role during the office/clinic visit. The patient can choose which portions of the visit are to be done without the parents in the room. The physician must clarify with the patient what must legally be shared with his or her parents. At this point, the physician should initiate discussion about the eventual transfer of care and why this is important. Teaching of self-management skills should start.

Ages 17–19
Patients should be able to do the following tasks:

- Gather information about IBD
- Book appointments, fill prescriptions, and contact the medical team directly
- In countries where it is applicable, name the insurance carrier and carry information in wallet

The providers should openly discuss potential barriers to transfer of care. The physician should identify potential adult providers and the patient should be encouraged to start exploring options for care. In many places, this will be possible in the same hospital in which pediatric care has been provided. The patient and family should be reminded that at age 18 the patient has the right to make his or her own healthcare decisions.

Ages 20–23

The patient should have:

- had telephone conversations with potential adult providers;
- a detailed medical summary provided by the pediatric gastroenterologist; and
- considered a final visit with the pediatric provider to discuss their experience with the adult provider and troubleshoot remaining concerns.

Transition is most likely to be successful if the actual transfer of care occurs at a time of relative medical and social stability. This may occur at different ages for various patients. For those who attend college, the transfer may be after graduation, when a job is secured, or graduate education has begun. For those who choose not to attend college, the transfer of care should occur when housing and employment arrangements are stabilized.

Conclusion

Having a well planned, gradual transition process promotes skills in self-advocacy, communication, and self-care. It is essential in order to provide uninterrupted healthcare to our young adult patients with IBD. While these guidelines provide a framework for transitioning patients, each patient's needs must be assessed individually.

References

1. Blum RW, Garell D, Hodgman CH, et al. Transition from child-centered to adult health-care systems for adolescents with chronic conditions. A position paper of the Society for Adolescent Medicine. *J Adolesc Health* 2003; **14**(7): 570–576.
2. Reiss JG, Gibson RW, Walker LR Health care transition: youth, family and provider perspectives. *Pediatrics* 2005; **115**(1): 112–120.
3. Tuchman LK, Slap GB, Britto MT Transition to adult care: experiences and expectations of adolescents with a chronic illness. *Child Care Health Dev* 2008; **34**(5): 557–563.
4. Viner RM. Transition of care from paediatric to adult services: one part of improved health services for adolescents. *Arch Dis Child* 2008; **93**(2): 160–163.
5. Freed GL, Hudson EJ. Transitioning children with chronic diseases to adult care: current knowledge, practices and directions. *J Pediatr* 2006; **148**(6): 824–827.
6. Hait E, Arnold JH, Fishman LN. Educate, communicate, anticipate–practical recommendations for transitioning adolescents with IBD to adult health care. *Inflamm Bowel Dis* 2006; **12**(1): 70–73.
7. Escher JC. Transition from pediatric to adult health care in inflammatory bowel disease. *Dig Dis* 2009; **27**(3): 382–386.
8. Baldassano R, Ferry G, Griffiths A, Mack D, Markowitz J, Winter H. Transition of the patient with inflammatory bowel disease from pediatric to adult care: recommendations of the North American Society for Pediatric Gastroenterology, Hepatology and Nutrition. *J Pediatr Gastroenterol Nutr* 2002; **34**(3: 245–248.

Other resources

The following Web sites have useful information for both patients and providers to help assist with the transition process:

NACC.org.uk: National Association for Crohns and Colitis provides accurate and relevant information as well as patient support. Based in the United Kingdom.

CCFA.org: Crohns and Colitis Foundation of America provides similar function for IBD patients in the United States.

www.ibdu.org: This Web site for college aged young adults with IBD produced by the Children's Digestive Health and Nutrition Foundation (CDHNF) provides practical tips for living with IBD in college.

http://hctransitions.ichp.ufl.edu/hct-promo/: This Web site was produced by the Institute for Child Health Policy at the University of Florida. It contains multimedia resources to help adolescent and young adults communicate more effectively with healthcare providers.

http://www.cdhnf.org/user-assets/documents/pdf/TransitionPatAndPhysCombo.pdf: This is a checklist for healthcare providers produced by the Children's Digestive Health and Nutrition Foundation (CDHNF) to help assist in transitioning young adults with IBD to an adult provider.

57 Medicolegal pitfalls in inflammatory bowel disease care

William J. Tremaine

Division of Gastroenterology and Hepatology, Mayo Clinic, Rochester, MN, USA

LEARNING POINTS

- It is important to document the rationale for recommending tests that have potential risks, such as colonoscopy, in addition to documenting discussion of risks and benefits of therapies.

- Changes in therapy made by telephone or email should also be documented in the medical record.

- When a medical error is discovered, the best approach for quality care, patient safety, and litigation risk reduction is to disclose the error to the patient and apologize.

- Physicians should not discuss a medical error with professional colleagues who were not involved with the patient's care without the agreement of his or her attorney.

- For IBD patients, failure to ensure that a patient does not have a latent infection prior to starting an immune suppressant might be considered negligence.

- The improper termination by a physician of a doctor–patient relationship might be considered abandonment.

Introduction

Providing quality medical care to patients with IBD, or for any other illness, requires not only knowledge and experience, but also attention to detail. Although many of the examples in this review are drawn from medical practice in the United States, the general principles apply to physicians and others who care for patients with IBD worldwide. Research shows that neglecting the details can harm both the patient and the physician. The 1999 Institute of Medicine report estimated that between 44,000 and 98,000 deaths each year in American hospitals were due to errors [1] and medical errors are prevalent in other countries as well [2]. Physicians pay the penalties for malpractice in terms of financial settlements, harm to reputation, and emotional stress. For physicians, the frightening aspect of the medicolegal system is its capriciousness: allegations of malpractice are sometimes erroneous, and physicians can be harmed even when they are doing all the right things. For example, a review led by medical experts determined that neither injury nor error was present in 40% of 1452 closed malpractice claims, but payment was awarded in over one-quarter of those claims that lacked merit [3]. Several instances of patient care carry a high risk for medicolegal consequences, all relevant to the care of IBD patients, as described below:

Pitfall number 1: failure to document

The necessity of documenting medical care is well understood, but the importance of documenting the rationale for choosing a particular diagnostic test or a particular treatment receives less emphasis. Tests and interventions have potential risks that can only be justified if they are performed for appropriate indications. Dr. Peter Cotton, a renowned endoscopist, reported his personal series of 59 allegations of endoscopic retrograde cholangiopancreatography (ERCP) malpractice against him and noted that the most common allegation, occurring in 54% of cases, was that the procedure or therapy was not indicated. He noted the importance of documenting the rationale for the

---

Clinical Dilemmas in Inflammatory Bowel Disease: New Challenges, Second Edition. Edited by P. Irving, C. Siegel, D. Rampton and F. Shanahan.
© 2011 Blackwell Publishing Ltd. Published 2011 by Blackwell Publishing Ltd.

procedure and discussing the risks and potential benefits [4]. Similarly, the rationale for higher risk care in IBD patients, such as endoscopic dilation of strictures or prescribing multiple simultaneous immunosuppressants, should be documented. IBD patients require frequent changes in therapies such as adjusting the dose of azathioprine, adding or stopping antibiotics, or escalating the dose of a biologic therapy. These changes are sometimes made via telephone calls or emails during a busy day when there is little time and the changes may not be documented, which is bad for patient's safety and adds liability for the clinician if there is litigation about a bad outcome. Documentation in the medical record of the rationale for using immune suppressants or biologics for treatment of IBD is sufficient and signed informed consent from the patient is unnecessary.

Pitfall number 2: failure to address medical errors appropriately

Several organizations, including the Centers for Medicare & Medicaid Services, have endorsed the importance of disclosing medical errors as a core component of quality healthcare, but physicians are uncertain about how much information can be shared with patients and others about adverse events without compromising their legal defense options [2]. For example, only 14% of 364 radiologists responded that they would definitely disclose that an error had been made in interpreting a mammogram in a hypothetical clinical vignette [5]. Physicians who treat IBD patients may miss the diagnosis of a complicating infection or malignancy, or make a prescribing error, or fail to monitor patients for adverse effects of therapy. When an error is discovered, the best approach for quality care, patient safety and to reduce the risk of litigation is to disclose to the patient and apologize. After initiating a program at the University of Michigan in 2002 to acknowledge medical error and compensate patients quickly and fairly, the claims and pending lawsuits at any given time dropped from 260 cases in 2001 to 114 in 2006 [6]. When an error occurs that causes harm, the physician should acknowledge that the event occurred and take responsibility, promptly inform the patient or, if the patient is vulnerable, inform his or her family, and show empathy and support, document the discussion in the medical record and stay in contact [7]. A physician who makes an error should discuss his or her feelings with personal confidants, such as his or her attorney, family members, and close friends to get emotional support to deal with the

psychological stress, but the physician should not discuss the medical details with professional colleagues without the agreement of his or her attorney [7].

Pitfall number 3: negligence

The legal term for malpractice is negligence, which is defined as acting unreasonably under certain circumstances, meaning failure to provide the standard of medical care [7]. For IBD patients, failure to ensure that a patient does not have active viral hepatitis prior to starting an anti-TNF-α antibody may be considered negligent. For example, in 2006, a Texas jury determined that the maker of infliximab negligently mislabeled and untruthfully advertised the biologic by not disclosing all of the risks, including the risk of hepatic injury, which caused harm to a patient who had both rheumatoid arthritis and hepatitis C infection. The patient and her husband were awarded $19,415,908 and the rheumatologist, who was unaware of the risk, settled out of court [8]. There have been several publications emphasizing the importance of vaccinating IBD patients for hepatitis, pneumonia, influenza, and HPV (see Chapter 10, and ruling out latent mycobacterial and fungal infection prior to starting a biologic: these safeguards might also be deemed standard care [9,10].

Pitfall number 4: terminating care improperly

Managing IBD is a partnership between the physician and the patient, with obligations for both. If a patient is unreliable and fails to return for regular follow-up visits, or to get blood tests to monitor therapy, or to take medications regularly, or to agree to therapy to stop smoking, the physician might choose to terminate the patient's care. As with other decisions in medicine, termination of the doctor–patient relationship should be thoroughly documented. Improperly terminating care is considered by the courts to be abandonment if all of the following are true: termination of care occurred when continued care was necessary; the termination was not by mutual consent; and the termination occurred without reasonable notice, such as at least 30 days [7]. The physician should notify the patient of the decision in writing and include the names of three other qualified physicians and continue to provide care for 30 days.

Conclusions

Providing high-quality care to patients with IBD requires not only cutting-edge testing and therapy, but also

LIBRARY, UNIVERSITY OF CHESTER

methods for dealing optimally with inevitable adverse events, medical errors, and physician–patient conflicts. In particular, it is just as important to document the rationale behind particular practices as to document the practices themselves.

References

1. Kohn L, Corrigan J, MS D, eds. *To Err Is Human: Building a Safer Health System.* Washington, DC: National Academy Press; 2000.

2. Gallagher TH, Studdert D, Levinson W. Disclosing harmful medical errors to patients. *N Engl J Med* 2007; **356**(26): 2713–2719.

3. Studdert DM, Mello MM, Gawande AA, Gandhi TK, Kachalia A, Yoon C. Claims, errors, and compensation payments in medical malpractice litigation. *N Engl J Med* 2006; **354**(19): 2024–2033.

4. Cotton PB. Analysis of 59 ERCP lawsuits; mainly about indications. *Gastrointest endosc* 2006; **63**(3): 378–382.

5. Gallagher TH, Cook AJ, Brenner RJ, Carney PA, Miglioretti DL, Geller BM. Disclosing harmful mammography errors to patients. *Radiology*; **253**(2): 443–452.

6. Clinton HR, Obama B. Making patient safety the centerpiece of medical liability reform. *N Engl JMed* 2006; **354**(21): 2205–2208.

7. Choctaw W. *Avoiding Medical Malpractice. A Physician's Guide to the Law,* 1st Ed. New York, NY: Springer; 2008, pp. 19–20.

8. Hamilton, et al. v. Centocor Inc., et al. No. 03-60526-4. Texas Ct at Law No 4, Nueces Cty. 2006.

9. Melmed GY. Vaccination strategies for patients with inflammatory bowel disease on immunomodulators and biologics. *Inflamm Bowel Dis* 2009; **15**(9): 1410–1416.

10. Rahier JF, Yazdanpanah Y, Colombel JF, Travis S. The European (ECCO) consensus on infection in IBD: what does it change for the clinician? *Gut* 2009; **58**(10): 1313–1315.

Index

Note: Page numbers with italicized *f*'s and *t*'s refer to figures and tables, respectively.

Clinical Dilemmas in Inflammatory Bowel Disease: New Challenges, Second Edition. Edited by P. Irving, C. Siegel, D. Rampton and F. Shanahan.
© 2011 Blackwell Publishing Ltd. Published 2011 by Blackwell Publishing Ltd.